T0200383

Myles
Survival Guide to
Midwifery

Senior Content Strategist: Alison Taylor
Content Development Specialist: Veronika Watkins
Project Manager: Julie Taylor
Designer: Margaret Reid
Illustration Manager: Nichole Beard

THIRD EDITION

Myles
Survival Guide to
Midwifery

Maureen Raynor MA PGCEA ADM RMN RN RM

Senior Lecturer in Midwifery, De Montfort University, Faculty of Health and Life Sciences, The Leicester School of Nursing and Midwifery, Division of Maternal and Child, Edith Murphy Building, Leicester, UK

Christine Catling RN RM MSc (Mid) PhD

Senior Lecturer in Midwifery, Centre for Midwifery, Child and Family Health, Faculty of Health, University of Technology Sydney, Sydney, Australia

ELSEVIER

Edinburgh London New York Oxford Philadelphia
St Louis Sydney Toronto 2017

ELSEVIER

© 2017 Elsevier Limited. All rights reserved.

First edition 2008
Second edition 2012

No part of this publication may be reproduced or transmitted in any form
or by any means, electronic or mechanical, including photocopying,
recording, or any information storage and retrieval system, without
permission in writing from the publisher. Permissions may be sought
directly from Elsevier's Rights Department: phone: (+1) 215 239 3804 (US)
or (+44) 1865 843830 (UK); fax: (+44) 1865 853333; e-mail:
healthpermissions@elsevier.com. You may also complete your request
online via the Elsevier website at http://www.elsevier.com/permissions.

ISBN 978-0-7020-7171-3

British Library Cataloguing in Publication Data
A catalogue record for this book is available from the British Library

Library of Congress Cataloging in Publication Data
A catalog record for this book is available from the Library of Congress

Notice
Knowledge and best practice in this field are constantly changing. As new
research and experience broaden our knowledge, changes in practice,
treatment and drug therapy may become necessary or appropriate. Readers
are advised to check the most current information provided (i) on
procedures featured or (ii) by the manufacturer of each product to be
administered, to verify the recommended dose or formula, the method and
duration of administration, and contraindications. It is the responsibility of
the practitioner, relying on their own experience and knowledge of the
patient, to make diagnoses, to determine dosages and the best treatment for
each individual patient, and to take all appropriate safety precautions. To
the fullest extent of the law, neither the Publisher nor the Editor assumes
any liability for any injury and/or damage to persons or property arising out
of or related to any use of the material contained in this book.

The Publisher

ELSEVIER your source for books,
journals and multimedia
in the health sciences

www.elsevierhealth.com

  Working together
to grow libraries in
developing countries

www.elsevier.com • www.bookaid.org

The
publisher's
policy is to use
paper manufactured
from sustainable forests

Printed in China

Contents

Contents

Preface

Feedback from midwives, student midwives and midwifery lecturers was pivotal to the genesis of this third edition of the *Survival Guide*. The foundations were already laid by Diane Fraser and Maggie Cooper, the editors of the second edition as well as all the chapter authors who contributed to the work, to whom we are truly grateful. This updated version of the text is thoroughly revised to reflect some of the key developments in contemporary midwifery practice from a local, national and global perspective.

WHAT'S NEW?

- Use of bullet points to make key information more readily accessible
- Some new illustrations
- Recommended further reading
- Useful websites

The guide is not intended to be used as a complete textbook, but to be accessed as a quick reference exemplar for key information whilst the midwife and student midwife are in midwifery practice areas. Chapter references are therefore not included, but as delineated above in the *'what's new'* list, it can be seen that suggested further reading and useful websites accompany each chapter to enable the reader to examine relevant topics in greater depth.

Maureen Raynor
Christine Catling

Acknowledgements

The editors wish to express their sincere gratitude to Diane Fraser and Maggie Cooper for all their efforts with the previous edition of the survival guide. Their passion and vision have been a creative force throughout the editorial process.

We also wish to thank all the reviewers (student midwives, midwives and midwifery lecturers) for their constructive comments and useful suggestions that made our work a lot easier.

Maureen Raynor
Christine Catling

Common Abbreviations Used Within the Guide

Use with caution, as some may have more than one meaning.

ACM	Australian College of Midwives
ACTH	Adrenocorticotrophic hormone
ADH	Antidiuretic hormone
AED	Antiepileptic drug
AFI	Amniotic fluid index
AFP	Alpha fetoprotein
AFV	Amniotic fluid volume
AID	Artificial insemination by donor
AIDS	Acquired immune deficiency syndrome
AIH	Artificial insemination by husband
AIMS	Association for Improvements in the Maternity Services
ALT	Alanine transaminase
ANA	Antinuclear antibody
ANC	Antenatal clinic
APH	Antepartum haemorrhage
APL	Antiphospholipid antibodies
APS	Antiphospholipid syndrome
ARM	Artificial rupture of membranes
ART	Antiretroviral therapy
ASB	Asymptomatic bacteriuria
ASD	Atrial septal defect
BBA	Born before arrival
BCG	Bacille Calmette–Guérin
BFI (UK)	Baby-Friendly Initiative or BFHI (Australia)
BGL	Blood glucose level
BMI	Body mass index
BMR	Basal metabolic rate
BP	Blood pressure
BPD	Biparietal diameter
bpm	Beats per minute
BTS	Blood Transfusion Service
BV	Bacterial vaginosis
CAM	Complementary and alternative medicine
CCT	Controlled cord traction
CDH	Congenital dislocation of hips
CEMACH	Confidential enquiry into maternal and child health

CF	Cystic fibrosis
CIN	Cervical intraepithelial neoplasia
CMV	Cytomegalovirus
CNS	Central nervous system
CNST	Clinical negligence scheme for trusts
CPAP	Continuous positive airways pressure
CPR	Cardiopulmonary resuscitation
CQC	Care Quality Commission
CRL	Crown–rump length
CS	Caesarean section
CSF	Cerebrospinal fluid
CTG	Cardiotocograph
CVP	Central venous pressure
CVS	Chorionic villus sampling
D&C	Dilatation and curettage
DI	Donor insemination
DIC	Disseminated intravascular coagulation
DM	Diabetes mellitus
DNA	Deoxyribonucleic acid
DVT	Deep vein thrombosis
DZ	Dizygotic
EBM	Expressed breast milk
ECG	Electrocardiogram
ECV	External cephalic version
EDB	Expected date of birth
EEG	Electroencephalogram
EFM	Electronic fetal monitoring
ELBW	Extremely low birth weight
ELISA	Enzyme-linked immunosorbent assay
ESR	Erythrocyte sedimentation rate
ET	Embryo transfer
EUA	Examination under anaesthetic
FACH	Forceps to aftercoming head
FASD	Fetal alcohol spectrum disorder
FBC	Full blood count
FBS	Fetal blood sampling
FDP	Fibrin degradation product
FFTS	Fetofetal transfusion syndrome
FGM	Female genital mutilation
FH	Fetal heart
FHH	Fetal heart heard

FIGO	International Federation of Gynaecologists and Obstetricians
FSE	Fetal scalp electrode
FSH	Follicle-stimulating hormone
FTA-abs	Fluorescent treponemal antibody absorption test
FVS	Fetal varicella syndrome
GA	General anaesthetic
GAS	Group A-haemolytic streptococcus
GBS	Group B-haemolytic streptococcus
GDM	Gestational diabetes mellitus
GFR	Glomerular filtration rate
GI	Gastrointestinal
GIFT	Gamete intrafallopian transfer
G6PD	Glucose 6-phosphate dehydrogenase
G&S	Group and save serum
GTT	Glucose tolerance test
GU	Genitourinary
GUM	Genitourinary medicine
HAART	Highly active antiretroviral therapy
Hb	Haemoglobin
HBV	Hepatitis B virus
HCG	Human chorionic gonadotrophin
HCV	Hepatitis C virus
HDN	Haemolytic disease of the newborn
HDU	High-dependency unit
HELLP	Haemolysis, elevated liver enzymes, low platelets
HIV	Human immunodeficiency virus
HPL	Human placental lactogen
HPV	Human papillomavirus
HSV	Herpes simplex virus
HVS	High vaginal swab
IADPSG	International Association of Diabetes in Pregnancy Study Groups
ICM	International Confederation of Midwives
ICP	Intrahepatic cholestasis of pregnancy
ICSI	Intracytoplasmic sperm injection
ICU	Intensive care unit
IG	Immunoglobulin
IHD	Ischaemic heart disease
IM	Intramuscular
IOL	Induction of labour

IUCD	Intrauterine contraceptive device
IU(F)D	Intrauterine (fetal) death
IUGR	Intrauterine growth restriction
IUI	Intrauterine insemination
IUT	Intrauterine fetal transfusion
IVF	In-vitro fertilization
IVIG	Intravenous immunoglobulin
IV	Intravenous
KMC	Kangaroo mother care
LAM	Lactational amenorrhoea method
LBW	Low birth weight
LDH	Lactate dehydrogenase
LFT	Liver function tests
LGA	Large for gestational age
LH	Luteinizing hormone
LMP	Last menstrual period
L:S	Lecithin:sphyngomyelin
LSA	Local Supervizing Authority
LSCS	Lower segment caesarean section
MAP	Mean arterial pressure
MCHC	Mean cell haemoglobin concentration
MCV	Mean cell volume
MSH	Melanocyte stimulating hormone
MSU	Midstream specimen of urine
MZ	Monozygotic
NEC	Necrotizing enterocolitis
NICE	National Institute for Health and Care Excellence
NICU	Neonatal intensive care unit
NIPE	Neonatal and infant physical examination
NIPT	Noninvasive prenatal testing
NMC	Nursing and Midwifery Council
NND	Neonatal death
NSAIDs	Nonsteroidal anti-inflammatory drugs
NT	Nuchal translucency
NTD	Neural tube defect
NTE	Neutral thermal environment
OASIS	Obstetric anal sphincter injuries
OGTT	Oral glucose tolerance test
PCIA	Patient-controlled intravenous analgesia
PCR	Polymerase chain reaction

PCV	Packed cell volume
PDA	Patent ductus arteriosus
PE	Pulmonary embolism (care – may also be used for pre-eclampsia)
PGD	Pre-implantation genetic diagnosis
PID	Pelvic inflammatory disease
PIH	Pregnancy-induced hypertension
PKU	Phenylketonuria
PND	Postnatal depression
PPH	Postpartum haemorrhage
PPROM	Preterm prelabour rupture of the membranes
PROM	Prelabour rupture of membranes
PTSD	Post traumatic stress disorder
PV	Per vaginam
RBC	Red blood cell
RCM	Royal College of Midwives
RCOG	Royal College of Obstetricians and Gynaecologists
RCT	Randomized controlled trial
RDA	Rectus abdominus diastasis
RDS	Respiratory distress syndrome
Rh	Rhesus
RPR	Rapid plasma reagin test
SB	Stillbirth
SCA	Sickle-cell anaemia
SCBU	Special care baby unit
SGA	Small for gestational age
SIDS	Sudden infant death syndrome
SLE	Systemic lupus erythematosus
SPD	Symphysis pubis dysfunction
SROM	Spontaneous rupture of membranes
STI	Sexually transmitted infection
TB	Tuberculosis
TED	Thromboembolic deterrent
TENS	Transcutaneous nerve stimulation
TEIA	Treponemal enzyme immunoassay
TIA	Transient ischaemic attack
TIBC	Total iron-binding capacity
TOP	Termination of pregnancy
TPHA	Treponema pallidum haemagglutination assay
TPN	Total parenteral nutrition

TPPA	Treponema pallidum particle agglutination assay
TRAP	Twin reversed arterial perfusion
TSH	Thyroid-stimulating hormone
TTTS	Twin-to-twin transfusion syndrome
UDCA	Ursodeoxycholic acid
UDT-GT	Uridine diphosphoglucuronyl transferase
U&E	Urea and electrolytes
UK	United Kingdom
UNICEF	United Nations Children's Fund
USS	Ultrasound scan
UTI	Urinary tract infection
UV	Ultra violet
VBAC	Vaginal birth after caesarean
VDRL	Venereal Disease Research Laboratory
VE	Vaginal examination
VKDB	Vitamin K deficiency bleeding
VLBW	Very low birth weight
VSD	Ventricular septal defect
WHO	World Health Organization
ZIFT	Zygote intrafallopian transfer

Section | 1 |

Anatomy and Reproduction

The Female Pelvis and the Reproductive Organs

THE FEMALE PELVIS

The normal pelvis is comprised of four pelvic bones:
- two innominate bones
- one sacrum
- one coccyx.

The innominate bones (Fig. 1.1)

Each innominate bone is composed of three fused parts:
- the ilium
- the ischium
- the pubic bone.

The ilium

- At the front of the iliac crest is a bony prominence known as the *anterior superior iliac spine*; below it is the *anterior inferior iliac spine*.
- Two similar points at the other end of the iliac crest are called the *posterior superior* and the *posterior inferior iliac spines*.
- The concave anterior surface of the ilium is the *iliac fossa*.

The ischium

The ischium is the thick lower part.
- The *ischial tuberosity* is the prominence on which the body rests when sitting.
- Behind and a little above the tuberosity is an inward projection, the *ischial spine*.

In labour the station of the fetal head is estimated in relation to the ischial spines.

The pubic bone

- This has a body and two oar-like projections: the *superior ramus* and the *inferior ramus*.

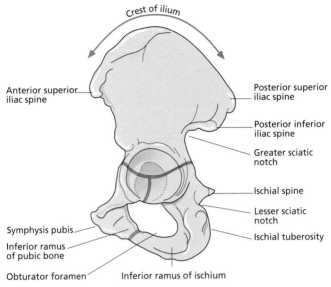

Fig. 1.1 Innominate bone showing important landmarks.

- The two pubic bones meet at the symphysis pubis and the two inferior rami form the *pubic arch,* merging into a similar ramus on the ischium.
- The space enclosed by the body of the pubic bone, the rami and the ischium is called the *obturator foramen.*
- The innominate bone contains a deep cup, the *acetabulum,* which receives the head of the femur.

On the lower border of the innominate bone are found two curves:

- One extends from the posterior inferior iliac spine up to the ischial spine and is called the *greater sciatic notch.* It is wide and rounded.
- The other lies between the ischial spine and the ischial tuberosity and is the *lesser sciatic notch.*

The sacrum

This is a wedge-shaped bone consisting of five fused vertebrae. The first sacral vertebra juts forward and is called the *sacral promontory.*

The coccyx

The coccyx consists of four fused vertebrae, forming a small triangular bone.

The pelvic joints

There are four pelvic joints:
- The *symphysis pubis* is formed at the junction of the two pubic bones, which are united by a pad of cartilage.
- Two *sacroiliac joints* join the sacrum to the ilium and thus connect the spine to the pelvis.
- The *sacrococcygeal joint* is formed where the base of the coccyx articulates with the tip of the sacrum. This joint moves backwards as the fetal head moves through the pelvis in the second stage of labour.

In the non-pregnant state, there is very little movement in these joints, but during pregnancy endocrine activity causes the ligaments to soften, which allows the joints to give.

The pelvic ligaments

Each of the pelvic joints is held together by ligaments:
- *interpubic* ligaments at the symphysis pubis
- *sacroiliac* ligaments
- *sacrococcygeal* ligaments.

Two other ligaments are important in midwifery:
- the *sacrotuberous* ligament
- the *sacrospinous* ligament.

The sacrotuberous ligament runs from the sacrum to the ischial tuberosity, and the sacrospinous ligament from the sacrum to the ischial spine. These two ligaments cross the sciatic notch and form the posterior wall of the pelvic outlet.

THE TRUE PELVIS

The true pelvis is the bony canal through which the fetus must pass during birth. It has a brim, a cavity and an outlet.

The pelvic brim

The fixed points on the pelvic brim are known as its landmarks (Fig. 1.2 and Box 1.1).

Fig. 1.2 Brim or inlet of female pelvis (see Box 1.1).

Box 1.1 **Landmarks of the pelvic brim (commencing posteriorly)**

See Fig. 1.2 for numbers
- Sacral promontory (1)
- Sacral ala or wing (2)
- Sacroiliac joint (3)
- Iliopectineal line: the edge formed at the inward aspect of the ilium (4)
- Iliopectineal eminence: a roughened area formed where the superior ramus of the pubic bone meets the ilium (5)
- Superior ramus of the pubic bone (6)
- Upper inner border of the body of the pubic bone (7)
- Upper inner border of the symphysis pubis (8)

Diameters of the brim

Three diameters are measured (Figs 1.3 and 1.4):
- anteroposterior
- oblique
- transverse.

The anteroposterior diameter

- This is a line from the sacral promontory to the upper border of the symphysis pubis.
  - The *anatomical conjugate* (12 cm) – a line taken to the uppermost point of the symphysis pubis.

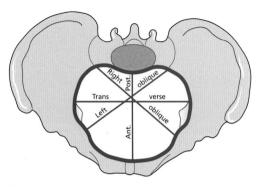

Fig. 1.3 View of pelvic inlet showing diameters.

	Anteroposterior	Oblique	Transverse
Brim	11	12	13
Cavity	12	12	12
Outlet	13	12	11

Fig. 1.4 Measurements of the pelvic canal in centimetres.

- The *obstetrical conjugate* (11 cm) – a line taken to the posterior border of the upper surface of the symphysis pubis.
- Both the **anatomical conjugate** and the **obstetrical conjugate** can be referred to as the obstetric conjugate.
- The *diagonal conjugate* is also measured anteroposteriorly from the lower border of the symphysis to the sacral promontory. It may be estimated on vaginal examination as part of a pelvic assessment and should measure 12–13 cm.

The oblique diameter

- This is a line from one sacroiliac joint to the iliopectineal eminence on the opposite side of the pelvis (12 cm).

The transverse diameter

- This is a line between the points furthest apart on the iliopectineal lines (13 cm).
- The *sacrocotyloid* (see Fig. 1.2) passes from the sacral promontory to the iliopectineal eminence on each side and measures 9–9.5 cm, which is important if the fetus is presenting posteriorly.

The pelvic cavity

- This extends from the brim above to the outlet below.
- The anterior wall is formed by the pubic bones and symphysis pubis and its depth is 4 cm.
- The posterior wall is formed by the curve of the sacrum, which is 12 cm in length.
- The cavity forms a curved canal; its lateral walls are the sides of the pelvis, which are mainly covered by the obturator internus muscle.
- The cavity is circular in shape and its diameters are all considered to be 12 cm (see Fig. 1.4).

The pelvic outlet

Two outlets are described: the *anatomical* and the *obstetrical*.

- *The obstetrical outlet* includes the narrow pelvic strait, through which the fetus must pass. This outlet is diamond shaped and its three diameters are as follows (see Fig. 1.4):
    - The *anteroposterior diameter* is a line from the lower border of the symphysis pubis to the sacrococcygeal joint and is the longest diameter (13 cm).
    - The *oblique diameter* is said to be between the obturator foramen and the sacrospinous ligament, although there are no fixed points (12 cm).
    - The *transverse diameter* is the smallest diameter (11 cm) and is measured between the two ischial spines.

THE FALSE PELVIS

This is the part of the pelvis situated above the pelvic brim. It is of no significance in obstetrics.

Fig. 1.5 Median section of the pelvis showing the inclination of the planes and the axis of the pelvic canal.

PELVIC INCLINATION

When a woman is standing in the upright position, her pelvis is on an incline; as can be seen in Fig. 1.5, the brim is tilted and forms an angle of 60° with the horizontal floor. The angles are important to understand when women are in different positions for an abdominal examination.

The pelvic planes

These are imaginary flat surfaces at the brim, cavity and outlet of the pelvic canal at the levels of the lines described previously.

The axis of the pelvic canal

A line drawn exactly half-way between the anterior wall and the posterior wall of the pelvic canal would trace a curve known as the *curve of Carus*. An understanding of this is necessary when assessing progress in labour.

Table 1.1 Features of the four types of pelvis

Features	Gynaecoid	Android	Anthropoid	Platypelloid
Brim	Rounded	Heart shaped	Long oval	Kidney shaped
Forepelvis	Generous	Narrow	Narrowed	Wide
Side walls	Straight	Convergent	Divergent	Divergent
Ischial spines	Blunt	Prominent	Blunt	Blunt
Sciatic notch	Rounded	Narrow	Wide	Wide
Subpubic angle	90°	< 90°	> 90°	> 90°
Incidence	50%	20%	25%	5%

THE FOUR TYPES OF PELVIS (Table 1.1)

Classically, the pelvis has been described according to the shape of the brim. If one of the important measurements is reduced by 1 cm or more from the normal, the pelvis is said to be contracted; this may give rise to difficulty in labour or necessitate caesarean section.

The *gynaecoid pelvis* is the ideal pelvis for childbearing. Its main features are:

- a rounded brim
- generous forepelvis (the part in front of the transverse diameter)
- straight side walls
- a shallow cavity with a broad, well-curved sacrum, blunt ischial spines, a rounded sciatic notch and a subpubic angle of 90°.

It is found in 50% of women of average build and height.

THE PELVIC FLOOR

This is formed by the soft tissues that fill the outlet of the pelvis, with the most important being the strong diaphragm of muscle slung like a hammock from the walls of the pelvis. Through it pass the urethra, the vagina and the anal canal. The pelvic floor comprises two muscle layers:

- the superficial layer (Fig. 1.6)
- the deep layer (Fig. 1.7).

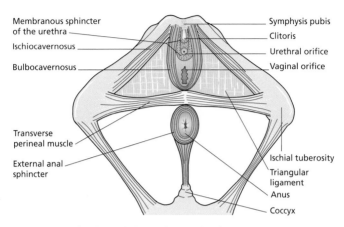

Membranous sphincter of the urethra

Ischiocavernosus

Bulbocavernosus

Transverse perineal muscle

External anal sphincter

Symphysis pubis

Clitoris

Urethral orifice

Vaginal orifice

Ischial tuberosity

Triangular ligament

Anus

Coccyx

Fig. 1.6 Superficial muscle layer of the pelvic floor.

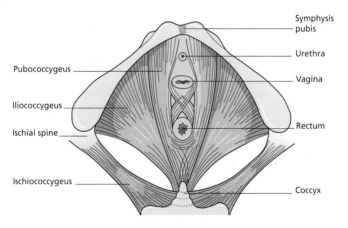

Pubococcygeus

Iliococcygeus

Ischial spine

Ischiococcygeus

Symphysis pubis

Urethra

Vagina

Rectum

Coccyx

Fig. 1.7 Deep muscle layer of the pelvic floor.

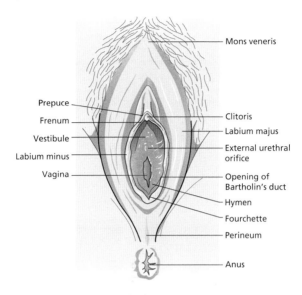

Fig. 1.8 Female external genital organs, or vulva.

THE VULVA

- The term 'vulva' applies to the external female genital organs (Fig. 1.8).

THE VAGINA

- This is a canal running from the vestibule to the cervix, passing upwards and backwards into the pelvis along a line approximately parallel to the plane of the pelvic brim (Figs 1.9 and 1.10).

THE UTERUS

The uterus is situated in the cavity of the true pelvis.

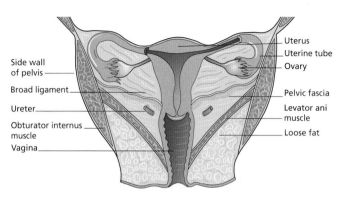

Fig. 1.9 Coronal section through the pelvis.

Fig. 1.10 Sagittal section of the pelvis.

Supports

The uterus is supported by the pelvic floor and maintained in position by several ligaments. These are:

- uterosacral ligaments
- cardinal ligaments
- round ligament
- broad ligament.

Structure

The non-pregnant uterus is a hollow, muscular, pear-shaped organ.

- It is 7.5 cm in length, 5 cm in width and 2.5 cm in depth, each wall being 1.25 cm thick.

- The cervix forms the lower third of the uterus and measures 2.5 cm in each direction.

The uterus consists of the following parts:

The body or corpus

This forms the upper two-thirds of the uterus.

The fundus

The fundus is the domed upper wall between the insertions of the uterine tubes.

The cornua

This is the upper outer angles of the uterus where the uterine tubes join.

The uterine tubes

- These extend laterally from the cornua of the uterus towards the side walls of the pelvis, and arch over the ovaries, the fringed ends hovering near the ovaries to receive the ovum.
- Each tube is 10 cm long.
- The lumen of the tube provides an open pathway from the outside to the peritoneal cavity.

The uterine tube has four portions:
- the interstitial portion
- the isthmus
- the ampulla
- the infundibulum (Fig. 1.11).

The cavity

- The cavity is a potential space between the anterior and posterior walls.
- It has a triangular shape with the base of the triangle being uppermost.

The isthmus

- The isthmus is a narrow area between the cavity and the cervix.
- It is 7 mm long but enlarges during pregnancy to form the lower uterine segment.

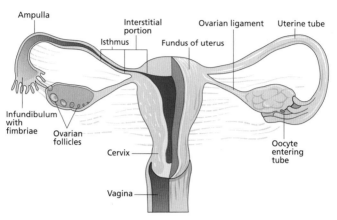

Fig. 1.11 The uterine tubes in section. Note the oocyte entering the fimbriated end of one tube.

The cervix

- Protrudes into the vagina.
- The *internal os* is the narrow opening between the isthmus and the cervix.
- The *external os* is a small round opening at the lower end of the cervix. After childbirth, it becomes a transverse slit.
- The *cervical canal* lies between these two ora and is a continuation of the uterine cavity.

Layers

The layers of the uterus are called:
- the endometrium
- the myometrium
- the perimetrium.

The endometrium

- It forms a lining of ciliated epithelium on a base of connective tissue or stroma.
- It is constantly changing in thickness throughout the menstrual cycle.
- The basal layer does not alter, but provides the foundation from which the upper layers regenerate.

- The epithelial cells are cubical in shape and dip down to form glands that secrete an alkaline mucus.

The *cervical endometrium* does not respond to the hormonal stimuli of the menstrual cycle to the same extent.

- Here the epithelial cells are tall and columnar in shape and the mucus-secreting glands are branching racemose glands.
- The cervical endometrium is thinner than that of the body of the uterus and is folded into a pattern known as the 'arbor vitae'.
- The portion of the cervix that protrudes into the vagina is covered with squamous epithelium similar to that lining the vagina.
- The point where the epithelium changes, at the external os, is termed the squamocolumnar junction.

The myometrium

- It is thicker in the upper part of the uterus but sparser in the isthmus and cervix.
- Its fibres run in all directions and interlace to surround the blood vessels and lymphatics that pass to and from the endometrium.
- The outer layer is formed of longitudinal fibres that are continuous with those of the uterine tube, the uterine ligaments and the vagina.
- In the cervix, the muscle fibres are embedded in collagen fibres, which enable it to stretch in labour.

The perimetrium

- It is a double serous membrane, an extension of the peritoneum, which is draped over the uterus, covering all but a narrow strip on either side of the uterus.
- It covers the anterior wall of the supravaginal cervix and is reflected up over the bladder.

Blood supply

- The uterine artery arrives at the level of the cervix and is a branch of the internal iliac artery.
- It sends a small branch to the upper vagina, and then runs upwards in a twisted fashion to meet the ovarian artery and form an anastomosis with it near the cornu.
- The ovarian artery is a branch of the abdominal aorta. It supplies the ovary and uterine tube before joining the uterine artery.
- The blood drains through corresponding veins.

Lymphatic drainage

Lymph is drained from the uterine body to the internal iliac glands and also from the cervical area to many other pelvic lymph glands.

Nerve supply

The nerve supply is mainly from the autonomic nervous system, sympathetic and parasympathetic, via the inferior hypogastric or pelvic plexus.

THE OVARIES

- These are situated within the peritoneal cavity.
- They are attached to the back of the broad ligaments but are supported from above by the ovarian ligament medially and the infundibulopelvic ligament laterally.
- Each ovary is composed of a medulla and cortex, covered with germinal epithelium. (See Chapter 3 for changes associated with the menstrual cycle.)

Useful website

TeachMeAnatomy info, available at: http://teachmeanatomy.info/pelvis/ (accessed April 10th 2016). This provides information and diagrams to enhance your understanding of the anatomy of the female pelvis and reproductive organs.

The Female Urinary Tract

The urinary system has important functions in connection with the control of water and electrolyte balance and of blood pressure.

THE KIDNEYS

The kidneys are two bean-shaped glands that have both endocrine and exocrine secretions.

Functions

Functions of the kidneys are shown in Box 2.1.

Position and appearance

- The kidneys are positioned at the back of the abdominal cavity, high up under the diaphragm. Each kidney is approximately 10 cm long, 6.5 cm wide and 3 cm thick.
- Each weighs approximately 120 g and is covered with a tough, fibrous capsule.

The inner border of the organ is indented at the hilum; here the large vessels enter and leave, and the ureter is attached by its funnel-shaped upper end to channel the urine away.

Inner structure

- The glandular tissue is formed of *cortex* on the outside and *medulla* within. The cortex is dark with a rich blood supply, whereas the medulla is paler.
- A collecting area for urine merges with the upper ureter and is called the *pelvis*. It is divided into branches or calyces.
- Each calyx forms a cup over a projection of the medulla known as a *pyramid*. There are some 12 pyramids in all and they contain bundles of tubules leading from the cortex.
- The tubules create a lined appearance and these are the *medullary rays*.
- The base of each pyramid is curved and the cortex arches over it and projects downwards between the pyramids, forming columns of tissue *(columns of Bertini)*.

Box 2.1 **Functions of the kidneys**

- Elimination of waste, particularly the breakdown products of protein, such as urea, urates, uric acid, creatinine, ammonia and sulphates
- Elimination of toxins
- Regulation of the water content of the blood and indirectly of the tissues
- Regulation of the pH of the blood
- Regulation of the osmotic pressure of the blood
- Secretion of the hormones renin and erythropoietin

The nephrons (Fig. 2.1)

The tissue of the kidney is made up of approximately 1 million nephrons, which are its functional units.

- Each nephron starts at a knot of capillaries called a *glomerulus*.
- It is fed by a branch of the renal artery, the *afferent arteriole*. (Afferent means 'carrying towards'.)
- The blood is collected up again into the *efferent arteriole*. (Efferent means 'carrying away'.)
- Surrounding the glomerulus is a cup known as the *glomerular capsule*, into which fluid and solutes are exuded from the blood.
- The glomerulus and capsule together comprise the *glomerular body*.
- The pressure within the glomerulus is raised because the afferent arteriole is of a wider bore than the efferent arteriole; this factor forces the filtrate out of the capillaries and into the capsule. At this stage, there is no selection; any substance with a small molecular size will filter out.
- The cup of the capsule is attached to a tubule, as a wine glass is to its stem. The tubule initially winds and twists, then forms a straight loop which dips into the medulla, rising into the cortex again to wind and turn before joining a *straight collecting tubule*, which receives urine from several nephrons.
- The first twisting portion of the nephron is the *proximal convoluted tubule*, the loop is termed the *loop of Henle* and the second twisting portion is the *distal convoluted tubule*.
- The whole nephron is approximately 3 cm in length.
- The straight collecting tubule runs from the cortex to a medullary pyramid; it forms a medullary ray and receives urine from over 4000 nephrons along its length.

Fig. 2.1 A nephron.

Juxtaglomerular apparatus

- The distal convoluted tubule returns to pass alongside granular cells of the afferent arteriole, and this part of the tubule is called the *macula densa*.
- The two are known as the *juxtaglomerular apparatus*. The granular cells secrete renin, whereas the macula densa cells monitor the sodium chloride concentration of fluid passing through.

Blood supply

- The renal arteries are early branches of the descending abdominal aorta and divert approximately a quarter of the cardiac output into the kidneys.
- Deoxygenated blood returns via the renal vein.

THE MAKING OF URINE

This takes place in three stages:
- filtration
- reabsorption
- secretion.

Filtration

- Water and the substances dissolved in it are passed from the glomerulus into the glomerular capsule as a result of the raised intracapillary pressure.
- Blood components such as corpuscles and platelets, as well as plasma proteins, which are large molecules, are kept in the blood vessel; water, salts and glucose escape through the filter as the *filtrate*.
- Fluid passes out at approximately 2 ml per second or 120 ml per minute. Ninety-nine per cent of this must be recovered.
- Filtration is increased in pregnancy, as it helps to eliminate the additional waste substances created by maternal and fetal metabolism.

Reabsorption

- The body selects from the filtrate those substances that it needs: water, salts and glucose.
- Normally, all the glucose is reabsorbed; only if there is already more than sufficient in the blood will any be excreted in the urine.
- The level of blood glucose at which this happens is the *renal threshold* for glucose:
    - in the non-pregnant woman, the threshold is 10 mmol/L.
    - in the pregnant woman, the threshold is 8.3 mmol/L.

It is more likely, therefore, that glucose will appear in the urine during pregnancy.

The water is almost all reabsorbed. The posterior pituitary gland controls the reabsorption of water by producing antidiuretic hormone (ADH). Minerals are selected according to the body's needs. The reabsorption of sodium is controlled by aldosterone, which is produced in the cortex of the adrenal gland. The interaction of aldosterone and ADH maintains water and sodium balance. The pH of the blood must be controlled and, if it is tending towards acidity, then acids will be excreted. However, if the opposite pertains, alkaline urine will be produced.

Secretion

Certain substances, such as creatinine and toxins, are added directly to the urine in the ascending arm of the loop of Henle.

ENDOCRINE ACTIVITY

The kidney secretes two hormones:
- *Renin* is produced in the afferent arteriole and is secreted when the blood supply to the kidneys is reduced and in response to lowered sodium levels. It acts on angiotensinogen, which is present in the blood, to form angiotensin, which raises blood pressure and encourages sodium reabsorption.
- *Erythropoietin* stimulates the production of red blood cells.

THE URINE

- An adult passes between 1 and 2 litres of urine daily, depending on fluid intake.
- Pregnant women secrete large amounts of urine because of the increased glomerular filtration rate.
- In the first day or two postpartum a major diuresis occurs and urine output is copious. This is due to decreased oestrogen levels, excretion of excess fluid (from increased pregnancy-related blood volume) and lower venous pressure in legs and feet following birth.
- The specific gravity of urine is 1.010–1.030. It is composed of:
  - 96% water
  - 2% urea
  - 2% other solutes.
- Urea and uric acid clearance are increased in pregnancy.
- Urine is usually acid and contains no glucose or ketones; nor should it carry blood cells or bacteria.
- Women are susceptible to urinary tract infection (UTI) but this is usually an ascending infection acquired via the urethra.

- A low count, less than 100 000 per ml, of bacteria in the urine (bacteriuria) is treated as insignificant.

THE URETERS

- The ureters convey urine from the kidneys to the bladder.
- They assist the passage of urine by the muscular peristaltic action of their walls.
- The upper end is funnel shaped and merges into the pelvis of the kidney, where the urine is received from the renal tubules.
- Each tube is approximately 25–30 cm long and runs from the renal hilum to the posterior wall of the bladder.
- In the abdomen, the ureters pass down the posterior wall, remaining outside the peritoneal cavity.
- On reaching the pelvic brim, they descend along the side walls of the pelvis to the level of the ischial spines and then turn forwards to pass beside the uterine cervix and enter the bladder from behind.
- They pass through the bladder wall at an angle, so that when the bladder contracts to expel urine the ureters are closed off and reflux is prevented.
- The hormones of pregnancy, particularly progesterone, relax the walls of the ureters and allow dilatation and kinking. In some women, this is quite marked and tends to result in a slowing down or stasis of urinary flow, making infection a greater possibility.

THE BLADDER

- It is the urinary reservoir, storing the urine until it is convenient for it to be voided.
- It is described as being pyramidal and its base is triangular.
- When it is full, however, it becomes more globular in shape as its walls are distended.
- Although it is a pelvic organ, it may rise into the abdomen when full.

Structure

- The base of the bladder is termed the *trigone*. It is situated at the back of the bladder, resting against the vagina.

- Its three angles are formed by the exit of the urethra below and the two slit-like openings of the ureters above.
- The apex of the trigone is at its lowest point, which is also termed the neck.
- The anterior part of the bladder lies close to the pubic symphysis and is termed the *apex* of the bladder. From it the urachus runs up the anterior abdominal wall to the umbilicus.
- The empty bladder is of similar size to the uterus; when full of urine, its capacity is approximately 600 ml but it can hold more, particularly under the influence of pregnancy hormones.

THE URETHRA

- The female urethra is 4 cm long and consists of a narrow tube buried in the outer layers of the anterior vaginal wall.
- It runs from the neck of the bladder and opens into the vestibule of the vulva as the urethral meatus.
- During labour the urethra becomes elongated, as the bladder is drawn up into the abdomen, and may become several centimetres longer.

MICTURITION

- The urge to pass urine is felt when the bladder contains approximately 200–300 ml of urine.
- Psychological and other external stimuli may also trigger a desire to empty the bladder.
- The sphincters relax, the detrusor muscle contracts and urine is passed.
- In summary, the bladder fills and then contracts as a reflex response.
- The internal sphincter opens by the action of Bell's muscles. If the urge is not resisted, the external sphincter relaxes and the bladder empties.
- The act of emptying may be speeded by raising intra-abdominal pressure either to initiate the process or throughout voiding. The act of micturition can be temporarily postponed.

Key points for practice are summarized in Box 2.2.

> **Box 2.2 Key points for practice**
>
> - Pregnant and postnatal women produce large amounts of urine
> - Glucose in the urine might be due to a temporary reduced reabsorption threshold or diabetes (pre-existing or gestational)
> - Protein in the urine might be due to contamination, UTI, pre-eclampsia or renal dysfunction
> - UTIs may present as asymptomatic bacteriuria, acute cystitis or pyelonephritis
> - Low birthweight and preterm birth are associated with asymptomatic bacteriuria
> - A full bladder can impede progress in labour and prevent contraction of the uterus following birth
> - Approximately 6 weeks after birth the hypotonia, dilated ureters and renal pelves return to the non-pregnant state.

FURTHER READING

Smaill, F.M., Vazquez, J.C., 2015. Antibiotics for asymptomatic bacteriuria in pregnancy. Cochrane Database Syst. Rev. (8): CD000490. doi: 10.1002/14651858.CD000490.pub3.

Useful website

TeachMeAnatomy info, available at: http://teachmeanatomy.info/abdomen/viscera/kidney/ (accessed April 10th 2016). This gives more information about the structure and function of the adult kidney.

Hormonal Cycles

FERTILIZATION AND EARLY DEVELOPMENT

The hypothalamus is the ultimate source of control, governing the anterior pituitary gland by hormonal pathways.

- The anterior pituitary gland in turn governs the ovary via hormones.
- The ovary produces hormones that control changes in the uterus. All these changes occur simultaneously and in harmony.
- A woman's moods may change along with the cycle, and emotional influences can alter the cycle because of the close relationship between the hypothalamus and the cerebral cortex.

THE OVARIAN CYCLE

- Under the influence of follicle-stimulating hormone (FSH) and, later, luteinizing hormone (LH) the Graafian follicle matures and moves to the surface of the ovary. At the same time, it swells and becomes tense, finally rupturing to release the secondary oocyte into the fimbriated end of the uterine tube; this is ovulation.
- The empty follicle, known as the corpus luteum, collapses, the granulosa cells enlarge and proliferate over the next 14 days, and the whole structure becomes irregular in outline and yellow in colour.
- Unless pregnancy occurs, the corpus luteum atrophies and becomes the *corpus albicans*.

Ovarian hormones

Oestrogen

It is produced under the influence of FSH by the granulosa cells and the theca in increasing amounts until the degeneration of the corpus luteum, when the level falls. The effects of oestrogen are as follows:

- It is responsible for the secondary female sex characteristics.
- It influences the production of cervical mucus and the structure of the vaginal epithelium.

- During the cycle, it causes the proliferation of the uterine endometrium.
- It inhibits FSH and encourages fluid retention.

Progesterone

This, with related compounds, is produced by the corpus luteum under the influence of LH. They act only on tissues that have previously been affected by oestrogen.

The effects of progesterone are mainly evident during the second half of the cycle:

- It causes secretory changes in the lining of the uterus, when the endometrium develops tortuous glands and an enriched blood supply in readiness for the possible arrival of a fertilized oocyte.
- It causes the body temperature to rise by 0.5 °C after ovulation and gives rise to tingling and a sense of fullness in the breasts prior to menstruation.

Relaxin

- This hormone is at its maximum level between weeks 38 and 42 of pregnancy. It originates in the corpus luteum.
- Relaxin is thought to relax the pelvic girdle, to soften the cervix and to suppress uterine contractions.

PITUITARY CONTROL

- Under the influence of the hypothalamus, which produces gonadotrophin-releasing hormone (GnRH), the anterior pituitary gland secretes two gonadotrophins: FSH and LH.
- The gonadotrophic activity of the hypothalamus and the pituitary is influenced by positive and negative feedback mechanisms from ovarian hormones.

FSH

- This hormone causes several Graafian follicles to develop and enlarge, one of them more prominently than all the others.
- FSH stimulates the secretion of oestrogen.
- The level of FSH rises during the first half of the cycle and when the oestrogen level reaches a certain point its production is stopped.

LH

- This is first produced a few days after the anterior pituitary starts producing FSH.
- Rising oestrogen causes a surge in both FSH and LH levels, the ripened follicle ruptures and ovulation occurs; levels of both gonadotrophins then fall rapidly.
- Progesterone inhibits any new rise in LH in spite of high oestrogen levels, but if no pregnancy occurs, the corpus luteum degenerates after 14 days.
- The negative feedback effect of progesterone ceases and FSH and LH levels rise again to begin a new cycle.

Prolactin

This is also produced in the anterior pituitary gland, but it does not play a part in the control of the ovary. If produced in excessive amounts, however, it will inhibit ovulation.

THE UTERINE CYCLE OR MENSTRUAL CYCLE

- The average cycle is taken to be 28 days long.
- The first day of the cycle is the day on which menstruation begins (Fig. 3.1).
- There are three main phases and they affect the tissue structure of the endometrium, controlled by the ovarian hormones.

FERTILIZATION

- Following ovulation, the oocyte passes into the uterine tube and is moved along towards the uterus. At this time, the cervix, under the influence of oestrogen, secretes a flow of alkaline mucus that attracts the spermatozoa.
- Sperm that reach the loose cervical mucus survive to propel themselves towards the uterine tubes, whilst the remainder are destroyed by the acid medium of the vagina. More will die en route.
- Spermatozoa that reach the uterine tube meet the oocyte, usually in the ampulla. During this journey the sperm finally become mature and capable of releasing the enzyme hyaluronidase, which allows penetration of the zona pellucida and the cell membrane surrounding the oocyte.

Fig. 3.1 The menstrual cycle and early pregnancy. Left: action of the gonadotrophic hormones on the ovary and of the ovarian hormones on the endometrium. Right: ovulation, fertilization, decidual reaction and embedding of the fertilized oocyte. FSH, Follicle-stimulating hormone; GnRH, gonadotrophin-releasing hormone; LH, luteinizing hormone.

- Only one sperm will enter the oocyte.
- The sperm and the oocyte each contribute half the complement of chromosomes to make a total of 46.
  - The sperm and oocyte are known as the male and female *gametes*.
  - The fertilized oocyte is known as the *zygote*.

Fertilization is most likely to occur when intercourse takes place not more than 48 hours before or 24 hours after ovulation.

Development of the zygote

When the oocyte has been fertilized, it continues its passage through the uterine tube and reaches the uterus 3 or 4 days later.

- During this time the zygote divides and subdivides to form a cluster of cells known as the *morula*.
- Next, a fluid-filled cavity appears in the morula, which now becomes known as the *blastocyst*.
- Around the outside of the blastocyst there is a single layer of cells known as the *trophoblast*.
- The remaining cells are clumped together at one end forming the *inner cell mass*.
- The trophoblast will form the placenta and chorion, whilst the inner cell mass will become the fetus, amnion and umbilical cord.

See Chapter 9 for calculation of the expected date of delivery based on menstrual history.

The decidua

- This is the name given to the endometrium during pregnancy. From the time of conception, the increased secretion of oestrogens causes the endometrium to grow to four times its non-pregnant thickness.
- The corpus luteum also produces large amounts of progesterone, which stimulate the secretory activity of the endometrial glands and increase the size of the blood vessels. This accounts for the soft, vascular, spongy bed in which the blastocyst implants.
- The three layers of the decidua are:
  - the basal layer
  - the functional layer
  - the compact layer.

The trophoblast

Small projections begin to appear all over the surface of the blastocyst, becoming most prolific at the area of contact. These trophoblastic cells differentiate into layers:

- the outer syncytiotrophoblast (syncytium)
- the inner cytotrophoblast.

> Box 3.1 **Problems of development**
>
> - Implantation bleeding – lighter than a period, not usually significant
> - Ectopic pregnancy – suspect when there is abdominal pain and amenorrhoea
> - Hydatidiform mole – gross malformation of the trophoblast
> - Miscarriage/abortion – threatened, inevitable, missed

See also Chapter 11

The inner cell mass

While the trophoblast is developing into the placenta, the inner cell mass is forming the fetus itself. The cells differentiate into three layers, each of which will form particular parts of the fetus:

- The *ectoderm* mainly forms the skin, some glands and nervous system.
- The *mesoderm* forms bone and muscle, as well as the heart and blood vessels, including those in the placenta. Certain internal organs also originate in the mesoderm.
- The *endoderm* forms epithelial membranes and some glands and organs.
- Two cavities appear in the inner cell mass:
  - The *amniotic cavity* is filled with fluid, and gradually enlarges and folds around the embryo to enclose it.
  - *The yolk sac* provides nourishment for the embryo until the trophoblast is sufficiently developed to take over.

The embryo

This name is applied to the developing offspring from day 15 after implantation until 8 weeks after conception when it measures approximately 3 cm from crown to rump. This is the most important time in the development of organs and main external features.

Problems of development are summarized in Box 3.1.

Useful website

Hill, M.A. (2016) Embryology Fertilization. Available at: https://embryology.med.unsw.edu.au/embryology/index.php/Fertilization (accessed April 10th 2016). This website has in-depth information about fertilization and videos depicting the process.

The Placenta

Originating from the trophoblastic layer of the fertilized oocyte, the placenta links closely with the mother's circulation to carry out functions that the fetus is unable to perform for itself during intrauterine life.

DEVELOPMENT

Initially, the zygote appears to be covered with a fine, downy hair, which consists of the projections from the trophoblastic layer. These proliferate and branch from approximately 3 weeks after fertilization, forming the *chorionic villi*. The villi become most profuse in the area where the blood supply is richest – that is, in the basal decidua.

- This part of the trophoblast is known as the *chorion frondosum* and it will eventually develop into the placenta.
- The villi under the capsular decidua, being less well nourished, gradually degenerate and form the *chorion laeve*, which is the origin of the chorionic membrane.

The villi erode the walls of maternal blood vessels as they penetrate the decidua, opening them up to form a lake of maternal blood in which they float. The maternal blood circulates slowly, enabling the villi to absorb food and oxygen and excrete waste. Each chorionic villus is a branching structure arising from one stem (Fig. 4.1). The placenta is completely formed and functioning from 10 weeks after fertilization.

Circulation through the placenta

- Fetal blood, low in oxygen, is pumped by the fetal heart towards the placenta along the umbilical arteries and transported along their branches to the capillaries of the chorionic villi.
- Having yielded up carbon dioxide and absorbed oxygen, the blood is returned to the fetus via the umbilical vein.
- The maternal blood is delivered to the placental bed in the decidua by spiral arteries and flows into the blood spaces surrounding the villi. It is thought that the direction of flow is similar to a fountain; the blood passes upwards and bathes the villus as it circulates around it and drains back into a branch of the uterine vein.

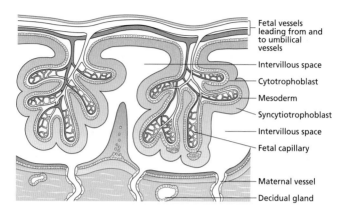

Fetal vessels leading from and to umbilical vessels

Intervillous space

Cytotrophoblast

Mesoderm

Syncytiotrophoblast

Intervillous space

Fetal capillary

Maternal vessel

Decidual gland

Fig. 4.1 Chorionic villi.

It is impossible for the maternal and fetal circulations to mix unless villi are damaged.

THE MATURE PLACENTA

Functions

The 'Green B' mnemonic (Box 4.1) can be helpful.

Box 4.1 **Functions of the mature placenta**

- Glycogen storage plus iron and fat-soluble vitamins
- Respiration
- Excretion
- Endocrine:
  - *Human chorionic gonadotrophin* (HCG) – is produced by the cytotrophoblastic layer of the chorionic villi
  - *Oestrogens* – as the activity of the corpus luteum declines, the placenta takes over the production of oestrogens
  - *Progesterone* – is made in the syncytial layer of the placenta
  - *Human placental lactogen* (HPL) – has a role in glucose metabolism in pregnancy
- Nutrition
- Barrier to some but not all infections

Appearance of the placenta at term

The placenta is a round, flat mass approximately 20 cm in diameter and 2.5 cm thick at its centre.

- *The maternal surface.* The surface is arranged in approximately 20 cotyledons (lobes), which are separated by sulci. The cotyledons are made up of lobules, each of which contains a single villus with its branches.

- *The fetal surface.* The amnion covering the fetal surface of the placenta gives it a white, shiny appearance. Branches of the umbilical vein and arteries are visible, spreading out from the insertion of the umbilical cord, which is normally in the centre. The amnion can be peeled off the surface, leaving the chorionic plate from which the placenta has developed and which is continuous with the chorion.

- *The fetal sac.* The fetal sac consists of a double membrane. The outer membrane is the chorion; this is a thick, opaque, friable membrane. The inner, smooth, tough, translucent membrane is the amnion, which contains the amniotic fluid.

AMNIOTIC FLUID

Functions

These are listed in Box 4.2.

Volume

- The total amount of amniotic fluid increases throughout pregnancy until 38 weeks' gestation, when there is approximately 1 litre.

Box 4.2 **Functions of the amniotic fluid**

- Distends the amniotic sac and allows for the growth and movement of the fetus
- Equalizes pressure and protects the fetus from jarring and injury
- Maintains a constant temperature for the fetus
- Provides small amounts of nutrients
- Protects the placenta and umbilical cord from the pressure of uterine contractions in labour, as long as the membranes remain intact. Also aids effacement of the cervix and dilatation of the uterine os, particularly where the presenting part is poorly applied

- It then diminishes slightly until term, when approximately 800 ml remains.
- If the total amount exceeds 1500 ml, the condition is known as *polyhydramnios*.
- If there is less than 300 ml, the term *oligohydramnios* is applied.

Constituents

Amniotic fluid is a clear, pale, straw-coloured fluid consisting of 99% water. The remaining 1% is dissolved solid matter, including food substances and waste products. In addition, the fetus sheds skin cells, vernix caseosa and lanugo into the fluid. Abnormal constituents of the liquor, such as meconium in the case of fetal distress, may give valuable diagnostic information about the condition of the fetus.

THE UMBILICAL CORD

The umbilical cord extends from the fetus to the placenta and transmits the umbilical blood vessels: two arteries and one vein (Fig. 4.2). These are enclosed and protected by *Wharton's jelly*. The whole cord is covered in a layer of amnion continuous with that covering the placenta. The length of the average cord is approximately 50 cm.

True knots should be noted on examination of the cord, but they must be distinguished from false knots, which are lumps of Wharton's jelly on the side of the cord and are not significant.

Anatomical variations of the placenta and the cord

These are listed in Box 4.3. Except for the dangers noted, these varieties of conformation have no clinical significance.

See Chapter 19 for inspection after birth.

Fig. 4.2 Three vessels in an umbilical cord. (Courtesy of Kellie Crosier.)

Box 4.3 **Anatomical variations of the placenta and the cord**

Succenturiate lobe of placenta

- A small extra lobe is present, separate from the main placenta but joined to it by blood vessels that run through the membranes to reach it
- A hole in the membranes with vessels running to it is likely to indicate a retained lobe

Circumvallate placenta

- An opaque ring is seen on the fetal surface of the placenta
- It is formed by a doubling back of the chorion and amnion and may result in the membranes leaving the placenta nearer the centre instead of at the edge as is usual

Battledore insertion of the cord

- The cord is attached at the very edge of the placenta in the manner of a table-tennis bat

Continued

35

Box 4.3 **Anatomical variations of the placenta and the cord – cont'd**

Velamentous insertion of the cord

- The cord is inserted into the membranes some distance from the edge of the placenta
- The umbilical vessels run through the membranes from the cord to the placenta
- If the placenta is normally situated, no harm will result to the fetus, but the cord is likely to become detached upon applying traction during active management of the third stage of labour
- If the placenta is low lying, the vessels may pass across the uterine os. The term applied to the vessels lying in this position is vasa praevia. In this case, there is great danger to the fetus when the membranes rupture and even more so during artificial rupture, as the vessels may be torn, leading to rapid exsanguination of the fetus

Bipartite placenta

- Two complete and separate parts are present, each with a cord leaving it
- The bipartite cord joins a short distance from the two parts of the placenta

Tripartite placenta

- This is similar to bipartite, but with three distinct parts

The Fetus

Knowledge of fetal development is needed to estimate the approximate age of a baby born before term and appreciate the ways in which developmental abnormalities arise.

TIME SCALE OF DEVELOPMENT

- For the first 3 weeks following conception the term *zygote* is used.
- From 3 to 8 weeks after conception it is known as the *embryo*.
- Following this it is called the *fetus* until birth. Development within the uterus is summarized in Box 5.1.

FETAL ORGANS

Blood

The fetal haemoglobin is termed HbF. It has a much greater affinity for oxygen and is found in greater concentration (18–20 g/dl at term); it carries 20–30% more oxygen than maternal blood. Towards the end of pregnancy, the fetus begins to make adult-type haemoglobin (HbA).

In utero, the red blood cells have a shorter lifespan, this being approximately 90 days by the time the baby is born.

The renal tract

The kidneys begin to function and the fetus passes dilute urine from 10 weeks' gestation. Oligohydramnious can be indicative due to renal dysfunction in the fetus.

The adrenal glands

The fetal adrenal glands produce the precursors for placental formation of oestriols. They are also thought to play a part in the initiation of labour.

The liver

The fetal liver is comparatively large in size. From the third to the sixth month of intrauterine life, it is responsible for the formation of

Box 5.1 **Summary of development**

0–4 weeks after conception

- Rapid growth
- Formation of the embryonic plate
- Primitive central nervous system forms
- Heart develops and begins to beat
- Limb buds form

4–8 weeks

- Very rapid cell division
- Head and facial features develop
- All major organs laid down in primitive form
- External genitalia present but sex not distinguishable
- Early movements
- Visible on ultrasound from 6 weeks

8–12 weeks

- Eyelids fuse
- Kidneys begin to function and fetus passes urine from 10 weeks
- Fetal circulation functioning properly
- Sucking and swallowing begin
- Sex apparent
- Moves freely (not felt by mother)
- Some primitive reflexes present

12–16 weeks

- Rapid skeletal development
- Meconium present in gut
- Lanugo appears
- Nasal septum and palate fuse

16–20 weeks

- 'Quickening' – mother feels fetal movements
- Fetal heart heard on auscultation
- Vernix caseosa appears
- Fingernails can be seen
- Skin cells begin to be renewed

Box 5.1 **Summary of development – cont'd**

20–24 weeks

- Most organs become capable of functioning
- Periods of sleep and activity
- Responds to sound
- Skin red and wrinkled

24–28 weeks

- Survival may be expected if born
- Eyelids reopen
- Respiratory movements

28–32 weeks

- Begins to store fat and iron
- Testes descend into scrotum
- Lanugo disappears from face
- Skin becomes paler and less wrinkled

32–36 weeks

- Increased fat makes body more rounded
- Lanugo disappears from body
- Head hair lengthens
- Nails reach tips of fingers
- Ear cartilage soft
- Plantar creases visible

36–40 weeks after conception (38–42 weeks after last menstrual period)

- Term is reached and birth is due
- Contours rounded
- Skull firm

red blood cells, after which they are mainly produced in the red bone marrow and the spleen. The liver stores glycogen (an important source of energy) and, towards the end of pregnancy, iron.

The alimentary tract

The digestive tract is mainly non-functional before birth. Sucking and swallowing of amniotic fluid containing shed skin cells and other debris begins approximately 12 weeks after conception. Digestive juices are present before birth and they act on the swallowed substances and discarded intestinal cells to form meconium. This is normally retained in the gut until after birth, when it is passed as the first stool of the newborn.

The lungs

It is mainly the immaturity of the lungs that reduces the chance of survival of infants born before 24 weeks' gestation, owing to the limited alveolar surface area, the immaturity of the capillary system in the lungs and the lack of adequate surfactant. Surfactant is a lipoprotein that reduces the surface tension in the alveoli and assists gaseous exchange. It is first produced from approximately 20 weeks' gestation and the amount increases until the lungs are mature at approximately 30–34 weeks. At term the lungs contain approximately 100 ml of lung fluid. Some of this is expelled during (a vaginal) birth and the rest is absorbed and carried away by the lymphatics and blood vessels within two hours.

There is some movement of the thorax from the third month of fetal life and more definite diaphragmatic movements from the sixth month.

The central nervous system

The central nervous system (CNS) development in a fetus is a complex process that occurs through a mix of genetic processes and environmental factors. During pregnancy, the fetus is able to perceive strong light and to hear external sounds. Periods of wakefulness and sleep occur.

The skin

- From 18 weeks after conception the fetus is covered with a white, protective, creamy substance called *vernix caseosa*.
- At 20 weeks, the fetus will be covered with a fine downy hair called *lanugo*; at the same time the head hair and eyebrows begin to form.
- Lanugo is shed from 36 weeks and a full-term infant has little left.
- Fingernails develop from approximately 10 weeks but the toenails do not form until approximately 18 weeks.

THE FETAL CIRCULATION

The key to understanding the fetal circulation (Fig. 5.1) is the fact that oxygen is derived from the placenta. At birth, there is a dramatic

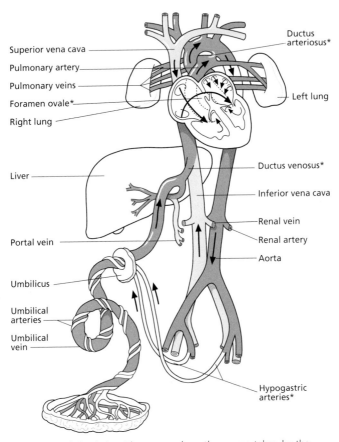

Superior vena cava

Pulmonary artery

Pulmonary veins

Foramen ovale*

Right lung

Liver

Portal vein

Umbilicus

Umbilical arteries

Umbilical vein

Ductus arteriosus*

Left lung

Ductus venosus*

Inferior vena cava

Renal vein

Renal artery

Aorta

Hypogastric arteries*

Fig. 5.1 Fetal circulation. The arrows show the course taken by the blood. The temporary structures are asterisked.

Box 5.2 **Temporary structures within the fetal circulation**

- Umbilical vein
- Ductus venosus
- Foramen ovale
- Ductus arteriosus
- Hypogastric arteries

alteration in this situation and an almost instantaneous change must occur. Several temporary structures, in addition to the placenta itself and the umbilical cord, enable the fetal circulation to function while allowing for the changes at birth (Box 5.2).

THE FETAL SKULL

The fetal skull (Fig. 5.2) contains the delicate brain, which may be subjected to great pressure as the head passes through the birth canal. At birth, the fetal head is one-fourth of the total length of the body.

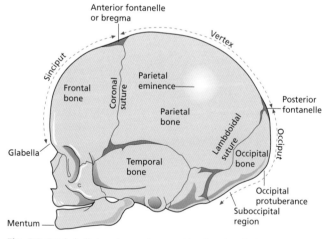

Fig. 5.2 Fetal skull showing regions and landmarks of obstetrical importance.

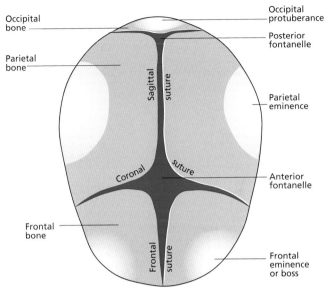

Fig. 5.3 View of fetal head from above (head partly flexed), showing bones, sutures and fontanelles.

Ossification

The bones of the fetal head originate in two different ways:

- The face is laid down in cartilage and is almost completely ossified at birth, the bones being fused together and firm.
- The bones of the vault are laid down in membrane and are much flatter and more pliable. They ossify from the centre outwards and this process is incomplete at birth, leaving small gaps which form the sutures and fontanelles. The ossification centre on each bone appears as a bony protuberance.

Bones of the vault (Fig. 5.3)

There are five main bones in the vault of the fetal skull:

- the occipital bone
- the two parietal bones
- the two frontal bones.

In addition to these five, the upper part of the *temporal bone* forms a small part of the vault.

> ### Box 5.3 **Sutures and fontanelles of significance in the fetal skull**
>
> - Lambdoidal suture
> - Sagittal suture
> - Coronal suture
> - Frontal suture
> - Posterior fontanelle or lambda
> - Anterior fontanelle or bregma

Sutures and fontanelles

Sutures are cranial joints and are formed where two bones adjoin. Where two or more sutures meet, a fontanelle is formed. There are several sutures and fontanelles in the fetal skull. Those of greatest obstetrical significance are shown in Box 5.3.

The sutures and fontanelles, because they consist of membranous spaces, allow for a degree of overlapping of the skull bones during labour and birth.

Regions and landmarks of the fetal skull

The skull is divided into the vault, the base and the face:
- The *vault* is the large, dome-shaped part above an imaginary line drawn between the orbital ridges and the nape of the neck.
- The *base* is composed of bones that are firmly united to protect the vital centres in the medulla.
- The *face* is composed of 14 small bones, which are also firmly united and non-compressible.

The regions of the skull are described in Box 5.4.

Diameters of the fetal skull

The measurements of the skull are important to understand the relationship between the fetal head and the mother's pelvis (Table 5.1 and Fig. 5.4). Some diameters are more favourable than others for easy passage through the pelvic canal.

Box 5.4 **Regions of the fetal skull**

Occiput

- Lies between the foramen magnum and the posterior fontanelle
- The part below the occipital protuberance is known as the suboccipital region

Vertex

- Bounded by the posterior fontanelle, the two parietal eminences and the anterior fontanelle

Sinciput or brow

- Extends from the anterior fontanelle and the coronal suture to the orbital ridges

Face

- Small in the newborn baby
- Extends from the orbital ridges and the root of the nose to the junction of the chin and the neck
- The point between the eyebrows is known as the glabella
- The chin is termed the mentum and is an important landmark

Table 5.1 Diameters of the fetal skull

Name of diameter	Measurement (cm)
Transverse diameters (Fig. 5.3)	
Biparietal	9.5
Bitemporal	8.2
Anteroposterior or longitudinal (Fig. 5.4)	
Suboccipitobregmatic (SOB)	9.5
Suboccipitofrontal (SOF)	10.0
Occipitofrontal (OF)	11.5
Mentovertical (MV)	13.5
Submentovertical (SMV)	11.5
Submentobregmatic (SMB)	9.5

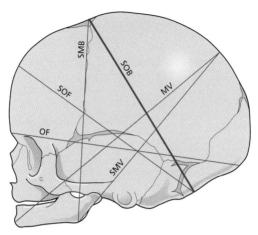

Fig. 5.4 Anteroposterior diameters of the fetal skull (see Table 5.1).

Attitude of the fetal head

This term is used to describe the degree of flexion or extension of the head on the neck. The attitude of the head determines which diameters will present in labour and therefore influences the outcome.

Presenting diameters

The diameters of the head, which are called the presenting diameters, are those that are at right angles to the curve of Carus. There are always two:
- an anteroposterior or longitudinal diameter
- a transverse diameter.

The diameters presenting in the individual cephalic or head presentations are as described in the following section.

Vertex presentation

When the head is well flexed, the suboccipitobregmatic diameter and the biparietal diameter present. As these two diameters are the same length, 9.5 cm, the presenting area is circular, which is the most favourable shape for dilating the cervix. The diameter that distends the vaginal orifice is the suboccipitofrontal diameter, 10 cm (see Chapter 18).

When the head is not flexed but erect, the presenting diameters are the occipitofrontal, 11.5 cm, and the biparietal, 9.5 cm. This situation often arises when the occiput is in a posterior position. If it remains so, the diameter distending the vaginal orifice will be the occipitofrontal, 11.5 cm.

Brow presentation

When the head is partially extended, the mentovertical diameter, 13.5 cm, and the bitemporal diameter, 8.2 cm, present. If this presentation persists, vaginal birth is extremely unlikely.

Face presentation

When the head is completely extended, the presenting diameters are the submentobregmatic, 9.5 cm, and the bitemporal, 8.2 cm.

The submentovertical diameter, 11.5 cm, will distend the vaginal orifice (see Chapter 21 for mechanisms in labour).

Moulding

This is the term applied to the change in shape of the fetal head that takes place during its passage through the birth canal. Alteration in shape is possible because the bones of the vault allow a slight degree of bending and the skull bones are able to override at the sutures. This overriding allows a considerable reduction in the size of the presenting diameters while the diameter at right angles to them is able to lengthen owing to the give of the skull bones.

In a normal vertex presentation, with the fetal head in a fully flexed attitude, the suboccipitobregmatic and the biparietal diameters will be reduced and the mentovertical will be lengthened. The shortening may amount to as much as 1.25 cm.

The intracranial membranes and sinuses (Fig. 5.5)

The skull contains delicate structures, some of which may be damaged if the head is subjected to abnormal moulding during delivery. Among the most important are the folds of dura mater and the venous sinuses associated with them (Box 5.5).

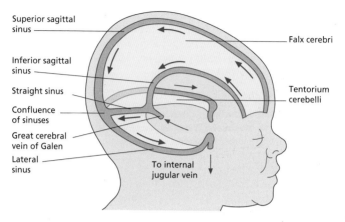

Fig. 5.5 Intracranial membranes and venous sinuses. Arrows show direction of blood flow.

Box 5.5 **Intracranial membranes and sinuses**

- Falx cerebri
- Tentorium cerebelli
- Superior sagittal sinus
- Inferior sagittal sinus
- Great cerebral vein of Galen
- Straight sinus
- Two lateral sinuses

Section | 2 |

Pregnancy

Chapter | 6 |

Preparing for Pregnancy

Preparing for pregnancy is a positive step towards enhancing pregnancy outcome and provides prospective parents with options that may not be available once a pregnancy is confirmed.

PRECONCEPTION CARE

The preconception period refers to a timespan of anything from 3 months to 1 year before conception. The aims of preconception care are:
- to ensure that the woman and her partner are in an optimal state of physical and emotional health at the onset of pregnancy
- to provide prospective parents with a series of options that may not be available once a pregnancy is confirmed.

Box 6.1 outlines the information and investigations that may be required.

GENERAL HEALTH AND FERTILITY

Body weight

- Fertility and obesity are closely linked, with subfertility-related problems occurring in women below and above the desirable range of body weight.
- The Quetelet index or body mass index (BMI) is calculated by dividing the weight in kilograms by the height in metres squared.
- The desirable or healthy range is between 18.5 and 24.9.

There is substantial evidence that shows an increased risk of pregnancy complications/adverse pregnancy outcomes in overweight or obese women. Overweight women should:
- be encouraged to lose weight before conception (this should be under supervision as consuming an energy-deficient diet immediately prior to conception may result in nutritional deficiencies that could disadvantage the fetus).
- be advised that dietary changes and weight loss should occur at least 3–4 months before attempting conception.

Box 6.1 **Information and investigations in a preconception programme**

History

- Family history
- Medical history
- Menstrual history
- Obstetric history
- Method of contraception
- Medication
- Occupation
- Diet
- Smoking
- Alcohol

Observations/investigations

- Height and weight
- Blood pressure
- Urinalysis
- Stool sample
- Blood tests:
  - haemoglobin
  - folic acid and vitamin levels
  - rubella immunity
  - venereal disease research laboratory (VDRL)
  - haemoglobinopathies
  - lead and trace elements
- Male – semen analysis
- Female – cervical smear, high vaginal swab (HVS)

Principles of a healthy diet

A simple and easy guide is to advise women to eat:
- fewer processed foods and less meat
- more starchy foods, such as cereals and bread (more wholegrains)
- at least five portions of fruit and vegetables daily
- fewer fatty, salty foods.

Folate, folic acid and neural tube defects

- Folic acid is a water-soluble vitamin belonging to the B complex.
- The term 'folates' is used to describe the folic acid derivatives that are found naturally in food.
- The term 'folic acid' is used to refer to the synthetic form found in vitamin supplements and fortified foods.
- Folates are vulnerable to heat and readily dissolve in water; therefore, considerable losses can occur as a result of cooking or prolonged storage.
- Folic acid is more stable and better absorbed than folate and is often added to many brands of bread and breakfast cereal.
- To reduce the risk of first occurrence of neural tube defects (NTDs), all women should increase their daily folate and folic acid intake by an additional 400 µg prior to conception and during the first 12 weeks of pregnancy.
- Women with a history of a previous child with NTD should take a daily dose of 5 mg of folic acid to reduce the risk of recurrence. This dose is also recommended in women with diabetes, those taking antiepileptic medication, and those who have malabsorption syndrome.

The main sources of folate are listed in Box 6.2.

Vitamin A

- Vitamin A is essential for embryogenesis, growth and epithelial differentiation, but a high intake of the retinol form of vitamin A is known to be teratogenic.
- Women who are pregnant or planning a pregnancy should avoid eating liver and liver products such as pâté or liver sausage, as these contain large amounts of retinol.

Box 6.2 **Principal sources of dietary folate**

- Dark green vegetables
- Potatoes
- Fruit and fruit juices
- Beans
- Yeast extract

PRE-EXISTING MEDICAL CONDITIONS AND DRUGS

Diabetes

- Infants of insulin-dependent diabetic women have ten times the general population risk of congenital malformation and five times the risk of stillbirth.
- Diabetic complications, such as retinopathy and nephropathy, may worsen during pregnancy, particularly if associated with hypertension.
- Women who have severe neuropathy or cardiovascular disease may be advised against pregnancy.
- The aim of preconception care is to achieve normoglycaemia both pre- and periconception, as many of the problems seen in insulin-dependent diabetic women are a direct result of hyperglycaemia.
- The safety of currently available oral hypoglycaemic agents in pregnancy is not well established.

Epilepsy

- The major anticonvulsant drugs used to treat epilepsy are known to have teratogenic effects, and the newer anti-epileptic drugs have not yet been sufficiently evaluated.
- Pregnancy alters the metabolism of anti-epileptic drugs, with approximately one-third of women experiencing an increase in the number of seizures.
- The aim of preconception care is to help the woman plan her pregnancies carefully and to keep her seizure free on the lowest possible dose of anticonvulsants. For some women, this may mean withdrawal of therapy and for others a reduction from polytherapy to monotherapy.
- Some anticonvulsant drugs are folate antagonists; therefore, folic acid supplements are needed.

Phenylketonuria

- Phenylketonuria (PKU) is an inborn error of metabolism.
- Some women with PKU discontinue treatment during middle childhood. However, unless they resume careful dietary control around the time of conception, the toxic effect of phenylalanine on the developing embryo/fetus results in a high rate of fetal abnormality.

Oral contraception

- Oral contraception should be stopped at least 3 months, and preferably 6 months, prior to planning a pregnancy to allow for the resumption of natural hormone regulation and ovulation.
- The oral contraceptive pill is also associated with vitamin and mineral imbalances that may need correcting.

Drug abuse

- Disruption of the menstrual cycle is common among women who use illegal drugs. Some of these drugs are:
  - Cocaine, ecstasy, methamphetamine, heroin, anabolic steroids and marijuana.
  - Women may also abuse prescription drugs (e.g. oxycodone, morphine and other medications with codeine).
- Drug abuse during pregnancy is associated with miscarriage, preterm labour, low birth weight, stillbirth and abnormalities.
- Women who abuse drugs need referral to specialist alcohol and other drug services. They also need non-judgemental care from midwives and all health professionals involved.
- A poor socioeconomic environment is a compounding factor.
- Women need to be prepared for their baby to require special care after birth due to the withdrawal symptoms they suffer. This is called neonatal abstinence syndrome.

ENVIRONMENTAL FACTORS

Smoking

- Fertility and pregnancy are adversely affected by smoking.
- Smoking can induce early menopause and menstrual problems, and in men it can cause abnormalities in sperm morphology and motility.
- During pregnancy, there is an increased risk of spontaneous abortion, preterm delivery, low birth weight and perinatal mortality because of antepartum haemorrhage and placental abruption.
- Nutritional status tends to be compromised in smokers.
- The aim of preconception care is to help the woman stop smoking, and partner involvement is known to enhance success.
- Health professionals should ask women about smoking at their first antenatal clinic visit and give advice and support for smoking cessation at every visit thereafter.

- Support should include directing women to specialized public health resources (e.g. local stop smoking services in the UK and the Quitline in Australia).

Alcohol

- High alcohol intakes in women have been associated with menstrual disorders and decreased fertility.
- Alcohol is a teratogen. Fetal alcohol spectrum disorder (FASD) is the term used to describe the congenital malformations associated with excessive maternal alcohol intake during pregnancy.
- No safe level of alcohol consumption during pregnancy has been determined; therefore, women should be directed to abstain from alcohol consumption in pregnancy.
- Women who drink alcohol regularly during their pregnancy will need specialist referral for treatment and support.

Exercise

Moderate exercise is known to be beneficial for health and the benefits of regular exercise for the healthy pregnant woman appear to outweigh the risks. However, exercise intensity should be modified according to maternal symptoms and should not continue to fatigue or exhaustion.

When women abuse drugs, smoke, drink alcohol or need help to change aspects of their lives either before or during pregnancy, health professionals can use techniques such as motivational interviewing to help women achieve their goals (see website following).

Workplace hazards and noxious substances

- Exposure to solvents, ionizing radiation and anaesthetic gases is known to be toxic and associated with central nervous system defects, microcephaly and an increased risk of miscarriage. Heavy metals are also known to be toxic.
- Employees are protected by governmental regulations that limit exposure to hazardous substances.
- There is no evidence that the use of computers during pregnancy increases risks of miscarriages or birth defects.

GENETIC COUNSELLING

Genetic counselling should be offered to the following women:
- Those with a family history of genetic disorders.

- Those who have had a previous baby affected with a congenital malformation.
- Those aged 35 or over.

Mendelian inheritance

Genetic disorders can occur as a result of Mendelian inheritance and are termed either dominant or recessive (see Chapter 34).

Chromosome abnormalities

- Chromosome aberrations include the *trisomies*, of which trisomy 21 (Down syndrome) is the most common; trisomy 13 and 18 are rarer.
- Age factors are significant, particularly in Down syndrome, for which the risk is 1% for a woman approximately 40 years of age.
- *Monosomies* are usually lethal and non-viable autosomal trisomies are extremely common in spontaneous abortions.
- Sex chromosome abnormalities, such as Turner syndrome (XO) and Klinefelter syndrome (XXY), have a rare recurrence rate in families.
- In *translocation*, extra chromosomal material is translocated onto another chromosome; it is regarded as balanced when the total amount of chromosome material is normal but only 45 chromosomes are present. Reciprocal translocations can also occur, in which there is an exchange of chromosome material but no change in chromosome number. The recurrence risk is low if neither parent is a balanced carrier for the translocation.

Non-Mendelian disorders

- The more common congenital malformations, such as NTDs and congenital heart disease, do not follow the Mendelian inheritance pattern, as there is no identified genetic locus; they are therefore referred to as *multifactorial*.
- These conditions arise as a result of a combination or interaction of environmental and genetic factors. The recurrence risk of such conditions depends upon the incidence of the disorder but is increased among close relatives.

Prenatal diagnosis

Ultimately, the goal of genetic counselling is to prevent or avoid a genetic disorder. Preconception care, involving a multidisciplinary team, is the way to achieve this.

INFERTILITY

- Infertility is categorized as *primary* if there has been no prior conception and *secondary* if there has been a previous pregnancy, irrespective of the outcome.
- Approximately one-third of cases of infertility involve problems with both partners, and in one-third of couples the causes of infertility remain unexplained. The most common causes are:
  - ovulation failure
  - sperm disorders.
- Much of the initial management of the infertile couple is via primary care. The investigative process is aimed at achieving:
  - an accurate diagnosis and definition of any cause
  - an accurate estimation of the chance of conceiving without treatment
  - a full appraisal of treatment options.
- Specialized investigations may need to be undertaken in a dedicated, specialist infertility clinic where there is access to appropriately trained staff and a multiprofessional team.

Assisted reproduction techniques

- A range of assisted reproduction techniques (ARTs) (Box 6.3) are available to treat the infertile couple and it is important for the appropriate treatment option to be offered.
- Midwives should have an understanding of the prolonged difficult journey couples have taken to achieve a pregnancy.
- Women may have a heightened anxiety regarding their baby's well-being during pregnancy.

Box 6.3 **Some assisted reproduction techniques**

- Ovulation induction
- Intrauterine insemination (IUI)
- Donor insemination (DI) or artificial insemination by donor (AID)
- In-vitro fertilization/embryo transfer (IVF/ET)
- Gamete intrafallopian transfer (GIFT)
- Zygote intrafallopian transfer (ZIFT)
- Intracytoplasmic sperm injection (ICSI)
- Pre-implantation genetic diagnosis (PGD)

SUGGESTED READING

Allot, L., Payne, D., Dann, L., 2013. Midwifery and assisted reproductive technologies. New Zealand College of Midwives Journal 47, 10–12. This article gives specific information on how midwifery care is important when caring for women who have had ART.

Useful website

Matulich, B., 2013. Introduction to Motivational Interviewing. Available at: https://www.youtube.com/watch?v=s3MCJZ7OGRk (accessed April 19th 2016). This video shows simple techniques to work with women towards making changes in their lives (e.g. reducing smoking, alcohol intake and taking exercise).

Change and Adaptation in Pregnancy

PHYSIOLOGICAL CHANGES IN THE REPRODUCTIVE SYSTEM

The body of the uterus

After conception, the uterus develops to provide a nutritive and protective environment in which the fetus will develop and grow.

Decidua

After embedding of the blastocyst there is thickening and increased vascularity of the lining of the uterus, or decidua.

- Decidualization, influenced by progesterone and oestradiol, is most marked in the fundus and upper body of the uterus.
- The decidua is believed to maintain functional quiescence of the uterus during pregnancy; spontaneous labour is thought to result from the activation of the decidua with resultant prostaglandin release following withdrawal of placental hormones.
- The decidua and trophoblast also produce relaxin, which appears to promote myometrial relaxation, and may have a role to play in cervical ripening and rupture of fetal membranes.

Myometrium

- Uterine growth is due to *hyperplasia* (increase in number due to division) and *hypertrophy* (increase in size) of myometrial cells under the influence of oestrogen (Table 7.1). The three layers of the myometrium become more clearly defined during pregnancy.
- The dimensions of the uterus vary considerably, however, depending on the age and parity of the woman.

Muscle layers
- The thin outer longitudinal layer of muscle fibres consists of a network of bundles of smooth muscles. These pass longitudinally

Table 7.1 Uterine growth during pregnancy		
	Prior to pregnancy	**At term**
Weight of uterus	60–80 g	1000 g
Size of uterus	7.5 × 5 × 2.5 cm	30 × 22.5 × 20 cm

from the front of the isthmus anteriorly over the fundus and into the vault of the vagina posteriorly, and extend into the round and transverse ligaments.

- The thicker middle layer comprises interlocked spiral myometrial fibres that are perforated in all directions by blood vessels. Each cell in this layer has a double curve so that the interlacing of any two gives the approximate form of a figure of eight.
- Due to this arrangement, contraction of these cells after birth causes constriction of the blood vessels, providing 'living ligatures'.
- The inner circular layer is arranged concentrically around the longitudinal axis of the uterus and bundle formation is diffuse. It forms sphincters around the openings of the uterine tubes and around the internal cervical os.

Uterine activity in pregnancy

- The myometrium is both contractile (can lengthen and shorten) and elastic (can enlarge and stretch) to accommodate the growing fetus and allow involution following the birth.
- The contractile ability of the myometrium is dependent on the interaction between two contractile proteins: actin and myosin.
- The interaction of actin and myosin brings about contraction, whereas their separation brings about relaxation under the influence of intracellular free calcium.
- The coordination of synchronous contractions across the whole organ is due to the presence of gap junctions that connect myometrial cells and provide connections for electrical activity.
- Promoted by oestrogens and prostaglandins, gap junctions are absent for most of the pregnancy but appear in significant numbers near term, manifesting themselves as *Braxton Hicks contractions*.
- Progesterone, prostacyclin and relaxin are all involved in inhibiting the formation of gap junctions by reducing cell excitability and cell connections and so limiting myometrial activity to small clumps of cells, thus maintaining uterine quiescence during pregnancy.

- Uterine activity can be measured as early as 7 weeks' gestation, when Braxton Hicks contractions can occur every 20–30 minutes and may reach a pressure of up to 10 mmHg.
- These contractions facilitate uterine blood flow through the intervillous spaces of the placenta, promoting oxygen delivery to the fetus. Braxton Hicks contractions are usually painless but may cause some discomfort when their intensity exceeds 15 mmHg.

In the last few weeks of pregnancy, *prelabour* occurs:

- Further increases in myometrial contractions cause the muscle fibres of the fundus to be drawn up.
- The actively contracting upper uterine segment becomes thicker and shorter in length and exerts a slow, steady pull on the relatively fixed cervix.
- This causes the beginning of cervical stretching and ripening known as effacement, and thinning and stretching of the passive lower uterine segment.

There is little rebound between contractions, however; hence there is no cervical dilatation at this time.

Perimetrium

The perimetrium is a thin layer of peritoneum that protects the uterus. It is deflected over the bladder anteriorly to form the uterovesical pouch, and over the rectum posteriorly to form the pouch of Douglas.

- The double folds of perimetrium (broad ligaments), hanging from the uterine tubes and extending to the lateral walls of the pelvis, become longer and wider with increasing tension exerted on them as the uterus enlarges and rises out of the pelvis.
- The anterior and posterior folds open out so that they are no longer in apposition and can therefore accommodate the greatly enlarged uterine and ovarian arteries and veins.
- The round ligaments (contained within the hanging folds of perimetrium) provide some anterior support for the enlarging uterus and undergo considerable hypertrophy and stretching during pregnancy, which may cause discomfort.

Blood supply

The uterine blood flow progressively increases from approximately 50 ml/min at 10 weeks' gestation to 450–750 ml/min at term.

Changes in uterine shape and size

For the first few weeks the uterus maintains its original pear shape, but as pregnancy advances the corpus and fundus assume a more globular form (Box 7.1).

Box 7.1 **Changes in the pregnant uterus**

10 weeks

- The uterus is approximately the size of an orange

12 weeks

- The uterus is approximately the size of a grapefruit
- It is no longer anteverted and anteflexed and has risen out of the pelvis and become upright
- The fundus may be palpated abdominally above the symphysis pubis
- The globular upper segment is sitting on an elongated stalk formed from the isthmus, which softens and which will treble in length from 7 mm to 25 mm between the 12th and 36th weeks

20 weeks

- The fundus of the uterus can be palpated at the level of the umbilicus
- As the uterus continues to rise in the abdomen, the uterine tubes become progressively more vertical, which causes increasing tension on the broad and round ligaments

30 weeks

- The fundus may be palpated midway between the umbilicus and the xiphisternum

38 weeks

- The uterus reaches the level of the xiphisternum
- As the upper segment muscle contractions increase in frequency and strength, the lower uterine segment develops more rapidly and is stretched radially; along with cervical effacement and softening of the tissues of the pelvic floor, this permits the fetal presentation to begin its descent into the upper pelvis
- This leads to a reduction in fundal height known as *lightening*, relieving pressure on the upper part of the abdomen but increasing pressure in the pelvis. In the majority of multiparous women, however, engagement rarely occurs prior to labour

---

The cervix

The cervix is composed of only approximately 10% muscular tissue, the remainder being collagenous tissue.

- During pregnancy the cervix remains firmly closed, acting as the gatekeeper of pregnancy as it provides a seal against external contamination and holding in the contents of the uterus.
- It remains 2.5 cm long throughout pregnancy but becomes softer and swollen under the influence of oestradiol and progesterone.
- Its increased vascularity makes it look bluish in colour.
- Under the influence of progesterone the mucous glands become distended and increase in complexity, resulting in the secretion of a thick, viscous, mucoid discharge. It forms a cervical plug called the *operculum*, which provides protection from ascending infection.
- As uterine activity builds up during pregnancy, the cervix gradually softens, or *ripens*, and the canal dilates.
- *Effacement* or *taking up of the cervix* normally occurs in the primigravida during the last 2 weeks of pregnancy but does not usually take place in the multigravida until labour begins.

Effacement of the cervix is a mechanism whereby the following occur:

- The connective tissue of the long firm cervix is progressively softened by prostaglandins and shortened from the top downwards.
- The softened muscular fibres at the level of the internal cervical os are pulled upwards or 'taken up' into the lower uterine segment and around the fetal presenting part and the forewaters.
- The canal that was approximately 2.5 cm long becomes a mere circular orifice with paper-thin edges.
- The operculum is expelled (called the 'show') as effacement progresses.

The vagina

During pregnancy the muscle layer hypertrophies and oestrogen causes the vaginal epithelium to become thicker and more vascular.

- The altered composition of the surrounding connective tissue increases the elasticity of the vagina, making dilatation easier during the birth of the baby.
- In pregnancy there is an increased rate of desquamation of the superficial vaginal mucosa cells. These epithelial cells release more glycogen, which is acted on by *Döderlein bacilli*, a normal commensal of the vagina, producing lactic acid and hydrogen peroxide.

63

- This leads to the increased and more acidic (pH 3.5–6.0) white vaginal discharge known as *leucorrhoea*.

CHANGES IN THE CARDIOVASCULAR SYSTEM

Understanding changes in the cardiovascular system is important in the care of women with normal pregnancies, as well as for the management of women with pre-existing cardiovascular disease.

The heart

- The heart enlarges by approximately 12% between early and late pregnancy.
- The growing uterus elevates the diaphragm, the great vessels are unfolded and the heart is correspondingly displaced upwards, with the apex moved laterally to the left by approximately 15°.
- By mid-pregnancy more than 90% of women develop an ejection systolic murmur, which lasts until the first week postpartum. If unaccompanied by any other abnormalities, it reflects the increased stroke output.
- 20% develop a transient diastolic murmur and 10% develop continuous murmurs, heard over the base of the heart, owing to increased mammary blood flow.
- Rotational and axis changes during pregnancy cause an inverted T wave to be apparent on the electrocardiogram (ECG) – essential to note if resuscitation is required.

NB: the changes to haemodynamic and cardiac function outlined are largely reversible postpartum.

Cardiac output

- The increase in cardiac output ranges from 35% to 50% in pregnancy, from an average of 5 L/min before pregnancy to approximately 7 L/min by the 20th week; thereafter the changes are less dramatic.
- The increased cardiac output is due to rises in both stroke volume and heart rate.
- The increase in heart rate begins in the 7th week and by the third trimester it has increased by 10–20%.
- Heart rates are typically 10–15 beats/min faster than those of the non-pregnant woman.

- The stroke volume increases by 10% during the first half of pregnancy, and reaches a peak at 20 weeks' gestation that is maintained until term.

Blood

Blood pressure

- Early pregnancy is associated with a marked decrease in diastolic blood pressure but little change in systolic pressure.
- With reduced peripheral vascular resistance, the systolic blood pressure falls an average of 5–10 mmHg below baseline levels, and the diastolic pressure falls 10–15 mmHg by 24 weeks' gestation.
- Thereafter blood pressure gradually rises, returning to pre-pregnant levels at term.
- Posture can have a major effect on blood pressure. The supine position can decrease cardiac output by as much as 25%.
- Compression of the inferior vena cava by the enlarging uterus during the late second and third trimesters results in reduced venous return, which in turn decreases stroke volume and cardiac output.

The pregnant woman may experience *supine hypotensive syndrome*, which consists of hypotension, bradycardia, dizziness, light-headedness, nausea and even syncope if she remains in the supine position too long. By rolling the woman onto her left side the cardiac output can be instantly restored.

Blood volume

- The total maternal blood volume increases 30–50% in singleton pregnancies.

Plasma

- The plasma volume, which corresponds with the increase in blood volume, increases by 50% over the course of the pregnancy.
- In a normal first pregnancy, it may increase by approximately 1250 ml above non-pregnant levels and in subsequent pregnancies it may increase by approximately 1500 ml.
- The increase starts in the first trimester, expands rapidly up until 32–34 weeks' gestation, and then in the last few weeks of pregnancy it plateaus with very little change.

- The increase in plasma volume reduces the viscosity of the blood and improves capillary flow.

Red blood cells

- Red cell mass increases during pregnancy in response to the extra oxygen requirements of maternal and placental tissue.
- Approximately 10–15% of women will have an increase in and reactivation of maternal fetal haemoglobin.
- The increase in red cell mass appears to be constant throughout pregnancy but it is most marked from approximately 20 weeks.
- In spite of the increased production of red blood cells, the marked increase in plasma volume causes dilution of many circulating factors.
- As a result, the red cell count, haematocrit and haemoglobin concentration all decrease (Table 7.2).

In healthy women with iron stores, the mean haemoglobin concentration:

- falls from 13.3 g/dl in the non-pregnant state to 11 g/dl in early pregnancy
- is at its lowest at approximately 32 weeks' gestation when plasma volume expansion is maximal
- after this time rises by approximately 0.5 g/dl, returning to 11 g/dl at approximately the 36th week of pregnancy.

Anaemia in pregnancy has been defined as a haemoglobin of less than 11 g/dl in the first and third trimesters and less than 10.5 g/dl in the second trimester.

Table 7.2 Falling haemoglobin and haematocrit in pregnancy despite rising blood volume and red cell mass

	Week of pregnancy			
	Non-pregnant	**20**	**30**	**40**
Plasma volume (ml)	2600	3150	3750	3850
Red cell mass (ml)	1400	1450	1550	1650
Total blood volume (ml)	4000	4600	5300	5500
Haematocrit (packed cell volume, PCV) (%)	35.0	32.0	29.0	30.0
Haemoglobin (g/dl)	13.3	11.0	10.5	11.0

Iron therapy is unnecessary unless:

- serial estimations show that the haemoglobin has fallen below 10 g/dl, *or*
- there is a progressive reduction in mean cell volume and low serum ferritin levels.

Iron metabolism

The increased red cell mass and the needs of the developing fetus and placenta lead to increased iron requirements in pregnancy.

- Iron demand increases from 2 to 4 mg daily.
- A healthy diet containing 10–14 mg of iron per day, 1–2 mg (5–10%) of which is absorbed, provides sufficient iron for most pregnant women.
- Caffeine interferes with iron absorption.

Plasma protein

The total serum protein content falls within the first trimester and remains reduced throughout pregnancy. Albumin plays an important role:

- as a carrier protein for some hormones, drugs, free fatty acids and unconjugated bilirubin
- because of its influence in decreasing colloid osmotic pressure, causing physiological oedema.

Clotting factors

Major changes in the coagulation system lead to the *hypercoagulable state* of normal pregnancy. The increased tendency to clot is caused by:

- reduced plasma fibrinolytic activity
- an increase in circulating fibrin degradation products in the plasma.

White blood cells (leucocytes)

- From 2 months, the total white cell count rises in pregnancy and reaches a peak at 30 weeks, mainly because of the increase in numbers of neutrophil polymorphonuclear leucocytes.
- This enhances the blood's phagocytic and bactericidal properties.

Table 7.3 is a summary of changes in blood values in pregnancy.

Table 7.3 Summary of common blood values and their changes

	Normal range (non-pregnant)	Change in pregnancy	Timing
Protein (total)	65–85 g/L	↓10 g/L	By 20 weeks then stable
Albumin	30–48 g/L	↓10 g/L	Most by 20 weeks then gradual
Fibrinogen	1.7–4.1 g/L	↑2 g/L	Progressively from third month
Platelets	150–400 × 10⁹ L	Slight decrease	No significant change until 3–5 days postpartum
Clotting time	6–12 min approx.	Little change	
White cell count	4–11 × 10⁹ L	9 × 10⁹ L	Peaks at 30 weeks then plateaus
Red cell count	4.5 × 10¹² L	3.8 × 10¹² L	Declines progressively to 30–34 weeks

Immunity

- Human chorionic gonadotrophin (HCG) and prolactin are known to suppress the immune response of pregnant women.
- Lymphocyte function is depressed.
- There is also decreased resistance to certain viral infections.
- Serum levels of immunoglobulins IgA, IgG and IgM decrease steadily from the 10th week of pregnancy, reaching their lowest level at 30 weeks and remaining at this level until term.

CHANGES IN THE RESPIRATORY SYSTEM

- Increased cardiac output in pregnancy leads to a substantial increase in pulmonary blood flow.
- The blood volume expansion and vasodilatation of pregnancy result in hyperaemia and oedema of the upper respiratory mucosa, which predispose the pregnant woman to nasal congestion, epistaxis and even changes in voice.
- As the uterus enlarges, the diaphragm is elevated by as much as 4 cm, and the ribcage is displaced upwards.

- Expansion of the ribcage causes the *tidal volume* to be increased by 30–40%.
- Although the respiratory rate is little changed in pregnancy from the normal 14 or 15 breaths per minute, breathing is deeper even at rest.
- Both the alveolar oxygen partial pressure and the arterial oxygen partial pressure (PaO_2) are increased from non-pregnant values of 98–100 mmHg to pregnant values of 101–104 mmHg.
- The rise in tidal volume and decrease in residual volume facilitates a 15–20% increase in oxygen consumption, which supports the additional metabolic requirements of mother and fetus.
- The 'hyperventilation of pregnancy' causes a 15–20% decrease in maternal arterial carbon dioxide partial pressure ($PaCO_2$) from an average of 5 kPa (35–40 mmHg) in the non-pregnant woman to 4 kPa (30 mmHg) or lower in late pregnancy.
- The fall in $PaCO_2$ is matched by an equivalent fall in plasma bicarbonate concentration from the non-pregnant values, resulting in mild alkalaemia.

CHANGES IN THE URINARY SYSTEM

- The kidneys increase in weight and lengthen by 1 cm.
- Under the influence of progesterone the calyces and renal pelves dilate.
- The ureters also dilate and lengthen and are thrown into curves of varying sizes.
- The right ureter is usually more dilated than the left, owing to the dextrorotation of the uterus, and as pregnancy advances the supine or upright posture may cause partial ureteric obstruction as the enlarged uterus compresses both ureters at the pelvic brim.
- All these factors can lead to urinary stasis and an increased risk of urinary tract infection in pregnancy.
- After the 4th month of pregnancy the bladder trigone is lifted and there is thickening of its intraureteric margin; this process continues until term, resulting in a deepened and widened trigone. Bladder pressure increases and may result in reduced bladder capacity. To compensate for this, the urethra lengthens and intraurethral pressure increases.
- The muscles of the internal urethral sphincter relax, which, along with pressure from the pregnant uterus on the bladder, causes a significant number of women to experience some degree of stress

69

incontinence. Antenatal teaching of pelvic floor exercises is important for helping to resolve this troublesome feature of pregnancy.

- Urgency of micturition and urge incontinence also increase in pregnancy, partly because of the effects of progesterone on the detrusor muscle. These all usually resolve spontaneously during the puerperium.
- Numerous factors affect renal function in pregnancy, including:
  - increased plasma volume
  - increased glomerular filtration rate (GFR)
  - increased renal plasma flow
  - alterations in hormones such as adrenocorticotrophic hormone (ACTH), antidiuretic hormone (ADH), aldosterone, cortisol, thyroid hormone and HCG.

Studies have shown:

- a 45% increase in creatinine clearance by 9 weeks' gestation
- a peak at approximately 32 weeks' gestation of approximately 50% above non-pregnant levels
- a significant decrease towards non-pregnant levels prior to birth.

The increased GFR means:

- Coupled with impaired tubular reabsorption capacity for filtered glucose, glucose will be excreted (*glycosuria*) at some time during pregnancy in 50% of women.
- There is a proportionate decrease in plasma levels of urea and creatinine.
- Many women with proteinuria before pregnancy experience a progressive increase in the amount of protein spilled during pregnancy; however, the upper limit of normal is considered to be 300 mg over 24 hours.

Other factors:

- The urine is more alkaline owing to the presence of glucose and to the increased renal loss of bicarbonate caused by the alkalaemia of pregnancy.
- Renin rises early in pregnancy and continues to increase until term. It acts on angiotensinogen to form increased amounts of angiotensin I and subsequently II (Fig. 7.1).
- Increased production of angiotensin II stimulates the release of increased levels of aldosterone.
- Aldosterone prevents the increased loss of sodium that could occur as a result of the increased GFR and the natriuretic effects of progesterone.

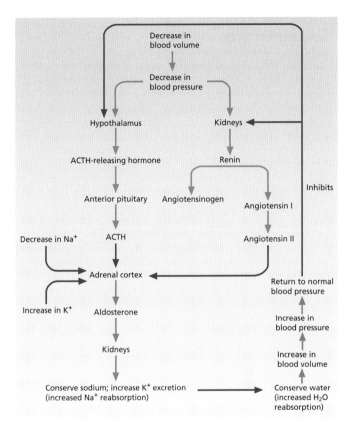

Fig. 7.1 The renin–angiotensin system. (From Wallace 2005 p. 232, with permission of Elsevier, London.)

- Despite elevated aldosterone levels, potassium excretion is decreased, possibly because of the effects of progesterone.

CHANGES IN THE GASTROINTESTINAL SYSTEM

- The gums become oedematous, soft and spongy during pregnancy, probably owing to the effect of oestrogen, which can lead to bleeding when the gums are mildly traumatized, as with a toothbrush.

71

- Occasionally a focal, highly vascular swelling known as *epulis* (or gingivitis) develops; it is caused by growth of the gum capillaries. It usually regresses spontaneously after birth.
- Profuse salivation, or ptyalism, is an occasional complaint in pregnancy.
- Dietary changes in pregnancy, such as aversion to coffee, alcohol and fried foods, are very common, as are cravings for salted and spiced foods.
- Pica, the term given to the bizarre craving for and compulsive, secret chewing of food or ingestion of non-food substances (e.g. ice, coal, disinfectants), is also reasonably common.
- Although in early pregnancy many women experience nausea, an increase in appetite may also be noticed, with the daily food intake increasing by up to 200 kcal.
- Many women notice an increase in thirst in pregnancy because of the resetting of osmotic thresholds for thirst and vasopressin.
- As pregnancy progresses, the enlarging uterus displaces the stomach and intestines. At term the stomach attains a vertical position rather than its normal horizontal one.
- These mechanical forces lead to increased intragastric pressure and a change in the angle of the gastro-oesophageal junction, leading to greater oesophageal reflux.
- Marked reduction of gastric and intestinal tone and motility plus relaxation of the lower oesophageal sphincter predispose to heartburn, constipation and haemorrhoids.

CHANGES IN METABOLISM

To provide for increased basal metabolic rate and oxygen consumption, as well as the needs of the rapidly growing uterus, fetus and placenta, the pregnant woman undergoes many metabolic changes.

- Protein metabolism is enhanced to supply substrate for maternal and fetal growth.
- Fat metabolism increases, as evidenced by elevation of all lipid fractions in the blood.
- Carbohydrate metabolism, however, demonstrates the most dramatic changes.

The continuous supply of glucose required by the growing fetus is met by:
- the intake of glucose when the mother eats
- the enhanced secretion of insulin in response to glucose.

Human placental lactogen (HPL) or other growth-related hormones may contribute to the process by reducing peripheral insulin sensitivity and there may be alterations in the characteristics of insulin binding to its receptor.

- Optimal blood glucose levels in the pregnant woman range between 4.4 and 5.5 mmol/L.
- In the pregnant woman hypoglycaemia is defined as a concentration below 3.3 mmol/L.
- It is recommended that pregnant women do not fast, skip meals or restrict their carbohydrate intake (Muslim women are exempt from fasting during Ramadan when pregnant).
- Maternal blood glucose levels are of critical importance for fetal wellbeing and prolonged fasting in pregnancy produces a more intense ketonaemia, which is dangerous to fetal health.

MATERNAL WEIGHT

Weight gain during pregnancy comprises:
- the products of conception (fetus, placenta and amniotic fluid)
- hypertrophy of several maternal tissues (uterus, breasts, blood, fat stores and extracellular and extravascular fluid) (Table 7.4).

An optimal weight gain for an average pregnancy is 12.5 kg.

- 9 kg of pregnancy weight is gained in the last 20 weeks.
- Appropriate weight gain for each individual woman is now based on the pre-pregnancy BMI, which reflects the mother's weight-to-height ratio.

SKELETAL CHANGES

- During pregnancy, relaxation of the pelvic joints results from hormonal changes.
- Oestrogen, progesterone and relaxin all appear to be implicated.
- This allows some expansion of the pelvic cavity during descent of the fetal head in labour.
- The increase in width of the symphysis pubis, which has been associated with severe pelvic pain, occurs more in multiparous

Table 7.4 Distribution of average increase in weight

	Weight gain (kg)	Percentage of total weight
Maternal		
Uterus	0.9	7.2
Breasts	0.4	3.2
Fat	4.0	32
Blood	1.2	9.6
Extracellular fluid	1.2	9.6
Total	7.7	61.6
Fetal		
Fetus	3.3	26.4
Placenta	0.7	5.6
Amniotic fluid	0.8	6.4
Total	4.8	38.4
Grand total	12.5	100

than in primigravid women, and returns to normal soon after birth.

- Posture usually alters to compensate for the enlarging uterus, particularly if abdominal muscle tone is poor.
- A progressive lordosis shifts the woman's centre of gravity back over her legs.
- There is also increased mobility of the sacroiliac and sacrococcygeal joints, which may contribute to the alteration in maternal posture, leading to low back pain in late pregnancy, particularly in the multiparous woman.

SKIN CHANGES

Pigmentation

From the 3rd month until term, some degree of skin darkening is observed in 90% of all pregnant women:

- The pigmented linea alba, now called the *linea nigra*, runs from the os pubis to above the umbilicus.
- Pigmentation of the face, which affects at least half of all pregnant women, is called *chloasma* or *melasma*, or 'mask of pregnancy'.

- Melasma is caused by melanin deposition into epidermal or dermal macrophages.
- Epidermal melanosis usually regresses postpartum but dermal melanosis may persist for up to 10 years in one-third of women.
- Chloasma can be minimized or prevented by avoiding sun exposure and using high-protection factor sun creams.

Stretch marks

As maternal size increases, stretching occurs in the collagen layer of the skin, particularly over the breasts, abdomen and thighs. In some women, the areas of maximum stretch become thin and stretch marks, *striae gravidarum*, appear as red stripes changing to glistening, silvery white lines approximately 6 months after the birth.

Itching

Although not common, itching of the skin in pregnancy (not due to liver disease) can be distressing. Obstetric cholestasis (see Chapter 12) must be excluded.

Hair

The proportion of growing hairs to resting hairs is increased in pregnancy so the woman reaches the end of pregnancy with many over-aged hairs. This ratio is reversed after birth so that sometimes alarming amounts of hair are shed during brushing or washing. Normal hair growth is usually restored by 6–12 months. Mild hirsutism is common during pregnancy, particularly on the face.

Other skin changes

A rise in temperature by 0.2–0.4 °C occurs as a result of the effects of progesterone and the increased basal metabolic rate (BMR). Angiomas or *vascular spiders* (minute red elevations on the skin of the face, neck, arms and chest) and *palmar erythema* (reddening of the palms) frequently occur, possibly as a result of the high levels of oestrogen. They are of no clinical significance and disappear after pregnancy.

CHANGES IN THE BREASTS

Major changes take place in the breasts during pregnancy owing to the increased blood supply; these changes are stimulated by secretion of oestrogen and progesterone from both corpus luteum and placenta.

Box 7.2 **Breast changes in chronological order**

3–4 weeks

- There may be a prickling, tingling sensation due to increased blood supply, particularly around the nipple

6–8 weeks

- Breasts increase in size, becoming painful, tense and nodular due to hypertrophy of the alveoli
- Delicate bluish surface veins become visible just beneath the skin

8–12 weeks

- Montgomery tubercles become more prominent on the areola; these hypertrophic sebaceous glands secrete sebum, which keeps the nipple soft and supple
- Pigmented areas around the nipple (the primary areola) darken, and may enlarge and become more erectile

16 weeks

- Colostrum can be expressed
- The secondary areola develops, with further extension of the pigmented areas that is often mottled in appearance

Late pregnancy

- Colostrum may leak from the breasts
- Progesterone causes the nipple to become more prominent and mobile

Among these changes is the formation of new ducts and acini cells (Box 7.2).

CHANGES IN THE ENDOCRINE SYSTEM

During pregnancy the intrauterine tissues can produce many of the peptide and steroid hormones that are produced by the endocrine glands in the non-pregnant state. Many hormones exert their actions indirectly by interacting with cytokines and chemokines. Early effects of placental hormones are described in Chapter 3. Later physiological effects caused by hormones have been highlighted throughout this chapter as they impact on the various systems, and are now summarized.

Placental hormones

These are listed in Box 7.3.

Pituitary gland and its hormones

- The pituitary gland enlarges during pregnancy owing to hypertrophy of the anterior lobe. Secretion of follicle-stimulating hormone (FSH) and luteinizing hormone (LH) is greatly inhibited during pregnancy by the negative feedback of progesterone and oestrogen.
- In contrast, there is increased secretion of hormones by the pituitary gland.

The anterior lobe secretes:
- thyroid-stimulating hormone (TSH)
- ACTH
- prolactin
- melanocyte-stimulating hormone (MSH).

The posterior lobe of the pituitary gland secretes:
- oxytocin
- antidiuretic hormone (ADH, vasopressin).

Box 7.3 **Placental hormones**

Human chorionic gonadotrophin
- Produced by the trophoblast
- Maintains the corpus luteum
- Forms the basis for the pregnancy test
- Suppresses the immune response

Human placental lactogen
- Detected in the trophoblast
- Participates in important metabolic processes

Oestrogens
- Stimulate the liver to produce serum cortisol, testosterone and thyroid-binding proteins
- Cause proliferation of the ductal system of the breasts, secretion of prolactin, growth of the uterus and onset of contractions

Progesterone
- Synthesized within the syncytiotrophoblast
- Maintains uterine quiescence
- Relaxes smooth muscle

Prolactin is essential for lactation and levels increase up to 10-fold during pregnancy and lactation. Its effect of producing milk is suppressed during pregnancy by high levels of oestrogen and progesterone.

- There is also intrauterine production of prolactin from cells within the decidua.
- The posterior pituitary gland releases oxytocin throughout pregnancy.
- Concentrations of oxytocin in the maternal circulation do not change significantly during pregnancy or prior to the onset of labour, but do rise late in the second stage of labour.
- There is, however, an increased uterine sensitivity to oxytocin during labour that is influenced by the ratio of oestrogen to progesterone.
- The pulsatile release produces more effective uterine contractions.
- Oxytocin is also important for successful lactation.

Thyroid function

- Alterations in the structure and function of the thyroid gland cause many thyroid symptoms to be mimicked in pregnancy, resulting in diagnostic confusion in the interpretation of thyroid function tests.
- Overall control of the thyroid gland, however, is unaltered during normal pregnancy.
- There is a moderate increase in size early in pregnancy.
- There is a marked increase in thyroid-binding globulin, and the bound forms of thyroxine (T_4) and tri-iodothyronine (T_3) peak at approximately 12 weeks' gestation.
- Circulating concentrations of unbound (inactive) T_3 and T_4 are essentially unaltered. Similarly, TSH shows no change in pregnancy.

Adrenal glands

- In early pregnancy the levels of ACTH are reduced, but from 3 months until term there is a significant rise, along with an increase in serum concentrations of circulating free cortisol.
- The placenta and the trophoblast cells also produce corticotrophin-releasing factor and ACTH. These hormones are important in relation to the priming of myometrial activity and may also influence the fetal adrenals.

- The raised levels of unbound cortisol are reflected in the excretion of double the amount of urinary cortisol.
- From 15 weeks' gestation until the third trimester there is a 10-fold increase in the secretion of aldosterone and deoxycorticosterone by the maternal adrenal glands, as well as by fetal intrauterine tissues, which is stimulated to a certain extent by the acute rise in ACTH.
- Its main means of control is via the renin–angiotensin system (see Fig. 7.1) with involvement of factors such as atrial natriuretic peptide and angiotensins.

DIAGNOSIS OF PREGNANCY

- Amenorrhoea, breast changes, nausea, changes in food and drink preference, overwhelming tiredness, frequency of micturition and backache often convince women that they are pregnant (Table 7.5).

Table 7.5 Signs of pregnancy

Sign	Time of occurrence (gestational age)	Differential diagnosis
Possible (presumptive) signs		
Early breast changes (unreliable in multigravida)	3–4 weeks +	Contraceptive pill
Amenorrhoea	4 weeks +	Hormonal imbalance Emotional stress Illness
Morning sickness	4–14 weeks	Gastrointestinal disorders Pyrexial illness Cerebral irritation, etc.
Bladder irritability	6–12 weeks	Urinary tract infections Pelvic tumour
Quickening	16–20 weeks +	Intestinal movement, 'wind'
Probable signs		
Presence of HCG in: Blood Urine	9–10 days 14 days	Hydatidiform mole Choriocarcinoma

Continued

Table 7.5 Signs of pregnancy – cont'd

Sign	Time of occurrence (gestational age)	Differential diagnosis
Softened isthmus (Hegar sign)	6–12 weeks	
Blueing of vagina (Chadwick sign)	8 weeks +	
Pulsation of fornices (Osiander sign)	8 weeks +	Pelvic congestion
Uterine growth	8 weeks +	Tumours
Changes in skin pigmentations	8 weeks +	
Uterine soufflé	12–16 weeks	Increased blood flow to uterus, as in large uterine myomas or ovarian tumours
Braxton Hicks contractions	16 weeks	
Ballottement of fetus	16–28 weeks	
Positive signs		
Visualization of gestational sac by: Transvaginal ultrasound Transabdominal ultrasound	4.5 weeks 5.5 weeks	
Visualization of heart pulsation by: Transvaginal ultrasound Transabdominal ultrasound	5 weeks 6 weeks	
Fetal heart sounds by: Doppler Fetal stethoscope	11–12 weeks 20 weeks +	
Fetal movements: Palpable Visible Fetal parts palpated	22 weeks + Late pregnancy 24 weeks +	
Visualization of fetus by: X-ray	16 weeks +	

- The fluttering movements of the fetus felt by the mother, known as *quickening*, are normally felt by a primigravid woman at 18–20 weeks, and a multigravid woman at 16–18 weeks.
- Using transvaginal ultrasound, the gestational sac can be visualized at 4.5 weeks and heart pulsation can be seen at 5 weeks.
- Using transabdominal ultrasound, visualization of the gestational sac and heart pulsation is possible 1 week later.
- Doppler can detect the fetal heart at 11–12 weeks' gestation.
- The palpation of fetal parts and fetal movements from approximately 22 weeks are good positive signs of pregnancy.
- Biochemical pregnancy tests depend on the detection of HCG, produced by the trophoblast.
- HCG can be detected in blood as early as 6 days after conception, and in urine 26 days after conception.
- Many different pregnancy tests are available, but the most popular over-the-counter home pregnancy test is the *enzyme-linked immunosorbent assay* (ELISA).

Common Disorders of and Exercises for Pregnancy

Common disorders experienced by some women because of the physiological changes occurring in their body are listed in Box 8.1. More information on caring for women with these disorders can be gained from accessing the website in the 'useful website' section.

RELIEF OF ACHES AND PAINS

Back and pelvic pain

- Backache can be eased by good posture and practice of the transversus and pelvic-tilting exercises in standing, sitting and lying positions (see later for a description of these exercises).
- Women complaining of severe pain involving more than one area of the pelvis (*pelvic arthropathy*) should be referred to a women's health physiotherapist for assessment, advice and possible manipulation.
- Sciatica-like pain may be relieved by lying on the side away from the discomfort so that the affected leg is uppermost. Pillows should be placed strategically to support the whole limb.
- Symphysis pubis dysfunction (SPD), formerly known as diastasis of the symphysis pubis, is covered in Chapter 12.

Midwives should be aware of necessary precautions and correct positions in relation to labour.

Cramp

- Women can help prevent cramp in pregnancy by practising foot and leg exercises. To relieve sudden cramp in the calf muscles while in the sitting position, the woman should hold the knee straight and stretch the calf muscles by pulling the foot upwards (dorsiflexing) at the same time.
- Alternatively, standing firmly on the affected leg and striding forwards with the other leg will stretch the calf muscles and solve the problem.

Box 8.1 **Common disorders of pregnancy**

- Nausea and vomiting
- Breast discomfort
- Backache and ligament pain
- Leg cramp
- Headaches
- Fatigue
- Constipation
- Emotional lability

ANTENATAL EXERCISES

Exercises must be adapted for different circumstances. The positions that pregnant women adopt for exercises should be carefully considered:

- Women should not lie flat in the later second and third trimesters because of the danger of supine hypotension.
- Instead, a half-lying position with the back raised to an angle of approximately 35° can be used.
- Foot and leg exercises and pelvic tilting can be performed in sitting or half-lying positions, whereas transversus and pelvic floor exercises can be carried out in any position.
- Muscles of good tone are more elastic and will regain their former length more efficiently and more quickly after being stretched than muscles of poor tone.
- Exercising the abdominal muscles antenatally will ensure a speedy postnatal return to normal, effective pushing in labour and the lessening of backache in pregnancy.
- An important function of the abdominal muscles is the control of pelvic tilt. As the ligaments around the pelvis stretch and no longer give such firm support to the joints, the muscles become the second line of defence, helping to prevent an exaggerated pelvic tilt and unnecessary strain on the pelvic ligaments.
- Overstretched ligaments and weakened abdominal muscles during pregnancy can lead to chronic skeletal problems postnatally, as well as backache antenatally. Exercises for the transversus muscles (transversus exercise) and rectus muscles (pelvic tilting) help to prevent this and maintain good abdominal tone.

- Exercises that involve the oblique abdominal muscles should be avoided in later pregnancy as they may cause diastasis recti.

Transversus exercise

To tone the deep transverse abdominal muscles and to help prevent backache:
- Sit comfortably or kneel on all fours with a level spine.
- Breathe in and out, then gently pull in the lower part of the abdomen below the umbilicus, keeping the spine still and breathing normally.
- Hold for up to 10 seconds then relax gently.
- Repeat up to 10 times.

Pelvic tilting or rocking

To encourage good posture and ease backache:
- Adopt a half-lying position, well supported with pillows, and the knees bent and feet flat.
- One hand should be placed under the small of the back and the other on top of the abdomen.
- Tighten the abdominals and buttocks, and press the small of the back down on to the hand underneath.
- Breathe normally; hold for up to 10 seconds then relax.
- Repeat up to 10 times.

Pelvic tilting can also be performed sitting, standing or kneeling.

Pelvic floor exercise

To maintain the tone of the muscles so they retain their functions and to help the muscles to relax during parturition and regain their former strength quickly during the puerperium:
- Sit, stand or half-lie with legs slightly apart.
- Close and draw up around the back passage as though preventing a bowel action then repeat around the front two passages as though preventing the flow of urine.
- Draw up inside and hold for as long as possible, up to 10 seconds, breathing normally, then relax.
- Repeat up to 10 times.

This simple exercise can be practised anywhere and at any time. It will build up the endurance of the postural slow-twitch fibres in the pelvic floor but can also be performed quickly up to 10 times without holding the contraction.

- This works the fast-twitch fibres, which need to work quickly to prevent leakage (e.g. when coughing).
- All women should practise this exercise very regularly antenatally, particularly after emptying the bladder.
- For those with diminished pelvic floor awareness, attempting to 'grip' on to an imaginary tampon that is slipping out or squeezing the pelvic floor muscles around the vagina and bladder, as if stopping the flow of urine, may assist the ability to contract the correct muscles. It was customary to inform women to practise their pelvic floor muscle exercises by trying to stop the flow of urine mid-stream. This is no longer seen as good practice as it could lead to urinary retention and have negative consequences for bladder function, especially if performed with regularity when the bladder is full.

Foot and leg exercises

To improve the circulation and prevent or alleviate cramp, oedema and varicose veins, each of the following should be repeated several times per day:
- bend and stretch the ankles
- circle feet at the ankles
- brace the knees and let go.

Additional information

- Advise pregnant women to avoid long periods of standing, which may increase oedema, but encourage walking.
- Discourage sitting or lying with legs crossed, which can impede the circulation.
- Describe how to relieve cramp.
- Advise on correct use of support tights.
- Stress the importance of supporting footwear of sensible height.
- Advise sitting with feet elevated whenever possible and with heels higher than hips if oedema is present.

STRESS, RELAXATION AND RESPIRATION

Tension manifests itself with muscle tightening and shows in the ways listed in Box 8.2.
- When tension increases, breathing often becomes shallow and rapid; when severe, breath holding may feature.

Box 8.2 **Signs of tension**

- Frowning face
- Tense jaw
- Hunched shoulders
- Elbows bent and close to sides
- Fingers gripping or tapping
- Trunk bent forward
- Crossed legs
- Feet pulled up or tapping

- The higher the stress level, the greater is the degree of postural change that will be evident. Mental tension often leads to physical tension and a vicious circle is established.
- Muscles can work singly but usually they work in groups and when any group of muscles is working, the opposite group relaxes. This is known as *reciprocal inhibition* or *reciprocal relaxation*.
- Reciprocal relaxation ensures that, when following a series of instructions for the whole body, one will be able to bring release of tension and relaxation to all areas.

Respiration

- Respiration is affected by stress and adapted breathing is one of the easiest ways of assisting relaxation.
- Breathing can be used to increase the depth of relaxation by varying its speed; slower breathing leads to deeper relaxation.
- Natural rhythmic breathing must not be confused with specific unnatural levels or rates of breathing. Women in labour frequently breathe very rapidly at the peak of a contraction but should be encouraged not to do so. Persistent rapid breathing or breath holding is usually a sign of panic.
- Very slow, deep breathing can cause hyperventilation, which produces tingling in the fingers and may proceed to carpopedal spasm and even tetany.
- Rapid, shallow breathing or panting is only tracheal and can lead to hypoventilation with subsequent oxygen deprivation.
- During pregnancy, labour and birth, emphasis should be placed on easy, rhythmic breathing and on avoiding very deep breathing, shallow panting or long periods of breath holding.

FURTHER READING

Liddle, S.D., Pennick, V., 2015. Interventions for preventing and treating low-back and pelvic pain during pregnancy. Cochrane Database Syst. Rev. (9): CD001139. doi: 10.1002/14651858.CD001139.pub4.

Useful website

National Institute for Health and Care Excellence, 2016. Antenatal care for uncomplicated pregnancies. Available at: https:// www.nice.org.uk/ guidance/cg62/chapter/1-Guidance (accessed July 27th 2016).

Chapter | 9 |

Antenatal Care

AIM OF ANTENATAL CARE

The aim is to monitor the progress of pregnancy in order to support maternal health and normal fetal development. The midwife critically evaluates the physical, psychological and sociological effects of pregnancy on the woman and her family by:

- developing a partnership with the woman
- providing a holistic approach to the woman's care that meets her individual needs
- promoting an awareness of the public health issues for the woman and her family
- exchanging information with the woman and her family and enabling them to make informed evidence-based choices about pregnancy and birth
- being an advocate for the woman and her family during her pregnancy, supporting her right to choose care that is appropriate for her own needs and those of her family
- recognizing complications of pregnancy and appropriately referring the woman within the multidisciplinary team
- assisting the woman and her family in their preparations to meet the demands of birth and making a birth plan
- assisting the woman in making an informed choice about methods of infant feeding and giving appropriate and sensitive advice to support her decision
- offering education for parenthood within a planned programme or on an individual basis
- working in partnership with other pertinent organizations.

THE INITIAL ASSESSMENT (BOOKING VISIT – IDEALLY BY 10 WEEKS' GESTATION)

The purpose of this visit is to:

- introduce the woman to the maternity service
- share information in order to discuss, plan and implement care for the duration of the pregnancy, the birth and postnatally.

The earlier the first contact is made with the midwife, the more appropriate and valuable the advice given relating to nutrition and care of the developing fetal organs. Medical conditions, infections, smoking, alcohol and drug taking may all have a profound and detrimental effect on the fetus during this time.

Models of midwifery care

Options for place of birth include:
- the home
- a birth centre
- a local maternity unit
- a tertiary hospital.

Most women receive antenatal care from midwives in the community, either in their own home, at a local health centre, or within a hospital setting. Hospital-based clinics are also available for women who receive care from an obstetrician or physician in addition to their midwife.

Introduction to the midwifery service

The woman's introduction to midwifery care is crucial in forming her initial impressions of the maternity service. The midwife can promote communication with the woman by:
- using gentle questioning
- using good listening skills
- making open-ended statements
- reflecting back key words used during the discussion to encourage and facilitate exploration of what is being said.

Communication encompasses the writing of accurate, comprehensive and contemporaneous records of information given and received and the plan of care that has been agreed.

Observations

Observation of physical characteristics is also important.
- Posture and gait can indicate back problems or previous trauma to the pelvis.
- The woman may be lethargic, which could be an indication of extreme tiredness, anaemia, malnutrition or depression.

Social history

- It is important to assess the response of the whole family to the pregnancy and to aim to improve health and reduce health inequalities in pregnant women and their young children.

- The midwife may, in partnership with the woman, advocate referral to a social worker or to other multiprofessional agencies.
- Routine questioning about domestic abuse needs to be included in antenatal care but requires discretion.

General health

General health should be discussed and advice given when required.

- The woman, her partner and other family members should be informed about the direct and passive effects of smoking on the baby.
- Drinking alcohol can cause fetal alcohol spectrum disorder. There is no proven safe amount of alcohol that women can drink during pregnancy. Therefore, it is recommended that women do not drink whilst pregnant.
- Nutritional supplements, food-acquired infections, prescribed medicines and complementary therapies should be discussed (see National Institute for Health and Care Excellence (NICE) guidelines in the 'useful website' section).

Menstrual history

The midwife needs to know how to determine the expected date of birth (referred to as EDB or, historically, EDD [expected date of delivery]).

- Abdominal assessment of uterine size can be made in conjunction with gestational age during the antenatal consultation.
- The midwife has a role in helping the woman to understand that an EDB is 1 day within a 5-week time frame during which her baby reaches term and may be born.
- The EDB is calculated by adding 9 calendar months and 7 days to the date of the first day of the woman's last menstrual period (LMP). This method assumes that:
  - the woman takes regular note of regularity and length of time between periods
  - conception occurred 14 days after the first day of the last period; this is true only if the woman has a regular 28-day cycle
  - the last period of bleeding was true menstruation; implantation of the zygote may cause slight bleeding.
- Naegele's rule suggests that the duration of a pregnancy is 280 days. However, controversy exists over the suitability of applying Naegele's rule to determine EDB; therefore, ultrasound scanning

has become the more accurate and commonly used method for predicting the EDB.

- This depends on an experienced ultrasonographer being both available and accessible, and also requires the woman's consent.
- Ultrasound before 14 weeks confirms the EDB; the 18–20-week scan identifies abnormalities.
- If the woman has taken oral contraceptives within the previous 3 months, this may also confuse estimation of dates because breakthrough bleeding and anovular cycles lead to inaccuracies.
- Some women become pregnant with an intrauterine contraceptive device (IUCD) still in place. Although the pregnancy is likely to continue normally, the position of the IUCD may be determined using ultrasound techniques.

Obstetric history

In order to give a summary of a woman's childbearing history, the descriptive terms -*gravida* and -*para* are used:

- 'Gravid' means 'pregnant', 'gravida' means 'a pregnant woman' and a subsequent number indicates the number of times she has been pregnant regardless of outcome.
- 'Para' means 'having given birth'; a woman's parity refers to the number of times that she has given birth to a child, live or stillborn, excluding miscarriages and abortions.
- A *grande multigravida* is a woman who has been pregnant five times or more irrespective of outcome.
- A *grande multipara* is a woman who has given birth five times or more.
- Any form of abortion occurring in a rhesus negative woman requires prophylactic administration of anti-D immunoglobulin to reduce the risk of rhesus incompatibility in a subsequent pregnancy (see Chapter 35).
- Confidential information may be recorded in a clinic-held summary of the pregnancy and not in the woman's hand-held record if she requests this.
- Repeated spontaneous abortion (miscarriage) may indicate conditions such as genetic abnormality, hormonal imbalance or incompetent cervix (also called cervical insufficiency). The woman may be more anxious about this pregnancy, minor disturbances in pregnancy may be exacerbated and preoccupation with the pregnancy may lead to other psychological, social or physical problems.

A risk assessment should be carried out based on the woman's obstetric and medical history and current pregnancy. This will enable the midwife and woman to:

- discuss the progress of the pregnancy
- determine the frequency of antenatal visits and the location of antenatal care (usually 10 visits for uncomplicated nulliparous women and 7 for uncomplicated parous women)
- identify appropriate screening techniques and other health professionals who may need to be involved
- make an informed choice about the place of birth, which will also be influenced by the risk assessment (Box 9.1). In all cases the ultimate decision is taken by the mother.

Medical history

During pregnancy both the mother and the fetus may be affected by a medical condition, or a medical condition may be altered by the pregnancy. If untreated, there may be serious consequences for the woman's health.

Family history

Certain conditions are genetic in origin, others are familial or related to ethnicity, and some are associated with the physical or social environment in which the family lives.

PHYSICAL EXAMINATION

Prior to the physical examination of a pregnant woman, her consent and comfort are primary considerations. Sophisticated biochemical assessments and ultrasound investigations can enhance clinical observations.

Weight

All women should be weighed or asked for a pre-pregnant weight at booking; if it is within the normal body mass index (BMI) range, repeated weighing is not recommended.

Women with a BMI of 30 or above, or 18 or under, should be carefully monitored and offered a referral to a dietician.

Blood pressure

Blood pressure is taken to ascertain normality and provide a baseline reading for comparison throughout pregnancy.

Box 9.1 **Factors that may require additional antenatal surveillance or advice**

Initial assessment
- Age less than 20 years or 40 years and over
- Grande multiparity (more than five previous births)
- Vaginal bleeding at any time during pregnancy
- Unknown or uncertain expected date of birth (EDB)
- Late booking

Past obstetric history
- Stillbirth or neonatal death
- Baby small or large for gestational age
- Congenital abnormality
- Rhesus isoimmunization
- Pregnancy-induced hypertension
- Two or more terminations of pregnancy
- Three or more spontaneous miscarriages
- Previous preterm labour
- Cervical cerclage in past or present pregnancy
- Previous caesarean section or uterine surgery
- Ante- or postpartum haemorrhage
- Precipitate labour
- Multiple pregnancy

Maternal health
- Previous history of deep vein thrombosis or pulmonary embolism
- Chronic illness, blood disorders
- Hypertension, cardiac disease
- History of infertility
- Uterine anomaly, including fibroids
- Substance abuse (drugs, alcohol, smoking)
- Family history of diabetes or genetic disorder
- Psychological or psychiatric disorders
- Complex social needs (including screening for female genital mutilation and domestic abuse)

Examination at the initial assessment
- Blood pressure 140/90 mmHg or above
- Maternal obesity or underweight according to BMI

- The systolic recording may be falsely elevated if a woman is nervous or anxious; long waiting times can cause additional stress. A full bladder can also cause an increase in blood pressure.
- The woman should be comfortably seated or resting in a lateral position on the couch when the blood pressure is taken. Brachial artery pressure is highest when sitting and lower when in the recumbent position.
- A systolic blood pressure of ≥ 140 mmHg or diastolic pressure of ≥ 90 mmHg at booking is indicative of hypertension and will need careful monitoring during pregnancy with both midwife and obstetrician support.

Urinalysis

At the first visit a midstream specimen should be sent to the laboratory for culture to exclude asymptomatic bacteriuria. Urinalysis for proteinuria is performed at every visit.

Blood tests in pregnancy

- The midwife should explain why blood tests are carried out to enable women to make informed choices.
- The midwife should be fully aware of the difference between screening and diagnostic tests, and of their accuracy, and should discuss these options with the women. Blood tests taken at the initial assessment include the ones listed in Box 9.2.
- Rhesus negative women who have threatened miscarriage, amnio-centesis or any other uterine trauma should be given anti-D gamma-globulin within a few days of the event.

Box 9.2 **Blood tests performed at initial assessment**

- ABO blood group and rhesus (Rh) factor
- Full blood count
- Venereal disease research laboratory (VDRL) test
- HIV antibodies
- Rubella immune status
- Hepatitis B screening
- Investigations for other blood disorders (in women and their partners of some ethnic groups – for example, sickle-cell disease, thalassaemia, vitamin D)

- In any event, many countries (such as the UK) recommend that women with rhesus D-negative blood type who are non-sensitized are routinely offered antenatal anti-D gamma-globulin prophylaxis during pregnancy.
- If the titration demonstrates a rising antibody response, then more frequent assessment will be made in order to plan management by an obstetrician and/or a specialist in rhesus disease.

The midwife's examination and advice

The midwife's general examination of the woman is holistic and should encompass her physical, social and psychological wellbeing and provide advice on the alleviation of common disorders.

Nausea and vomiting

Over 50% of women will suffer from nausea and vomiting which is thought to be because of hormonal changes during pregnancy.

The midwife may suggest remedies such as:
- eating a dry biscuit or cracker with a drink before rising in the morning
- avoiding spicy or pungent odours
- eating little and often (helps to maintain the body's blood sugar levels); drinking small amounts of fluid between meals will help to maintain hydration.

Other suggested remedies have included:
- the use of neurological devices, which transmit electrical stimulation via the wrist and are thought to trigger sensory and neurological impulses that control vomiting
- complementary therapies, such as acupuncture and homeopathic and herbal remedies, which may be of benefit in minimizing discomfort.
- pharmacological remedies, such as antihistamines.

Nausea and vomiting generally improve at approximately 16 weeks' gestation, although many women suffer for longer. A small proportion of affected women will develop a more serious condition known as hyperemesis gravidarum, which requires urgent referral to a doctor.

Bladder and bowel function

- Bladder and bowel function may be discussed.
- Dietary advice may be necessary at this visit or later in the pregnancy, with reference to how hormonal changes may alter normal bowel and kidney function.

- Advice can be given on how to avoid constipation, for example, by taking a high-fibre diet and maintaining an adequate fluid intake.
- If constipation persists, then haemorrhoids may develop, caused by straining at defaecation.

Vaginal discharge

- Vaginal discharge increases in pregnancy; the woman may discuss any increase or changes with the midwife. Once the woman has identified what is normal she will then be able to report any changes to the midwife during subsequent visits.
- If the discharge is itchy, causes soreness, is any colour other than creamy-white or has an offensive odour, then infection is likely and should be investigated further.
- Later in pregnancy the woman may report a change from leucorrhoea to a heavier mucous discharge. Mucoid loss is evidence of cervical changes, and if it occurs before the 37th week, may be an early sign of preterm labour.
- The obstetrician will investigate vaginal bleeding during pregnancy; however, in early pregnancy spotting may occur at the time when menstruation would have been due.
- Early bleeding is not uncommon; the midwife should advise the woman to rest at this time and to avoid sexual intercourse until the pregnancy is more stable.

Abdominal examination

This should be performed at each antenatal visit (see later).
- At the initial assessment, the midwife will observe for signs of pregnancy.
- It is unlikely that the uterus will be palpable abdominally before the 12th week of gestation.
- If it has previously been retroverted, it may not be palpable until the 16th week.

Oedema

This is not likely to be in evidence during the initial assessment but may occur as the pregnancy progresses.
- Physiological oedema occurs after rising in the morning and worsens during the day; it is often associated with daily activities or hot weather.
- At visits later in pregnancy, the midwife should observe for oedema and ask the woman about symptoms.

Varicosities

These are more likely to occur during pregnancy and are a predisposing cause of deep vein thrombosis. The woman should be asked to report any tenderness that she feels either during the examination or at any time during the pregnancy. Advice about support tights can be offered.

ABDOMINAL EXAMINATION

The abdominal examination is carried out to establish and affirm that fetal growth is consistent with gestational age during the progression of pregnancy.

Preparation

- The bladder should be emptied.
- Privacy is essential.
- The woman should be lying comfortably with her arms by her sides to relax the abdominal muscles.
- After the examination, the woman should sit up to discuss the findings with the midwife.

Method

Inspection

- The size of the uterus is assessed approximately by observation.
- The shape of the uterus is longer than it is broad when the lie of the fetus is longitudinal. If the lie is transverse, the uterus is low and broad.
- The multiparous uterus may lack the snug ovoid shape of the primigravid uterus. Often it is possible to see the shape of the fetal back or limbs.
- If the fetus is in an occipitoposterior position, a saucer-like depression may be seen at or below the umbilicus.
- The midwife may observe fetal movements or they may be felt by the mother; this can help the midwife determine the position of the fetus.
- Lax abdominal muscles in the multiparous woman may allow the uterus to sag forwards; this is known as *pendulous abdomen* or anterior obliquity of the uterus. In the primigravida it is a serious sign, as it may be due to pelvic contraction.

Skin changes

- Stretch marks known as *striae gravidarum* from previous pregnancies appear silvery and recent ones appear pink.
- A *linea nigra* may be seen; this is a normal dark line of pigmentation running longitudinally in the centre of the abdomen below and sometimes above the umbilicus.
- Scars may indicate previous obstetric or abdominal surgery.

Palpation

- To determine the height of the fundus the midwife places one hand just below the xiphisternum.
- Pressing gently, the hand is moved down the abdomen until the curved upper border of the fundus is felt, noting the number of fingerbreadths that can be accommodated between the two.
- Alternatively, the distance between the fundus and the symphysis pubis can be determined with a tape measure.
- The height of the fundus correlates well with gestational age, especially during the earlier weeks of pregnancy (Fig. 9.1).
- If the uterus is unduly big the fetus may be large, but multiple pregnancy or polyhydramnios may be suspected.
- When the uterus is smaller than expected, the LMP date may be incorrect, or the fetus may be small for gestational age.
- If there is a greater than 2 cm discrepancy from the fundal height measurement, the midwife should discuss this with the obstetrician.

Fundal palpation

- This determines the presence of the breech or the head. This information will help to diagnose the lie and presentation of the fetus.
- Watching the woman's reaction to the procedure, the midwife lays both hands on the sides of the fundus, fingers held close together and curving round the upper border of the uterus.
- Gentle yet deliberate pressure is applied using the palmar surfaces of the fingers to determine the soft consistency and indefinite outline that denotes the breech. Sometimes the buttocks feel rather firm but they are not as hard, smooth or well defined as the head.
- With a gliding movement, the fingertips are separated slightly in order to grasp the fetal mass, which may be in the centre or deflected

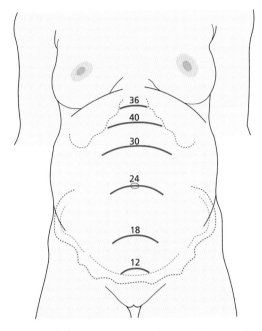

Fig. 9.1 Growth of the uterus, showing the fundal heights at various weeks of pregnancy.

to one side, to assess its size and mobility. The breech cannot be moved independently of the body, as the head can.

- The head is much more distinctive in outline than the breech, being hard and round; it can be balloted (moved from one hand to the other) between the fingertips of the two hands because of the free movement of the neck.

Lateral palpation

- This is used to locate the fetal back in order to determine position.
- The hands are placed on either side of the uterus at the level of the umbilicus.
- Gentle pressure is applied with alternate hands to detect which side of the uterus offers the greater resistance.

99

- More detailed information is obtained by feeling along the length of each side with the fingers. This can be done by sliding the hands down the abdomen while feeling the sides of the uterus alternately.
- Some midwives prefer to steady the uterus with one hand and, using a rotary movement of the opposite hand, to map out the back as a continuous smooth resistant mass from the breech down to the neck; on the other side the same movement reveals the limbs as small parts that slip about under the examining fingers.
- 'Walking' the fingertips of both hands over the abdomen from one side to the other is an excellent method of locating the back. The fingers should be dipped deeply into the abdominal.
- The firm back can be distinguished from the fluctuating amniotic fluid and the receding knobbly small parts. To make the back more prominent, fundal pressure can be applied with one hand and the other used to 'walk' over the abdomen.
- Palpating from the neck upwards and inwards can locate the anterior shoulder.

Pelvic palpation

- Pelvic palpation will identify the fetal presentation; however, as this can cause discomfort to the woman it is not recommended before 36 weeks.
- Ask the woman to bend her knees slightly to relax the abdominal muscles.
- Suggest that she breathe steadily; relaxation may be helped if she sighs out slowly.
- The sides of the uterus just below umbilical level are grasped snugly between the palms of the hands with the fingers held close together, and pointing downwards and inwards.
- If the head is presenting, a hard mass with a distinctive round, smooth surface will be felt. The midwife should also estimate how much of the fetal head is palpable above the pelvic brim to determine engagement.
- The two-handed technique appears to be the more comfortable for the woman and gives the most information.
- Pawlik's manoeuvre is sometimes used to judge the size, flexion and mobility of the head but the midwife must be careful not to apply undue pressure. It should be used only if absolutely necessary. The midwife grasps the lower pole of the uterus between her fingers

Fig. 9.2 Auscultation of the fetal heart.

and thumb, which should be spread wide enough apart to accommodate the fetal head.

Auscultation

Although the antenatal care guidelines issued by NICE in the UK for the care of women with uncomplicated pregnancy states that routine auscultation of the fetal heart is not recommended, hearing their baby's heartbeat provides great reassurance to women. When using a Pinard stethoscope:

- Place on the mother's abdomen, at right angles to it over the fetal back (Fig. 9.2).
- The ear of the midwife must be in close, firm contact with the stethoscope but the hand should not touch it while listening.
- The stethoscope should be moved about until the point of maximum intensity is located where the fetal heart is heard most clearly.
- The midwife should count the beats per minute, which should be in the range of 110–160.
- Taking the woman's pulse at the same time as listening to the fetal heart enables the midwife to distinguish between the two.

Ultrasound equipment (e.g. a Sonicaid or Doppler) is often used for auscultation, so that the woman may also hear the fetal heartbeat.

Findings

The midwife assesses all the information which she has gathered and critically evaluates the wellbeing of the mother and the fetus. Deviation from the expected growth and development should be referred to the obstetrician.

Gestational age

- During pregnancy the uterus is expected to grow at a predicted rate and in early pregnancy uterine size will usually equate with the gestation estimated by dates.
- Later in pregnancy, increasing uterine size gives evidence of continuing fetal growth but is less reliable as an indicator of gestational age.
- Multiple pregnancy increases the overall uterine size and should be diagnosed by 24 weeks' gestation.
- In a singleton pregnancy, the fundus reaches the umbilicus at 22–24 weeks and the xiphisternum at 36 weeks.
- In the last month of pregnancy lightening occurs as the fetus sinks down into the lower pole of the uterus. The uterus becomes broader and the fundus lower.
- In the primigravida, strong, supportive abdominal muscles encourage the fetal head to enter the brim of the pelvis.

Lie

The lie of the fetus is the relationship between the long axis of the fetus and the long axis of the uterus. In the majority of cases the lie is *longitudinal* owing to the ovoid shape of the uterus; the remainder are oblique or transverse.

Attitude

Attitude is the relationship of the fetal head and limbs to its trunk. The attitude should be one of flexion.

Presentation

Presentation refers to the part of the fetus that lies at the pelvic brim or in the lower pole of the uterus. Presentations can be:
- vertex
- breech

- shoulder
- face
- brow.

Vertex, face and brow are all head or cephalic presentations.

Denominator

The denominator is the name of the part of the presentation, which is used when referring to fetal position. Each presentation has a different denominator and these are as follows:

- In the vertex presentation, it is the occiput.
- In the breech presentation, it is the sacrum.
- In the face presentation, it is the mentum.
- Although the shoulder presentation is said to have the acromion process as its denominator, in practice the dorsum is used to describe the position.
- In the brow presentation, no denominator is used.

Position

The position is the relationship between the denominator of the presentation and six points on the pelvic brim. In addition, the denominator may be found in the midline either anteriorly or posteriorly, especially late in labour. This position is often transient and is described as *direct anterior* or *direct posterior.*

Anterior positions are more favourable than posterior positions because, when the fetal back is in front, it conforms to the concavity of the mother's abdominal wall and can therefore flex more easily. When the back is flexed, the head also tends to flex and a smaller diameter presents to the pelvic brim. There is also more room in the anterior part of the pelvic brim for the broad biparietal diameter of the head.

The positions in a vertex presentation are summarized in Box 9.3 and Figs 9.3–9.8.

Engagement

- Engagement is said to have occurred when the widest presenting transverse diameter has passed through the brim of the pelvis.
- In cephalic presentations, this is the biparietal diameter, and in breech presentations it is the bitrochanteric diameter.
- Engagement in a cephalic presentation demonstrates that the maternal pelvis is likely to be adequate for the size of the fetus and that the baby will birth vaginally.

Box 9.3 **Positions in a vertex presentation**

Left occipitoanterior (LOA)

- The occiput points to the left iliopectineal eminence
- The sagittal suture is in the right oblique diameter of the pelvis (Fig. 9.3)

Right occipitoanterior (ROA)

- The occiput points to the right iliopectineal eminence
- The sagittal suture is in the left oblique diameter of the pelvis (Fig. 9.4)

Left occipitolateral (LOL)

- The occiput points to the left iliopectineal line midway between the iliopectineal eminence and the sacroiliac joint
- The sagittal suture is in the transverse diameter of the pelvis (Fig. 9.5)

Right occipitolateral (ROL)

- The occiput points to the right iliopectineal line midway between the iliopectineal eminence and the sacroiliac joint
- The sagittal suture is in the transverse diameter of the pelvis (Fig. 9.6)

Left occipitoposterior (LOP)

- The occiput points to the left sacroiliac joint; the sagittal suture is in the left oblique diameter of the pelvis (Fig. 9.7)

Right occipitoposterior (ROP)

- The occiput points to the right sacroiliac joint; the sagittal suture is in the right oblique diameter of the pelvis (Fig. 9.8)

Direct occipitoanterior (DOA)

- The occiput points to the symphysis pubis; the sagittal suture is in the anteroposterior diameter of the pelvis

Direct occipitoposterior (DOP)

- The occiput points to the sacrum; the sagittal suture is in the anteroposterior diameter of the pelvis

In breech and face presentations the positions are described in a similar way using the appropriate denominator.

Fig. 9.3 Left occipitoanterior.

Fig. 9.4 Right occipitoanterior.

Fig. 9.5 Left occipitolateral.

Fig. 9.6 Right occipitolateral.

Fig. 9.7 Left occipitoposterior.

Fig. 9.8 Right occipitoposterior.

$\frac{5}{5}$	$\frac{4}{5}$	$\frac{3}{5}$	$\frac{2}{5}$	$\frac{1}{5}$	$\frac{0}{5}$
Sinciput and occiput above the brim	Sinciput prominent, occiput descending	Sinciput rising, occiput can be tipped	Sinciput not so prominent	Sinciput and occiput not felt	Head on pelvic floor

Fig. 9.9 Descent of the fetal head estimated in fifths palpable above the pelvic brim.

- In a primigravid woman the head normally engages at any time from approximately 36 weeks of pregnancy, but in a multipara may not occur until after the onset of labour.
- When the vertex presents and the head is engaged the following will be evident on clinical examination:
  - only two-fifths to three-fifths of the fetal head is palpable above the pelvic brim (Fig. 9.9)
  - the head is not mobile
  - on rare occasions the head is not palpable abdominally because it has descended deeply into the pelvis.
- If the head is not engaged, the findings are as follows:
  - more than half of the head is palpable above the brim
  - the head may be high and freely movable (ballotable) or partly settled in the pelvic brim and consequently immobile.
- If the head does not engage in a primigravid woman at term, there is a possibility of a malposition or cephalopelvic disproportion. Referral to an obstetrician should be made.

ONGOING ANTENATAL CARE

The information gathered during the antenatal visits will enable the midwife and pregnant woman to determine the appropriate pattern of antenatal care. The following schedule is based on guidelines from the UK's NICE.

16 weeks

- Review, discuss and document results of screening tests undertaken at initial assessment.
- Investigate a haemoglobin level below 11 g/dl and consider iron supplementation.
- Measure blood pressure.
- Urinalysis for proteinuria.
- Information exchange and review of care plan.

18–20 weeks

- Ultrasound scan to detect fetal anomalies.

25 weeks

- Measure fundal height.
- Measure blood pressure.
- Urinalysis for proteinuria.
- Information exchange and review of care plan.

28 weeks

- Offer repeat screening for anaemia and atypical red-cell alloantibodies.
- Investigate a haemoglobin level below 10.5 g/dl and consider iron supplementation.
- Offer anti-D to rhesus negative women.
- Measure fundal height.
- Measure blood pressure.
- Urinalysis for proteinuria.
- Information exchange and review of care plan.

31 weeks (nulliparous women)

- Measure fundal height.
- Measure blood pressure.
- Urinalysis for proteinuria.

- Review, discuss and document results of screening tests undertaken at 28-week assessment.
- Information exchange and review of care plan.

34 weeks

- Offer a second dose of anti-D to rhesus negative women.
- Measure fundal height.
- Measure blood pressure.
- Urinalysis for proteinuria.

Multiparous women – review, discuss and document results of screening tests undertaken at 28-week assessment.

- Information exchange and review of care plan.

36 weeks

- Measure blood pressure.
- Urinalysis for proteinuria.
- Measure fundal height.
- Check presentation of fetus; refer to obstetrician if breech.
- Information exchange and review of care plan.

38 weeks

- Measure blood pressure.
- Urinalysis for proteinuria.
- Measure fundal height.
- Information exchange and review of care plan.

40 weeks (nulliparous women)

- Measure blood pressure.
- Urinalysis for proteinuria.
- Measure fundal height.
- Information exchange and review of care plan.

41 weeks

- Measure blood pressure.
- Urinalysis for proteinuria.
- Measure fundal height.
- Information exchange and review of care plan.
- Offer a membrane sweep.
- Offer induction of labour.

FURTHER READING

Dowswell, T., Carroli, G., Duley, L., et al., 2015. Alternative versus standard packages of antenatal care for low-risk pregnancy. Cochrane Database Syst. Rev. (7): CD000934. doi: 10.1002/14651858.CD000934.pub3.

Useful website

National Institute for Care and Excellence, 2016. Antenatal care for uncomplicated pregnancies. Available at: https:// www.nice.org.uk/ guidance/cg62/chapter/1-Guidance (accessed July 27th 2016).

Specialized Fetal Investigations

Advances in technology mean that assessment of the fetus during pregnancy has become increasingly sophisticated and more widespread. Biochemical tests on maternal serum are commonly performed to identify which pregnancies carry a high risk of Down syndrome (trisomy 21) and ultrasound scanning is continually being refined.

PSYCHOLOGICAL ASPECTS OF PRENATAL TESTING

Prenatal testing is a two-edged sword. Whereas it enables midwives and doctors to give people choices, it may also increase the amount of anxiety and psychological trauma experienced in pregnancy.

Anxiety caused by consideration of possible fetal abnormality may be accompanied by moral or religious dilemmas. For instance, tests that can diagnose chromosomal or genetic abnormalities also carry a risk of procedure-induced miscarriage. Many parents agonize about whether to subject a potentially normal fetus to this risk in order to obtain a diagnosis. Parents may then need to consider whether they wish to terminate or continue with an affected pregnancy. Informed consent must be given (Box 10.1).

TESTS FOR FETAL ABNORMALITY

Broadly speaking, there are two types of test for fetal anomaly:
- screening tests
- diagnostic tests.

Screening for fetal abnormality

- Screening tests aim to identify a proportion of individuals (often approximately 5% of a population) who have the highest chances of a named disorder. This makes it possible to target further investigations towards those with the best indication.
- Mothers who undergo screening tests will be classified as above or below an action limit, whereby they are recalled and offered follow-up procedures.

Box 10.1 **Information required for obtaining informed consent**

- Purpose of the procedure
- All risks and benefits to be reasonably expected
- Details of all possible future treatments that could arise as a consequence of testing
- Disclosure of all appropriate techniques that may be advantageous
- The option of refusing any tests
- The offer to answer any queries

Box 10.2 **Performance criteria for screening tests**

Detection rate/sensitivity

- The proportion of affected pregnancies that would be identified as high risk

False-positive rate

- The proportion of unaffected pregnancies with a high-risk classification
- The higher the specificity, the fewer the false positives

False-negative rate

- The proportion of affected pregnancies that would not be identified as high risk
- The higher the sensitivity, the fewer the false negatives

- The performance criteria for a screening test are defined in several ways (Box 10.2).

THE USE OF ULTRASOUND IN MATERNITY CARE

- Most mothers undergo at least one ultrasound scan during pregnancy. This procedure can enable assessment and monitoring of many aspects of the pregnancy and is often presented as 'routine'.
- It can be used to screen for and to diagnose fetal malformations.
- Ultrasound works by transmitting sound at a very high pitch, via a probe, in a narrow beam. When the sound waves enter the body

111

and encounter a structure, some of that sound is reflected back. The amount of sound reflected varies according to the type of tissue encountered.

- Generally, pictures are transmitted in 'real time', which enables fetal movements to be seen.

First trimester pregnancy scans

Many areas offer mothers a scan in early pregnancy. The purpose of this is to establish:

- that the pregnancy is viable and intrauterine
- gestational age
- fetal number (and chorionicity or amnionicity in multiple pregnancies)
- detection of gross fetal malformations, such as anencephaly.

Ultrasound scans can:

- reduce the need to induce labour for postmaturity
- show a gestation sac from 5 weeks' gestation and a small embryo from 6 weeks.
- show accurate gestational age until 13 weeks through crown–rump length (CRL) measurement.

Mothers are asked to attend with a full bladder, as this aids visualization of the uterus at an early gestation.

Measurement of nuchal translucency at 10–14 weeks as a screen for Down syndrome

- Information about the fetus can be gained by observation of the nuchal translucency (NT) at 10–14 weeks' gestation.
- This involves measuring the thickness of the subcutaneous collection of fluid at the back of the neck.
- Increased NT is used as a basis upon which to screen for Down syndrome.
- Increased NT is also associated with other structural (mainly cardiac) and genetic syndromes, and this enables increased pregnancy surveillance to be arranged.
- However, a disadvantage of this knowledge is that parents may suffer considerable anxiety until later scans offer some degree of reassurance.

Second trimester ultrasound scans

- After 13 weeks of pregnancy, gestational age is primarily assessed using the biparietal diameter (BPD).

- This measurement becomes less accurate towards the end of pregnancy because the shape of the head may alter. Limbs are also measured, most notably the femur.

The detailed fetal anomaly scan

- This scan is usually performed at 18–22 weeks of pregnancy. Visualization of fetal anatomy is more difficult before that time, although some ultrasound departments have very sophisticated equipment which can identify anomalies much earlier.
- The purpose of this scan is to reassure the mother that the fetus has no obvious structural abnormalities.
- Detection rates vary considerably, but it is thought that approximately 50% of significant abnormalities are identified at this time.

It is important to note that some structural problems do not have associated sonographic signs and some fetal abnormalities may not appear until later in pregnancy. Diagnosis may therefore be missed.

Markers for chromosomal abnormality

- Markers are minor sonographic signs that increase the chance that the fetus has a chromosomal abnormality (most are associated with Down syndrome).
- The strength of association between each individual marker and Down syndrome varies considerably.
- When markers are identified, it is important to consider whether there are other risk factors, such as advancing maternal age or increased NT measurement at 10–14 weeks.
- The mother's aggregate risk for Down syndrome can then be calculated, taking all these factors into account.

Third trimester pregnancy scans

- In general, late pregnancy scans are performed in response to a specific clinical need and not as a screen of the low-risk pregnant population.
- However, fetal abnormalities may come to light or be reassessed at this time.
- Many late scans are performed as a means of monitoring fetal wellbeing, growth and development.

Fetal growth

- Many scans are performed to detect instances when growth deviates from normal.

- In order to assess fetal growth, the gestational age must be accurately assessed on scan before 24 weeks.
- Women at high risk of having an abnormally grown fetus should have serial scans – often at 28, 32 and 36 weeks. Where there is a particular concern, growth may be measured every 2 weeks.
- The most important measurements are head circumference and abdominal circumference. In this way, trends in fetal growth can be assessed.
- Fetuses with excessive growth (*macrosomia*) have increased perinatal mortality and morbidity.
- Fetuses may be small because they are preterm or because they are small for gestational age. Sometimes, these two problems overlap.

In general, growth-restricted fetuses can have either symmetrical growth restriction or asymmetrical growth restriction.

- Most symmetrically small fetuses are entirely normal and may be genetically predetermined to be small.
- In some instances, this may be caused by chromosomal malformations, infection or environmental factors such as maternal substance misuse.

Asymmetrical growth restriction

- These fetuses have a head size appropriate for gestational age, but thin bodies. This is generally caused by placental insufficiency.
- Glycogen stores in the liver are reduced, so there are fewer energy reserves for the fetus during labour.
- Asymmetrically growth-restricted fetuses are therefore more likely to suffer antenatal or perinatal asphyxia, or both.
- Other potential problems include hypoglycaemia, hypothermia and premature birth.

Doppler ultrasonography

In recent years, there have been major developments in the use of Doppler ultrasound techniques for the study of maternal and fetal circulation. Abnormalities in Doppler measurements may be detected before growth becomes impaired and can be used as a prognostic indicator.

Biophysical profiling

Another ultrasound measure of fetal wellbeing is the fetal biophysical profile. This is used to determine whether there are signs of fetal

---

Box 10.3 **Criteria used in biophysical profiling**

- Fetal breathing movements
- Fetal movements
- Fetal tone
- Fetal reactivity
- Qualitative amniotic fluid volume

---

hypoxia or compromised placental function, or both. A score is calculated on the basis of five criteria (Box 10.3).

Findings from growth scans, biophysical profile scores and cardiotocography (CTG) recordings should be considered collectively, taking into account the full clinical picture and obstetric history.

SCREENING FOR FETAL ABNORMALITY

It is important to relay to women that screening tests do not diagnose conditions, but they identify women who should be offered further testing to detect if their baby is affected.

There are two different screening options that test for Down syndrome. These consist of:

- First trimester screening (the 'combined' test).
  - Performed between 9–13 weeks and 6 days' gestation.
- Second trimester screening (the 'triple' or 'quadruple' test). This also provides information on the risk of having a baby with neural tube defects.
  - Performed between 15 to 20 weeks' gestation.

The combined test analyses results from a blood test and NT scan. The blood test analyses two biochemical markers:

- Human chorionic gonadotrophin (HCG).
- Pregnancy-associated plasma protein A (PAPP-A).

The triple test is a blood test that analyses markers:

- Alfa fetoprotein (AFP) (when fetuses have an open neural tube defect, AFP can be detected in maternal serum).
- HCG.
- Unconjugated oestriol (one of the three oestrogens produced by the body).

The quadruple test is a blood test that involves the triple test markers, as well as inhibin-A (a protein complex).

115

Accuracy of tests:
- Because the AFP varies with gestational age, it is important to accurately assess gestational age in order to get reliable results.
- There is a 95% accuracy rate.
- The levels of biochemical markers are considered in conjunction with maternal age. A combined risk is then calculated. If this risk is greater than a specified limit, the woman is considered to be in a high-risk group and is offered further diagnostic tests.

Noninvasive prenatal testing (NIPT)
- This is a DNA-based blood test that has been shown to identify > 99% babies with Down syndrome.
- It also detects the sex of the baby and other genetic conditions such as trisomy 18 and trisomy 13.
- This test can be performed at any gestation over 10 weeks.

INVASIVE DIAGNOSTIC TESTS

If women are found to have an increased risk of chromosomal or genetic problems, they may wish to undergo a diagnostic procedure. The two most frequently used tests are:
- chorionic villus sampling (CVS)
- amniocentesis.

These tests provide the opportunity to examine the fetal karyotype (the number and structure of chromosomes, visible through a microscope during mitotic metaphase) or for DNA analysis for particular gene mutations, or both.

Chorionic villus sampling

- CVS is the acquisition of chorionic villi (placental tissue) under continuous ultrasound guidance. This may be performed at any stage after 10 weeks of pregnancy.
- Access may be achieved transcervically (until 13 weeks' gestation) or via the transabdominal route.
- The main advantage of CVS is that this is the earliest way mothers can obtain definitive information about the chromosomal/genetic status of the fetus.
- The main disadvantage with CVS is the procedure-induced risk of miscarriage, which is 0.5–2%.

Amniocentesis

- This is usually performed after 15 weeks' gestation, as early amniocentesis has a higher loss rate than early CVS.
- The procedure involves transabdominal insertion of a fine needle into the amniotic fluid cavity, under continuous ultrasound guidance; 15 ml of amniotic fluid is aspirated.
- Cytogenetic, molecular (DNA) and biochemical analyses are possible. Amniocytes are often examined. These comprise cells that have been shed from several fetal sites, including skin, lungs and renal tract.
- The risk of procedure-induced miscarriage is 1%.
- Recent advances in cytogenetic techniques mean that women can obtain an initial set of results (usually for Down syndrome) and then a full culture result after 2–3 weeks.

Fetal blood sampling

- The use of this technique has declined in recent years because improved molecular and cytogenetic techniques allow more diagnoses to be made from chorionic villi or amniotic fluid.
- However, fetal blood may be advantageous when there are ambiguous findings from placental tissue.
- In addition, when there is rhesus isoimmunization, it may be necessary to determine the fetal haemoglobin. When this is low, an intrauterine transfusion may be performed.
- Blood can be sampled from the umbilical cord or intrahepatic umbilical vein; the latter is less risky.
- Fetal loss rate depends upon the gestation and condition of the fetus, but in uncomplicated procedures after 20 weeks' gestation, the loss rate is approximately 1%.

SUGGESTED READING

Woolcock, J., Grivell, R., 2014. Noninvasive prenatal testing. Aust. Fam. Physician 43, 432–434. Available at: http://www.racgp.org.au/afp/2014/july/noninvasive-prenatal-testing/.

Useful websites

National Screening Committee (NSC) UK: https://www.gov.uk/guidance/fetal-anomaly-screening-programme-overview

NICE guidelines: https://www.nice.org.uk/guidance/cg62/chapter/1-Guidance#screening-for-fetal-anomalies

Abnormalities of Early Pregnancy

For the purposes of this chapter, 'early' pregnancy is defined as the first trimester.

BLEEDING IN PREGNANCY

Vaginal bleeding during pregnancy is abnormal. If the woman presents with a history of bleeding in the current pregnancy, it is important to establish:

- when it occurred
- how much blood was lost
- the colour of the loss
- whether it was associated with any pain
- if the symptoms have subsided (important to advise the woman to report any recurrence)
- the fetal condition. This will depend on gestation:
  - First trimester: ultrasound scanning can confirm viability of the pregnancy before heart sounds are audible or movements felt.
  - Second trimester: the use of ultrasound equipment can elicit the heart sounds, and note of fetal movements may also be made.

Implantation bleeding

- As the trophoblast erodes the endometrial epithelium and the blastocyst implants, a small vaginal blood loss may be apparent to the woman.
- It occurs around the time of expected menstruation and may be mistaken for a period, although lighter.
- It is of significance if the estimated date of birth is to be calculated from menstrual history.

Cervical ectropion

This condition (commonly and erroneously known as a cervical erosion) is a physiological response to the hormonal changes in pregnancy.

- High levels of oestrogen cause proliferation of columnar epithelial cells, found in the cervical canal.
- These occupy a wider area, including the vaginal aspect of the cervix, encroaching on the squamous epithelial cells (metaplasia).
- As the cells are vascular they may cause intermittent blood-stained loss, or spontaneous bleeding particularly following sexual intercourse.
- Normally, treatment is not required in pregnancy and the ectropion will usually disappear during the puerperium.

Cervical polyps

These are small, vascular pedunculated growths attached to the cervix and may bleed during pregnancy. They can be visualized on speculum examination and no treatment is required during pregnancy, unless bleeding is profuse or a cervical smear suggests malignancy.

Carcinoma of the cervix

Carcinoma of the cervix is the most frequently diagnosed cancer in pregnancy. It is a treatable condition if detected early.

- *Cervical intraepithelial neoplasia* (CIN) is the precursor to invasive cancer of the cervix. If the condition is detected at this stage, treatment can be given and the cytology reverts to normal. The principal screening test used is the Papanicolaou smear (Pap smear).

Types

There are two main types of cervical cancer:
- squamous cell carcinoma
- adenocarcinoma (less common).

Clinical presentation

- Bleeding is the most common symptom.
- Vaginal discharge is the next most common.

As symptoms may be mistakenly diagnosed as symptoms of pregnancy, there may be delay in diagnosis.

Investigation

- A Papanicolaou smear test will detect atypical cells on the surface of the cervix, or within the endocervix.
- When changes are detected, a repeat smear test, followed by colposcopy, is indicated.

- Biopsies can be taken to reveal the extent of the lesion.

The woman and her partner should be fully informed about any tests and treatments that are offered and when and from whom results will be available. A positive test result following a smear test will cause anxiety to the woman and her family and it is important that accurate information is available, along with supportive counselling.

Treatment

Treatment depends on the stage of the disease and gestation.

- Laser treatment or cryotherapy following colposcopy can be carried out on an outpatient basis and will result in the destruction of the abnormal area of cells.
- Cone biopsy under general anaesthesia involves excision of cervical tissue and is both a diagnostic tool and a treatment, but it may increase the risk of miscarriage. The cervix is highly vascular in pregnancy and the risk of haemorrhage is high.
- Delaying treatment until the end of pregnancy is an option for women who are found to have early changes in cervical cytology.

If the changes to the cervix are advanced and diagnosis is made in the first or second trimester, the woman may have to make a choice as to whether to terminate the pregnancy in order to undergo treatment. If diagnosis is made later in pregnancy, a decision to induce birth may be taken to allow the woman to commence treatment.

SPONTANEOUS MISCARRIAGE

Spontaneous miscarriage is defined as the involuntary loss of the products of conception prior to 24 weeks' gestation.

Incidence

Approximately 15% of all confirmed pregnancies are said to result in miscarriages, the majority of which happen in the first trimester. The different outcomes of potential miscarriage (abortion) have varying signs and symptoms (Fig. 11.1 and Table 11.1).

Sequelae to early pregnancy loss

- Language should be appropriate, avoiding terms such as 'products' or 'scrape', recognizing that most women will be grieving for their lost baby.

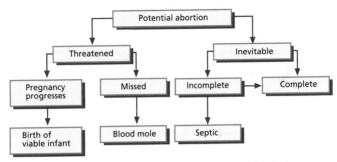

Fig. 11.1 Possible outcomes of potential miscarriage (abortion).

- Regardless of gestation, the parents may want to see and hold the baby. Some parents may want to see the loss when there is no body.
- Creation of memories is important for the grieving process, and midwives can assist by taking photographs of the baby for the parents, and by providing a letter or certificate to confirm the loss.
- Parents need information on how the remains will be disposed of. Whilst there is no legal requirement to have a funeral or cremation after a miscarriage, respectful disposal is nevertheless paramount. At no time should any fetal remains be included with hospital clinical waste. Note that miscarriage is defined differently in different countries, for example, under 24 weeks' gestation in the UK, and under 20 weeks in Australia.
- Parents may wish to take the remains home; burial in a garden is not precluded in this instance.
- If cremation is considered, then midwives should be aware that the size of the fetus may result in few ashes, if any.
- Full written consent must be given by the woman for postmortem or any other investigations involving fetal tissue.
- Follow-up after miscarriage is needed, with parents being given the opportunity to receive further information about their loss and to be offered advice regarding future pregnancies.

INDUCED ABORTION

Legal termination of pregnancy occurs before 24 weeks' gestation (in the UK) and 20 weeks (in Australia). Other countries will have different definitions in terms of their current legislation.

Table 11.1 Signs of miscarriage

Signs and symptoms	Threatened miscarriage	Inevitable miscarriage	Incomplete miscarriage	Complete miscarriage	Delayed miscarriage	Septic miscarriage
Pain	Variable	Severe/rhythmical	Severe	Diminishing/none	None	Severe/variable
Bleeding	Scanty	Heavy/clots	Heavy profuse	Minimal/none	Some spotting possible Brown loss	Variable May smell offensive
Cervical os	Closed	Open	Open	Closed	Closed	Open
Uterus (if palpable)	Soft, no tenderness	Tender, may be smaller than expected	Tender/painful	Firm, contracted	Smaller than expected	Bulky/tender/painful
Additional signs and symptoms			Tissue present in cervix Shock			

Methods

- Abortion can be carried out in the first trimester, using vacuum aspiration, dilatation and evacuation under general anaesthetic.
- Medical methods using medications such as mifepristone (Mifegyne), misoprostol (Cytotec), methotrexate and prostaglandin can be used to help the body expel the fetus and placental tissue.
- In the second trimester, medical methods such as extrauterine prostaglandin, accompanied by large doses of oxytocin, are used to promote uterine contractions. The woman experiences labour pains and the process may be protracted.
- Prophylactic antibiotics may be given following termination, and for non-sensitized rhesus negative women, anti-D immunoglobulin is recommended.

RECURRENT MISCARRIAGE

Recurrent miscarriage is defined as the loss of three or more consecutive pregnancies.

- The incidence of recurrent miscarriage suggests that there are significant underlying causes and the loss of the pregnancy is not chance.
- In many cases, no causative factor is identified, however, some factors are listed in Box 11.1.
- Women should be referred to specialist clinics where a screening service is available.

CERVICAL INSUFFICIENCY

- Cervical insufficiency (which used to be called 'cervical incompetence') describes painless dilatation of the cervix in the second or early third trimester, allowing bulging membranes through the cervical os into the vagina.

Box 11.1 **Some factors associated with recurrent miscarriage**

- Genetic causes
- Immunological factors
- Hypersecretion of luteinizing hormone
- Infection
- Structural anomalies

123

- Miscarriage or preterm birth may occur if the membranes rupture.
- Cervical insufficiency recurs in subsequent pregnancies.

Causes

- Trauma to the cervix during dilatation and curettage or induced abortion.
- Cone biopsy or congenital weakness of the cervix.

Treatment

- Treatment for subsequent pregnancies by cervical cerclage remains controversial.
- If undertaken, it is carried out after the risk of early miscarriage is thought to be past.
- At 14 weeks' gestation a non-absorbable suture may be inserted at the level of the internal os.
- This remains in situ until 38 weeks or the onset of labour, when it is removed.

ECTOPIC PREGNANCY

An ectopic pregnancy is one where implantation occurs at a site other than the uterine cavity. Sites can include:
- the uterine tube
- an ovary
- the cervix
- the abdomen.

Women require prompt, appropriate treatment for this life-threatening condition. Midwives need to consider the possibility of ectopic pregnancy being responsible for unexplained abdominal pain and bleeding in early pregnancy.

Risk factors for ectopic pregnancy

Any of the alterations of the normal function of the uterine tube in transporting the gametes listed in Box 11.2 contributes to the risk of ectopic pregnancy.

Clinical presentation (Box 11.3)

Tubal pregnancy rarely remains asymptomatic beyond 8 weeks.
- Severe pelvic pain occurs as the result of tubal rupture and relates to the degree of haemorrhage there has been.

Box 11.2 **Risk factors for ectopic pregnancy**

- Previous ectopic pregnancy
- Previous surgery on the uterine tube
- Exposure to diethylstiboestrol in utero
- Congenital abnormalities of the tube
- Previous infection including chlamydia, gonorrhoea and pelvic inflammatory disease
- Use of intrauterine contraceptive devices
- Assisted reproductive techniques

Box 11.3 **Signs of ectopic pregnancy**

Typical signs
- Localized/abdominal pain
- Amenorrhoea
- Vaginal bleeding or spotting

Atypical signs
- Shoulder pain
- Abdominal distension
- Nausea, vomiting
- Dizziness, fainting

- Ultrasound enables an accurate diagnosis of tubal pregnancy, making management more proactive.
- Vaginal ultrasound, combined with the use of sensitive blood and urine tests which detect the presence of human chorionic gonadotrophin (HCG), aids diagnosis.
- If the tube ruptures, shock may ensue; therefore, resuscitation, followed by laparotomy, is needed.
- The woman should be offered follow-up support and information regarding subsequent pregnancies.

GESTATIONAL TROPHOBLASTIC DISEASE

Gestational trophoblastic disease is a general term covering:
- hydatidiform mole (benign)
- choriocarcinoma (malignant).

Hydatidiform mole

- Hydatidiform mole applies to a gross malformation of the trophoblast in which the chorionic villi proliferate and become avascular.
- They are found in the cavity of the uterus and, very rarely, within the uterine tube.
- Two forms of mole have been identified:
  - complete hydatidiform mole
  - partial mole.
- As the complete form can lead to the development of choriocarcinoma, accurate diagnosis, treatment and follow-up are essential.

Clinical presentation

See Box 11.4. Diagnosis is confirmed by ultrasound scan and serum HCG levels.

Treatment

- The aim of treatment is to remove all trophoblast tissue.
- In some cases, the hydatidiform mole aborts spontaneously.
- Where this does not occur, vacuum aspiration or dilatation and curettage is necessary.
- Spontaneous expulsion of the mole carries less risk of malignant change.
- Follow up care:
  - All women who have been treated for hydatidiform mole in the UK (and some states in Australia) are recorded on a central register.

Box 11.4 **Clinical presentation of hydatidiform mole**

- Exaggerated signs of pregnancy, appearing by 6–8 weeks due to high levels of HCG
- Bleeding or a blood-stained vaginal discharge after a period of amenorrhoea
- Ruptured vesicles, resulting in a light pink or brown vaginal discharge, or detached vesicles, which may be passed vaginally
- Anaemia as a result of the gradual loss of blood
- Early-onset pre-eclampsia
- On examination, uterine size exceeding that expected for gestation; on palpation, a uterus that feels 'doughy' or elastic

---

- Women confirmed as having a complete mole require follow-up over a 2-year period during which pregnancy should be avoided.
- Intrauterine contraceptive devices are contraindicated and hormonal methods of contraception should not be used until levels of HCG have returned to normal.

Administration of anti-D immunoglobulin in early pregnancy

Significant fetomaternal haemorrhage can occur following early pregnancy loss; therefore, anti-D immunoglobulin should be administered to reduce the risk of isoimmunization in rhesus negative women.

RETROVERSION OF THE UTERUS

- When the long axis of the uterus is directed backwards during pregnancy, the uterus is said to be retroverted.
- In most cases it corrects spontaneously, the uterus rising out of the pelvis into the abdomen as pregnancy progresses, and there are no further problems.
- If the retroverted uterus fails to rise out of the pelvic cavity by the 14th week, it is said to be incarcerated.

FIBROIDS (LEIOMYOMAS)

These are firm, benign tumours of muscular and fibrous tissue, ranging in size from very small to very large.

Effect of pregnancy on fibroids

Fibroids do not significantly increase in size during pregnancy; however, they may become more vascular and oedematous, making them softer and more difficult to detect on palpation. Some women may experience mild abdominal pain.

Effect of fibroids on pregnancy

The outcome of pregnancy is dependent on the position of the fibroid.
- Early pregnancy loss is associated with submucosal fibroids.
- Fibroids located in the lower segment or on the cervix can prevent descent of the fetal head, causing malpresentation and obstructed labour and resulting in the need for caesarean section.
- Severe postpartum haemorrhage may be caused if the fibroids prevent the complete separation of the placenta or contraction of

the uterus. In anticipation of this, blood should be available for urgent cross-matching.

- Removal of fibroids during caesarean section should be avoided because of the risk of profuse haemorrhage.

Red degeneration of fibroids

Degeneration of a fibroid occurs if a rapidly growing fibroid exceeds the available blood supply.

HYPEREMESIS GRAVIDARUM

- Defined as excessive nausea and vomiting that start between 4 and 10 weeks' gestation, resolve before 20 weeks and require intervention.
- The aetiology of hyperemesis is uncertain, although endocrine and gastrointestinal factors are likely. Rising levels of oestrogen and HCG appear to be significant.
- Causes of vomiting not due to pregnancy need to be excluded.
- A woman suspected of suffering from hyperemesis presents as being unable to retain food or fluids. She may have lost weight, and be distressed and debilitated by her symptoms.
- The impact of nausea and vomiting on the woman and her daily life should not be underestimated. The woman requires admission to hospital for assessment and for management of symptoms.

Clinical presentation

- A history of the frequency and severity of the bouts of vomiting is taken.
- The woman's appearance is noted, including any dryness or inelasticity of the skin (signs of marked dehydration). In severe cases jaundice may be apparent.
- Additional signs of dehydration, such as rapid pulse, low blood pressure and dry furred tongue, may be seen. Other signs of dehydration include an elevated haematocrit, alterations in electrolyte levels and ketonuria.
- The woman's breath may smell of acetone, a sign of ketosis.

Management

- Initially nothing is given by mouth, to allow time for the vomiting to be controlled, usually with anti-emetics.

- Fluids and diet are gradually reintroduced as the woman's condition improves, but this is closely monitored.
- Hypovolaemia and electrolyte imbalance are corrected by intravenous infusion.
- Vitamin supplements can be given parenterally, particularly where hyperemesis has been prolonged.

Useful websites

Royal College of Obstetricians and Gynaecologists, 2016. The Management of Nausea and Vomiting of Pregnancy and Hyperemesis Gravidarum (Green-top Guideline No.69). Available at: https://www.rcog.org.uk/en/guidelines-research-services/guidelines/gtg69/

Breeze, C., 2016. Early Pregnancy Bleeding. Available at: http://www.racgp.org.au/afp/2016/may/early-pregnancy-bleeding/

Problems of Pregnancy

ABDOMINAL PAIN IN PREGNANCY

Abdominal pain is a common complaint in pregnancy. It is probably suffered by all women at some stage, and therefore presents a problem for the midwife of how to distinguish between the:

- physiologically normal (e.g. mild indigestion or muscle stretching)
- pathological but not dangerous (e.g. degeneration of a fibroid)
- dangerously pathological requiring immediate referral to the appropriate medical practitioner for urgent treatment (e.g. ectopic pregnancy or appendicitis).

The midwife should take a detailed history and perform a physical examination in order to reach a decision about whether to refer the woman. Treatment will depend on the cause (Box 12.1) and the maternal and fetal conditions.

Uterine fibroid degeneration

Uterine fibroid degeneration may cause recurrent acute pain during pregnancy and is due to a diminished blood supply that may cause central core necrosis of a fibroid or fibroids.

Management

- Rest and analgesia are required.
- Be aware that enlargement of the fibroid may occasionally impede the progress of labour and lead to rupture of the uterus.

Severe uterine torsion

Severe uterine torsion refers to rotation of the uterus by more than 90°, which may cause pain in the latter half of pregnancy.

Management

- Bed rest is necessary, altering the maternal position to correct the torsion spontaneously.

Box 12.1 Causes of abdominal pain in pregnancy

Pregnancy-specific causes

Physiological

- Heartburn, excessive vomiting, constipation
- Round ligament pain
- Severe uterine torsion
- Braxton Hicks contractions
- Miscellaneous discomfort in late pregnancy

Pathological

- Ectopic pregnancy
- Miscarriage
- Uterine fibroids
- Placental abruption
- Preterm labour
- Severe pre-eclampsia
- Uterine rupture

Incidental causes (consider domestic abuse)

Common pathology

- Appendicitis
- Intestinal obstruction
- Cholecystitis
- Inflammatory bowel disease
- Peptic ulcer
- Renal disease
- Ovarian pathology, e.g. torsion
- Acute pancreatitis
- Urinary tract infection
- Malaria
- Tuberculosis (may be associated with HIV infection)

Rare pathology

- Rectus haematoma
- Sickle-cell crisis
- Porphyria
- Arteriovenous haemorrhage
- Malignant disease

Fig. 12.1 Types of uterine fibroids.

- Analgesia is required.
- In severe cases a laparotomy will need to be performed in order for a clear diagnosis to be made.
- Depending on the location of the fibroid (see Fig. 12.1 for types of fibroids), a caesarean section may be performed, either preceded or followed by manipulation of the uterus.

Symphysis pubis dysfunction (pelvic girdle pain [PGP])

This refers to abnormal relaxation of ligaments, causing increased mobility of the pubic joint. The woman may complain of pain at any time from the 28th week of pregnancy.

Management

- Reduce non-essential weight-bearing activities and avoid straddle movements that abduct the hips, e.g. squatting.
- A supportive panty girdle or 'tubigrip' and comfortable shoes may help with the woman's mobility.
- Refer to an obstetric physiotherapist for advice and treatment.
- In severe cases, bed rest on a firm mattress may be necessary.
- Postnatal physiotherapy will aid the strengthening and stabilization of the joint.

ANTEPARTUM HAEMORRHAGE

Antepartum haemorrhage (APH) is bleeding from the genital tract after the 24th week of gestation and before the onset of labour.

Effect on the fetus

- Fetal mortality and morbidity are increased as a result of severe vaginal bleeding in pregnancy.
- Stillbirth or neonatal death may occur.
- Premature placental separation and consequent hypoxia may result in severe neurological damage in the baby.

Effect on the woman

If bleeding is severe, it may be accompanied by shock and disseminated intravascular coagulation (DIC). The woman may die or be left with permanent ill health.

Types of APH (Table 12.1)

- Bleeding from local lesions of the genital tract (*incidental causes*).
- Placental separation due to *placenta praevia* or *placental abruption*.

Initial appraisal of a woman with APH

- APH is unpredictable and the woman's condition can deteriorate rapidly at any time.
- A rapid decision about the urgency of need for a medical or paramedic presence, or both, must be made, often at the same time as observing and talking to the woman and her partner.
- Because APH can result from domestic abuse, sensitive enquiry should be made as part of the history taking.

Assessment of physical condition

Maternal condition

- Take a history from the woman.
- Observe pulse rate, respiratory rate, blood pressure and temperature.
- Look for any pallor or breathlessness.
- Assess the amount of blood lost.
- Perform a gentle abdominal examination, observing for signs that the woman is going into labour.

Table 12.1 Causes of bleeding in late pregnancy

Cause	Incidence (%)
Placenta praevia	31.0
Placental abruption	22.0
'Unclassified bleeding', e.g.	47.0
Marginal	
Show	
Cervicitis	
Trauma	
Vulvovaginal varicosities	
Genital tumours	
Genital infections	
Haematuria	
Vasa praevia	
Other	

On no account must any vaginal or rectal examination be done; nor may an enema or suppository be given to a woman suffering from an APH.

Fetal condition

The woman should be asked if the baby has been moving as much as normal.

Attempt to auscultate the fetal heart; ultrasound apparatus may be used in order to obtain information.

Factors to aid differential diagnosis

- The location of the placenta is perhaps the most critical piece of information that will be needed to make a correct diagnosis.
- If this is initially unknown, eliciting the information listed in Box 12.2 and talking to the woman and her partner, will help her to arrive at a provisional diagnosis.

Supportive treatment

- Provide emotional reassurance.
- Give rapid fluid replacement (warmed) with a plasma expander, and later with whole blood if necessary.

Box 12.2 **Diagnosis of antepartum haemorrhage**

Pain
- Did the pain precede bleeding and is it continuous or intermittent?

Onset of bleeding
- Was this associated with any event such as abdominal trauma or sex?

Amount of visible blood loss
- Is there any reason to suspect that some blood has been retained in utero?

Colour of the blood
- Is it bright red or darker in colour?

Degree of shock
- Is this commensurate with the amount of blood visible or more severe?

Consistency of the abdomen
- Is it soft or tense and board-like?

Tenderness of the abdomen
- Does the woman tense on abdominal palpation?

Lie, presentation and engagement
- Are any of these abnormal when account is taken of parity and gestation?

Audibility of the fetal heart
- Is the fetal heart heard?

Ultrasound scan
- Does a scan suggest that the placenta is in the lower uterine segment?

- Give analgesia.
- If at home, arrange transfer to hospital.

Subsequent management depends on the definite diagnosis and reason for the APH.

Placenta praevia

- In this condition the placenta is partially or wholly implanted in the lower uterine segment on either the anterior or posterior wall.

> **Box 12.3 Degrees of placenta praevia**
>
> **Type 1 placenta praevia**
> - The majority of the placenta is in the upper uterine segment.
> - Blood loss is usually mild and the woman and fetus remain in good condition.
> - Vaginal birth is possible.
>
> **Type 2 placenta praevia**
> - The placenta is partially located in the lower segment near the internal cervical os.
> - Blood loss is usually moderate, although the conditions of the woman and fetus can vary.
> - Vaginal birth is possible, particularly if the placenta is anterior.
>
> **Type 3 placenta praevia**
> - The placenta is located over the internal cervical os but not centrally.
> - Bleeding is likely to be severe.
> - Vaginal birth is inappropriate.
>
> **Type 4 placenta praevia**
> - The placenta is located centrally over the internal cervical os.
> - Torrential haemorrhage is very likely.
> - Caesarean section is essential.

- The lower uterine segment grows and stretches progressively after the 12th week of pregnancy. In later weeks this may cause the placenta to separate and severe bleeding can occur.

Degrees of placenta praevia

See Box 12.3 and Figs 12.2–12.9.

Indications of placenta praevia

- Painless bleeding from the vagina is the only sign. The uterus is not tender or tense.
- The presence of placenta praevia should be considered when:
  - the fetal head is not engaged in a primigravida (after 36 weeks)
  - there is a malpresentation, especially breech
  - the lie is oblique or transverse
  - the lie is unstable, usually in a multigravida.

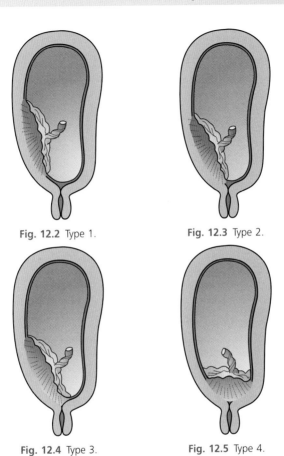

Fig. 12.2 Type 1.

Fig. 12.3 Type 2.

Fig. 12.4 Type 3.

Fig. 12.5 Type 4.

Figs 12.2–12.5 Types of placenta praevia.

Localization of the placenta using ultrasound will confirm the existence of placenta praevia and establish its degree.

Management of placenta praevia

The management of placenta praevia depends on:
- the amount of bleeding
- the condition of woman and fetus

Fig. 12.6 Type 1

Fig. 12.7 Type 2.

Fig. 12.8 Type 3.

Fig. 12.9 Type 4.

Figs 12.6–12.9 Relation of placenta praevia to cervical os.

- the location of the placenta
- the stage of the pregnancy.

Placental abruption

Premature separation of a normally situated placenta occurring after the 24th week of pregnancy is referred to as *placental abruption*. The aetiology is not always clear; some predisposing factors are listed in Box 12.4.

Blood loss may be:
- revealed
- concealed
- mixed.

Management of different degrees of placental abruption

Mild separation of the placenta

- In this case the placental separation and the haemorrhage are slight.
- Woman and fetus are in a stable condition. There is no indication of maternal shock and the fetus is alive with normal heart sounds.
- The consistency of the uterus is normal and there is no tenderness on abdominal palpation.
- An ultrasound scan can determine the placental location and identify any degree of concealed bleeding.

> **Box 12.4 Predisposing factors in placental abruption**
>
> - Pregnancy-induced hypertension
> - A sudden reduction in uterine size: e.g. when the membranes rupture or after the birth of a first twin
> - Direct trauma to the abdomen
> - High parity
> - Previous caesarean section
> - Cigarette smoking

- Fetal condition should be assessed while bleeding persists by frequent or continuous monitoring of the fetal heart rate. Subsequently, cardiotocography (CTG) should be carried out once or twice daily.
- If the woman is not in labour and the gestation is less than 37 weeks, she may be cared for in an antenatal ward for a few days. She may then go home if there is no further bleeding and the placenta has been found to be in the upper uterine segment.
- Women who are greater than 37 weeks' gestation may be offered induction of labour, especially if there has been more than one episode of mild bleeding.
- Further heavy bleeding or evidence of fetal compromise may indicate that a caesarean section is necessary.

Moderate separation of the placenta

This describes placental separation of approximately one-quarter. A considerable amount of blood may be lost, some of which will escape from the vagina and some of which will be retained as a retroplacental clot or an extravasation into the uterine muscle.

- The woman will be shocked, with altered respirations, a raised pulse rate and a lowered blood pressure.
- There will be a degree of uterine tenderness and abdominal guarding.
- The fetus may be alive, although hypoxic; intrauterine death is also a possibility.

The immediate aims of care are to reduce shock and to replace blood loss:

- Fluid replacement should be monitored with the aid of a central venous pressure line.

- The fetal condition should be assessed with continuous CTG monitoring if the fetus is alive, in which case immediate caesarean section may be indicated once the woman's condition is stabilized.
- If the fetus is in good condition or has already died, vaginal birth may be contemplated.
- Such a birth is advantageous because it enables the uterus to contract and control the bleeding.
- The spontaneous onset of labour frequently accompanies moderately severe placental abruption, but if it does not, then amniotomy is usually sufficient to induce labour.
- Oxytocin may be used with great care, if necessary. Birth is often quite sudden after a short labour.
- The use of drugs to attempt to stop labour is usually inappropriate.

Severe separation of the placenta

This is an acute obstetric emergency; at least two-thirds of the placenta has become detached and 2000 ml of blood or more are lost from the circulation.

- Most or all the blood can be concealed behind the placenta.
- The woman will be severely shocked, perhaps to a degree far beyond what might be expected from the amount of visible blood loss.
- The blood pressure will be lowered; however, the reading may lie within the normal range if there has been a preceding hypertension.
- The fetus will almost certainly be dead.
- The woman will have very severe abdominal pain with excruciating tenderness; the uterus has a board-like consistency.
- Features associated with severe haemorrhage are:
  - coagulation defects (e.g. DIC)
  - renal failure
  - pituitary failure.

Treatment is the same as for moderate haemorrhage, which requires a skilled multidisciplinary approach (midwives, obstetricians, anaesthetist, neonatologist, theatre team and laboratory facilities).

- Blood samples are needed for full blood count, coagulation profile and cross-matching. In addition, urea and electrolytes and liver function tests will be required. The Kliehauer test will also be necessary in Rh D negative women to both the degree of feto-maternal haemorrhage and the dose of Ant-D immunoglobulin to be administered.

- Whole blood should be transfused rapidly and subsequent amounts calculated in accordance with the woman's central venous pressure.
- Labour may begin spontaneously in advance of amniotomy and the midwife should be alert for signs of uterine contraction causing periodic intensifying of the abdominal pain.
- However, if bleeding continues or a compromised fetal heart rate is present, caesarean section may be required as soon as the woman's condition has been adequately stabilized.
- The woman requires constant explanation and psychological support, despite the fact that, because of her shocked condition, she may not be fully conscious.
- Pain relief must also be considered.
- The woman's partner will also be very concerned, and should not be forgotten in the rush to stabilize the woman's condition.

Complications

See Box 12.5.

BLOOD COAGULATION FAILURE

Disseminated intravascular coagulation

- This is a situation of inappropriate coagulation within the blood vessels, which leads to the consumption of clotting factors.
- As a result, clotting fails to occur at the bleeding site.
- DIC is rare when the fetus is alive and it usually starts to resolve when the baby is born.
- DIC is never a primary disease – it always occurs as a response to another disease process.

Box 12.5 **Complications of placental abruption**

- Disseminated intravascular coagulation
- Postpartum haemorrhage
- Renal failure
- Pituitary necrosis

141

- Events that trigger DIC include:
  - placental abruption
  - intrauterine fetal death, including delayed miscarriage
  - amniotic fluid embolism
  - intrauterine infection, including septic abortion
  - pre-eclampsia and eclampsia.

Management

- The midwife should be alert for signs that clotting is abnormal, and the assessment of the nature of the clot should be part of her routine observation during the third stage of labour.
- Oozing from a venepuncture site or bleeding from the mucous membrane of the woman's mouth and nose must be noted and reported.
- Blood tests should include full blood count and blood grouping, clotting studies and the levels of platelets, fibrinogen and fibrin degradation products (FDPs).
- Treatment involves the replacement of blood cells and clotting factors in order to restore equilibrium. This is usually done by the administration of fresh frozen plasma and platelet concentrates. Banked red cells will be transfused subsequently.

HEPATIC DISORDERS AND JAUNDICE IN PREGNANCY

Some liver disorders are specific to pregnant women, and some pre-existing or coexisting disorders may complicate the pregnancy (Box 12.6).

Box 12.6 **Hepatic disorders of pregnancy**

Specific to pregnancy

- Intrahepatic cholestasis of pregnancy
- Acute fatty liver in pregnancy
- Pre-eclampsia and eclampsia (see Ch. 14)
- Severe hyperemesis gravidarum (see Ch. 11)

Pre-existing or coexisting in pregnancy

- Gall bladder disease
- Hepatitis

Intrahepatic cholestasis of pregnancy

- Intrahepatic cholestasis of pregnancy (ICP) is an idiopathic condition that begins in pregnancy, usually in the third trimester but occasionally as early as the first trimester.
- It resolves spontaneously following birth, but has a 60–80% recurrence rate in subsequent pregnancies.
- It is not a life-threatening condition for the woman, but she is at increased risk of preterm labour and fetal compromise and her stillbirth risk is increased by 15% unless there is active management of her pregnancy.

Clinical presentation

- There is pruritus, particularly at night.
- Fifty per cent of women affected will develop mild jaundice.
- Fever, abdominal discomfort and nausea and vomiting may occur.
- Urine may be darker and stools paler than usual.

Investigation

The woman will need blood tests to look for an increase in bile acids, serum alkaline phosphatase, bilirubin and transaminases. Other tests for a differential diagnosis include hepatic viral studies, an ultrasound scan of the hepatobiliary tract and an autoantibody screen.

Management

- Give antipruritic agents, such as ursodeoxycholic acid (UDCA).
- Give vitamin K supplements to the woman.
- Monitor fetal wellbeing.
- Consider an induction of labour when the fetus is mature, or earlier if the fetal condition appears to be compromised by the intrauterine environment.
- Give sensitive psychological care.
- Research is ambivalent regarding adverse effects for women who have had ICP and their use of hormonal contraception. Hence, careful counselling regarding future contraception use is necessary.

Gall bladder disease

Pregnancy appears to increase the likelihood of gallstone formation but not the risk of developing acute cholecystitis.

143

Diagnosis

This will include the woman's previous history and an ultrasound scan of the hepatobiliary tract.

Treatment

Provide symptomatic relief of biliary colic by analgesia, hydration, nasogastric suction and antibiotics. Surgery should be avoided, if possible.

Viral hepatitis B (HBV)

- Viral hepatitis is the most common cause of jaundice in pregnancy. Acute infection affects approximately 1 in 1000 pregnancies and has an incubation period of 1–6 months.
- In healthy adults 90% of cases resolve completely within 6 months.
- In the remaining 10%, hepatitis B surface antigen (HBsAg) remains in the serum and the woman is considered to be a chronic carrier.
- The main means of spread is via blood, blood products and sexual activity.
- The virus can also be transmitted across the placenta.

Clinical presentation

- Nausea, vomiting, anorexia
- Pain over the liver
- Mild diarrhoea
- Jaundice lasting several weeks
- Malaise.

Diagnosis

This will include the woman's history of her symptoms and lifestyle, and serological studies.

Management

- Provide relief of symptoms.
- Implement infection control measures if the woman is considered to be infectious.
- Provide information about the disease, nutrition and sexual health.
- Monitor liver function/fetal wellbeing.

- Assess fetal wellbeing.
- Offer immunization to household contacts once their HBsAg seronegativity is established.
- Sexual partners should be traced and offered testing and vaccination.
- All infants born to HBV-infected mothers should receive hepatitis B immune globulin and the first dose of hepatitis B vaccine within 12 hours of birth.
- There are no contraindications to breastfeeding, however, if nipples are damaged and bleeding, breastfeeding should be temporarily suspended until they are healed.

SKIN DISORDERS

Many women suffer from physiological pruritus in pregnancy, especially over the abdomen.

Management

Give reassurance and apply calamine lotion over the affected area. If pruritus is generalized, exclude other causes, e.g. intrahepatic cholestasis.

DISORDERS OF THE AMNIOTIC FLUID

There are two chief abnormalities of amniotic fluid:
- polyhydramnios (or hydramnios) and
- oligohydramnios.

Polyhydramnios

- The amount of liquor present in a pregnancy is estimated by measuring 'pools' of liquor around the fetus with ultrasound scanning.
- The single deepest pool is measured to calculate the amniotic fluid volume (AFV).
- However, where possible, a more accurate diagnosis may be gained by measuring the liquor in each of four quadrants around the fetus in order to establish an amniotic fluid index (AFI).
- Polyhydramnios is said to be present when the AFV exceeds 8 cm, or the calculated AFI is more than 24 cm.

145

Causes

These include:

- oesophageal atresia
- open neural tube defect, anencephaly
- multiple pregnancy, especially in the case of monozygotic twins
- maternal diabetes mellitus
- rarely, an association with rhesus isoimmunization
- chorioangioma, a rare tumour of the placenta
- in many cases, an unknown cause.

Types

Chronic polyhydramnios

This is gradual in onset, usually starting from approximately the 30th week of pregnancy. It is the most common type.

Acute polyhydramnios

This is very rare. It usually occurs at approximately 20 weeks and comes on very suddenly. The uterus reaches the xiphisternum in approximately 3 or 4 days. It is frequently associated with monozygotic twins or severe fetal abnormality.

Diagnosis

- The woman may complain of breathlessness and discomfort.
- If the polyhydramnios is acute in onset, she may have severe abdominal pain.
- The condition may cause exacerbation of symptoms associated with pregnancy, such as indigestion, heartburn and constipation.
- Oedema and varicosities of the vulva and lower limbs may be present.

Abdominal examination

On inspection:

- The uterus is larger than expected for the period of gestation and is globular in shape.
- The abdominal skin appears stretched and shiny with marked striae gravidarum and obvious superficial blood vessels.

On palpation:

- The uterus feels tense and it is difficult to feel the fetal parts, but the fetus may be balloted between the two hands.

- A fluid thrill may be elicited by placing a hand on one side of the abdomen and tapping the other side with the fingers.

Ultrasonic scanning is used to confirm the diagnosis of polyhydramnios and may also reveal a multiple pregnancy or fetal abnormality.

Complications

These include:
- maternal ureteric obstruction
- increased fetal mobility leading to unstable lie and malpresentation
- cord presentation and prolapse
- prelabour (and often preterm) rupture of the membranes
- placental abruption when the membranes rupture
- preterm labour
- increased incidence of caesarean section
- postpartum haemorrhage
- raised perinatal mortality rate.

Management

Care will depend on the condition of the woman and fetus, the cause and degree of the polyhydramnios and the stage of pregnancy.
- The presence of fetal abnormality will be taken into consideration in choosing the mode and timing of the birth.
- If gross abnormality is present, labour may be induced; if the fetus is suffering from an operable condition such as oesophageal atresia, it may be appropriate to arrange transfer to a neonatal surgical unit.
- Mild asymptomatic polyhydramnios is managed expectantly.
- For a woman with symptomatic polyhydramnios, an upright position will help to relieve any dyspnoea and she may be given antacids to relieve heartburn and nausea.
- If the discomfort from the swollen abdomen is severe, then therapeutic amniocentesis, or amnioreduction (involving withdrawing no more than 500 ml at any one time), may be considered.
  - However, this is at best a temporary relief as the fluid will rapidly accumulate again and the procedure may need to be repeated.
  - It involves increased risks of infection and may provoke the onset of labour.

147

- Acute polyhydramnios managed by amnioreduction has a poor prognosis for the baby.
- Labour may need to be induced in late pregnancy if the woman's symptoms become worse.
- The lie must be corrected if it is not longitudinal and the membranes should be ruptured cautiously, allowing the amniotic fluid to drain out slowly in order to avoid altering the lie and to prevent cord prolapse.
- Placental abruption is also a hazard if the uterus suddenly diminishes in size.
- Labour is usually normal but the midwife should be prepared for the possibility of postpartum haemorrhage.
- The baby should be carefully examined for abnormalities and the patency of the oesophagus ascertained by passing a nasogastric tube.

Oligohydramnios

Oligohydramnios is an abnormally small amount of amniotic fluid. At term, it may be 300–500 ml but amounts vary and it can be even less.

- When diagnosed in the first half of pregnancy the condition is often found to be associated with renal agenesis (absence of kidneys) or Potter syndrome, in which the baby also has pulmonary hypoplasia.
- When diagnosed at any time in pregnancy before 37 weeks, it may be due to fetal abnormality or to preterm premature rupture of the membranes where the amniotic fluid fails to reaccumulate.
- The lack of amniotic fluid reduces the intrauterine space and over time will cause compression deformities. The baby has a squashed-looking face, flattening of the nose, micrognathia and talipes. The skin is dry and leathery in appearance.
- Oligohydramnios sometimes occurs in the post-term pregnancy.

Diagnosis

- On inspection, the uterus may appear smaller than expected for the period of gestation.
- Women who have had a previous normal pregnancy may notice a reduction in fetal movements.
- Upon palpation, the uterus is small and compact and fetal parts are easily felt.

- Ultrasonic scanning will enable differentiation of oligohydramnios from intrauterine growth restriction. Renal abnormality may be visible on the scan.

Management

- If the ultrasound scan demonstrates renal agenesis, the baby will not survive.
- Liquor volume will also be estimated from the ultrasound scan, and if renal agenesis is not present, then further investigations will include careful questioning of the woman to check the possibility of preterm rupture of the membranes.
- Placental function tests will also be performed.
- Where fetal anomaly is not considered to be lethal, or the cause of the oligohydramnios is not known, prophylactic amnioinfusion with normal saline, Ringer lactate (similar to Hartmann solution) or 5% glucose may be performed in order to prevent compression deformities and hypoplastic lung disease, and prolong the pregnancy.
- Labour may occur spontaneously or be induced because of the possibility of placental insufficiency.
- Epidural analgesia may be indicated because uterine contractions are often unusually painful.
- Continuous fetal heart rate monitoring is desirable.

PRETERM PRELABOUR RUPTURE OF THE MEMBRANES

Preterm prelabour rupture of the membranes (PPROM) occurs before 37 completed weeks of gestation where rupture of the fetal membranes takes place without the onset of spontaneous uterine activity resulting in cervical dilatation.

Risks of PPROM

See Box 12.7.

Management

If PPROM is suspected, the woman will be admitted to the labour suite. A careful history is taken and rupture of the membranes confirmed by a sterile speculum examination of any pooling of liquor in the posterior fornix of the vagina. A fetal fibronectin immunoenzyme test may be used to confirm rupture of the membranes.

149

> Box 12.7 **Some risks involved in preterm prelabour rupture of the membranes (PPROM)**
>
> - Labour, which may result in a preterm birth
> - Chorioamnionitis, which may be followed by fetal and maternal systemic infection if not treated promptly
> - Oligohydramnios if prolonged PPROM occurs
> - Psychosocial problems resulting from uncertain fetal and neonatal outcome and long-term hospitalization
> - Cord prolapse
> - Malpresentation associated with prematurity
> - Primary antepartum haemorrhage

- Digital vaginal examination should be avoided to reduce the risk of introducing infection.
- Observations must also be made of the fetal condition from the fetal heart rate (an infected fetus may have a tachycardia) and maternal infection screen, temperature and pulse, uterine tenderness and any purulent or offensively smelling vaginal discharge. A decision on future management will then be made.
- If the woman is less than 32 weeks' gestation, the fetus appears to be uncompromised, and APH and labour have been excluded, she will be managed expectantly.
- Offer frequent ultrasound scans to check the growth of the fetus and the extent and complications of any oligohydramnios.
- Administer corticosteroids.
- If labour intervenes, consider tocolytic drugs to prolong the pregnancy.
- Treat known vaginal infection with antibiotics. Prophylactic antibiotics may be offered to women without symptoms of infection.

If the woman is more than 32 weeks pregnant, the fetus appears to be compromised and APH or intervening labour is suspected or confirmed, active management will ensue.

MALIGNANT DISEASE IN PREGNANCY

- If cancer is discovered before pregnancy is embarked upon, it should be treated and followed up before pregnancy is attempted.

- Once successfully treated, and as long as the reproductive organs are not damaged, pregnancy is rarely contraindicated for medical reasons.
- However, cancer discovered during pregnancy leads to a host of management dilemmas. The options involve balancing the effects of the treatment, the disease and birth on both the woman and the fetus.

OBESITY OR FAILURE TO GAIN WEIGHT IN PREGNANCY

The amount of weight gained during pregnancy can affect the health of women and their babies. See Appendix 3 for body mass index (BMI) recommendations during pregnancy.

A woman who is obese at the beginning of pregnancy, or puts on an excessive amount of weight during pregnancy, is at greater risk of:
- hypertensive disorders
- gestational diabetes
- urinary tract infection
- uncertain fetal position
- postpartum haemorrhage
- thrombophlebitis
- having a caesarean section
- giving birth to a baby who is either small or large for gestational age
- wound infection following operative birth.

Obesity may also be associated with malnourishment from essential nutrient deficiency, or a symptom of another disease. Ideally, all women should be given the opportunity to discuss diet, as well as other general lifestyle factors, from as early on in their pregnancy as possible, and at regular intervals thereafter. Referral to a dietitian may be helpful.

Necessary observations include:
- blood pressure measurements taken accurately with a correctly sized cuff
- screening for gestational diabetes and urinary tract infection.

Routine weighing is rarely of any practical benefit (e.g. it does not detect fetal growth restriction or macrosomia) and may only reduce a woman's self-esteem and make her dread her antenatal appointments. However, routine weighing in the context of helping obese and overweight women to maintain a healthy weight gain in pregnancy should be considered.

Conversely, if the woman's BMI is less than 18.5 at the beginning of her pregnancy and the midwife notices a lack of weight gain, detailed discussion should attempt to elicit the quality and quantity of the woman's diet and her weight pattern over previous years.

Where a woman is suffering from nutritional deprivation she is at greater risk of:

- anaemia
- preterm birth
- intrauterine growth restriction and its sequelae, including birth asphyxia and perinatal death.

FURTHER READING

Jana, N., Barik, S., Arora, N., 2014. Unexplained antepartum haemorrhage – a risk factor for preterm labour and delivery. BJOG 121, 1446. doi: 10.1111/1471-0528.12814.

Useful websites

Diet and exercise interventions for preventing excessive weight gain during pregnancy. Available at: http://www.cochrane.org/CD007145/PREG_diet -and-exercise-interventions-for-preventing-excessive-weight-gain-during -pregnancy.

Antepartum Haemorrhage (Green-top Guideline No. 63). Available at: https://www.rcog.org.uk/en/guidelines-research-services/guidelines/gtg63/. A useful guideline on the management of antepartum haemorrhage.

Planned home versus hospital care for rupture of the membranes before 37 weeks' gestation. Available at: http://www.cochrane.org/CD008053/ PREG_planned-home-versus-hospital-care-for-rupture-of-the-membranes -before-37-weeks-gestation.

Common Medical Disorders Associated with Pregnancy

CARDIAC DISEASE

In most pregnancies, heart disease is diagnosed before pregnancy. There is, however, a small but significant group of women who will present at an antenatal clinic with an undiagnosed heart condition. Those more likely to be seen in pregnancy are:

- rheumatic heart disease
- congenital heart disease.

The most common congenital heart defects found in pregnancy are shown in Box 13.1. Some acquired heart conditions are listed in Box 13.2.

Changes in cardiovascular dynamics during pregnancy

- In normal pregnancy, the haemodynamic profile alters to meet the increasing demands of the growing fetoplacental unit. Although this increases the workload of the heart quite significantly, normal, healthy pregnant women are able to adjust to these physiological changes easily.
- In women with coexisting heart disease, however, the added workload can precipitate complications. The haemodynamic changes commence early in pregnancy and gradually reach their maximum effect between 28 and 32 weeks.
- During labour there is a significant increase in cardiac output as a result of uterine contractions.
- In the 12–24 hours following birth there is further alteration with the shift of blood (approximately 1 litre) from the uterine to the systemic circulation.

Diagnosis

The recognition of heart disease in pregnancy may be difficult, as many of the symptoms of normal pregnancy resemble those of heart

Box 13.1 **Common congenital heart defects in pregnancy**

- Atrial septal defect (ASD)
- Ventricular septal defect (VSD)
- Patent ductus arteriosus (PDA)
- Pulmonary stenosis
- Aortic stenosis
- Tetralogy of Fallot
- Eisenmenger syndrome
- Marfan syndrome

Box 13.2 **Some acquired heart conditions**

- Aortic dissection (acute)
- Rheumatic heart disease
- Ischaemic heart disease (IHD)
- Endocarditis
- Peripartum cardiomyopathy

Box 13.3 **Common signs and symptoms of cardiac compromise in pregnancy**

- Fatigue
- Shortness of breath (dyspnoea)
- Difficulty in breathing unless upright (orthopnoea)
- Palpitations
- Bounding/collapsing pulse
- Chest pain
- Development of peripheral oedema
- Distended jugular veins
- Progressive limitation of physical activity

disease. The signs and symptoms of cardiac compromise are listed in Box 13.3.

Laboratory tests can assist with the diagnosis of cardiac disease and determine the type of lesion, together with giving an assessment of current functional capacity. Tests include:

- full blood count (FBC)
- electrocardiography (ECG)
- chest radiograph to assess cardiac size and outline, pulmonary vasculature and lung fields
- clotting studies
- echocardiography.

Risks to the woman and fetus

The majority of pregnancies complicated by maternal heart disease can be expected to have a favourable outcome for both woman and fetus. The risk for morbidity and mortality depends on:
- the nature of the cardiac lesion
- its effect on the functional capacity of the heart
- pregnancy, infection, thrombosis and haemorrhage.

Preconception care

Women with known heart disease should seek advice from a cardiologist and an obstetrician before becoming pregnant, so that the risks of the condition can be discussed.

Antenatal care

The symptoms of normal pregnancy, together with the haemodynamic changes, can mimic the signs and symptoms of heart disease. Maternal investigations should be carried out prior to and at the onset of pregnancy to gain baseline referral points.

Management

- All pregnant women with heart disease should be managed in obstetric units via a multidisciplinary approach involving midwives, obstetricians, cardiologists and anaesthetists.
- The aim is to maintain a steady haemodynamic state and prevent complications, as well as promote physical and psychological wellbeing.
- Visits to a joint clinic run by a cardiologist and obstetrician are usually made every 2 weeks until 30 weeks' gestation and weekly thereafter until birth.
- At each visit, functional grading is made according to the New York Heart Association classification and the severity of the heart lesion is assessed by clinical examination.

- Evaluation of fetal wellbeing will include:
  - ultrasound examination to confirm gestational age and assess for congenital abnormality
  - assessment of fetal growth and amniotic fluid volume, both clinically and by ultrasound
  - monitoring the fetal heart rate by cardiotocography (CTG)
  - measurement of fetal and maternal placental blood flow indices by Doppler ultrasonography.

Intrapartum care

The first stage of labour

- Vaginal birth is preferred unless there is an obstetric indication for caesarean section.
- Optimal management involves monitoring the maternal condition closely. This will include the measurement of:
  - temperature
  - pulse
  - respiration
  - blood pressure
  - urine output
  - pulse oximetry
  - insertion of a central venous pressure (CVP) catheter, and ECG monitoring may also be utilized.

Fluid balance

- Women with significant heart disease require care to be taken concerning fluid balance in labour.
- Indiscriminate use of intravenous crystalloid fluids will lead to an increase in circulating blood volume, which women with heart disease will find difficult to cope with and they may easily develop pulmonary oedema.

Pain relief

It is important to consult a doctor before administering any form of pain-relieving drug to a woman with a heart condition. In the majority, an epidural would be the analgesia of choice.

Positioning

Cardiac output is influenced by the position of the labouring woman. It is preferable for an upright or left lateral position to be adopted.

Preterm labour

If a woman with heart disease should go into labour prematurely, then beta-sympathomimetic drugs, i.e. tocolytic agents (e.g. ritodrine) are contraindicated, because they encourage migration of potassium into cells. The net result is hypokalaemia and fluid retention due to their antidiuretic effect.

Induction

The least stressful labour for a woman with cardiac disease will be spontaneous in onset; induction is considered safe only if the benefits outweigh the disadvantages.

The second stage of labour

- This should be short without undue exertion on the part of the woman.
- The midwife should encourage the woman to breathe normally and follow her natural desire to push, giving several short pushes during each contraction.
- Forceps or ventouse may be used to shorten the second stage if the maternal condition deteriorates.
- Care should be taken when the woman is in the lithotomy position, as this produces a sudden increase in venous return to the heart, which may result in heart failure.

The third stage of labour

- This is usually actively managed owing to the increased risk of postpartum haemorrhage (PPH).
- Oxytocin is the drug of choice but its use in the prevention of PPH must be balanced against the risk of oxytocin-induced hypotension and tachycardia in women with cardiovascular compromise.
- Ergot-containing preparations such as ergometrine are contraindicated.

Postnatal care

- During the first 48 hours following birth the heart must cope with the extra blood from the uterine circulation.
- Close observation should identify early signs of infection, thrombosis or pulmonary oedema.
- Breastfeeding is not contraindicated.
- Discharge planning is particularly important for women with heart disease. The woman and her partner will need to discuss the

implications of a future pregnancy with the cardiologist and obstetrician.

RESPIRATORY DISORDERS

Asthma

Pregnancy does not consistently affect the maternal asthmatic status; some women experience no change in symptoms whereas others have a distinct worsening of the disease.

Antenatal care

- The main anxiety for women and those providing care is generated by the use of medication and the fear that this may harm the fetus.
- To date all medications commonly used in the treatment of asthma, including systemic steroids, are considered safe and it is crucial that therapy is maintained during pregnancy to prevent deterioration of the condition and precipitation of adverse pregnancy events.
- The lynchpin of management is the use of peak expiratory flow rates (PEFR) to monitor the level of resistance in the airways caused by inflammation or bronchospasm, or both.

Intrapartum care

- If an asthma attack does occur, it should be treated with the same rapidity and medication as an attack outside of pregnancy.
- Intravenous, intraamniotic and transcervical prostaglandins should be avoided in pregnancy and labour because of their bronchospasmic action.
- Any woman who has received corticosteroids in pregnancy should have increased doses for the stress of labour.

Postnatal care

Breastfeeding should be encouraged, particularly as it may protect infants from developing certain allergic conditions.

Cystic fibrosis

Cystic fibrosis (CF) is an autosomal recessive disorder affecting the exocrine glands that causes production of excess secretions with abnormal electrolyte concentrations, resulting in the obstruction of the ducts and glands.

Pre-pregnancy care

- When planning a pregnancy, a woman with CF and her partner should have genetic counselling.
- Although pregnancy appears to be well tolerated in women with pre-existing mild pulmonary dysfunction, morbidity and mortality are increased in women with pancreatic insufficiency or moderate to severe lung disease, or both.

Antenatal care

Once pregnancy is confirmed, a multidisciplinary approach combining midwifery, obstetric, dietetic, medical, nursing and physiotherapy expertise is essential.

Intrapartum care

- During labour close monitoring of cardiorespiratory function will be required and an anaesthetist should be involved at an early stage.
- Fluid and electrolyte management requires careful attention, as women with CF may easily become hypovolaemic from the loss of large quantities of sodium in sweat.
- Epidural analgesia is the recommended form of pain relief in labour and general anaesthesia should be avoided.

Postnatal care

- Women should be cared for in a high-dependency unit and should be closely monitored, as studies have highlighted that cardiorespiratory function often deteriorates following birth.
- Breastfeeding is not contraindicated; however, in order for this to be successful, women need to be well nourished and maintain an adequate calorie intake.

Pulmonary tuberculosis

Tuberculosis (TB) is caused by the tubercle bacillus, *Myobacterium tuberculosis*. The lungs are the organ most commonly affected, although the disease may involve any organ.

Management

- Standard antituberculous therapy should be used to treat TB in pregnancy.
- TB is treated in two phases:

- In the first phase, rifampicin, isoniazid and pyrazinamide are given daily for the first 2 months.
- In the second (continuation) phase, rifampicin and isoniazid are taken for a further 4 months.
- Attention should also be given to rest, good nutrition and education with regard to preventing the spread of the disease.
- TB is usually rendered noninfectious after 2 weeks of treatment.

Postnatal care

- Babies born to mothers with infectious TB should be protected from the disease by the prophylactic use of isoniazid syrup 5 mg/kg per day for 6 weeks and should then be tuberculin tested.
- If the tuberculin test is negative, Bacille Calmette–Guérin (BCG) vaccination should be given and drug therapy discontinued.
- If the test is positive, the baby should be assessed for congenital or perinatal infection, and drug therapy should be continued if these are excluded.
- There are very small concentrations of antituberculosis drugs in breast milk. Therefore, breastfeeding should not be discouraged in women who are taking first-line medications for TB.
- It is advisable for a woman with TB to avoid further pregnancies until the disease has been quiescent for at least 2 years.
- The woman needs to be aware that rifampicin reduces the effectiveness of oral contraception.

RENAL DISEASE

Asymptomatic bacteriuria

- A diagnosis of asymptomatic bacteriuria (ASB) is made when there are more than 100 000 bacteria per millilitre of urine.
- All women should be screened for bacteriuria using a clean voided specimen of urine at their first antenatal visit.
- If ASB is not identified and treated with antibiotics, 20–30% of affected women will develop a symptomatic urinary tract infection such as cystitis or pyelonephritis.
- These infections represent a significant risk for both woman and fetus and there is evidence to suggest that they may play a role in the onset of preterm labour.

> Box 13.4 **Clinical presentation of pyelonephritis**
>
> - Pyrexia, rigours and tachycardia
> - Nausea and vomiting; dehydration
> - Pain and tenderness over the loin area; muscle guarding
> - Urine cloudy; infecting organism often found to be *Escherichia coli*

Pyelonephritis

Clinical presentation

See Box 13.4.

Management

- Refer to a doctor; admit to hospital.
- Obtain a midstream specimen of urine (MSU) to test for culture and sensitivity.
- Give intravenous antibiotics followed by oral antibiotics once the pyrexia has settled.
- Record fluid balance; intravenous fluids may be required.
- Maintain 4-hourly observation of temperature and pulse.
- Monitor uterine activity.
- Prevent complications of immobility, e.g. deep vein thrombosis.
- Repeat cultures 2 weeks after completion of antibiotics and monthly until birth.

Chronic renal disease

- In order to determine the impact of pregnancy on a woman with chronic renal disease, the following factors need to be considered:
  - type of pre-existing renal disease
  - general health status of the woman
  - presence or absence of hypertension
  - current renal function
  - pre-pregnancy drug therapy.
- If renal disease is under control, the maternal and fetal outcome is usually good.
- In some instances, renal function may deteriorate and the chance of pregnancy complications subsequently rises.

Care and management

- The aim of pregnancy care is to prevent deterioration in renal function. This will necessitate more frequent attendance for antenatal care and close liaison between the midwife, obstetrician and nephrologist.
- Renal function is assessed on a regular basis by measuring serum urate levels, serum electrolyte and urea, and serum creatinine.
- It is also necessary to screen for glycosuria, proteinuria, haematuria, urinary tract infection and anaemia.
- Monitor for the emergence and severity of hypertension and pre-eclampsia.
- Fetal surveillance includes fortnightly ultrasound scans from 24 weeks' gestation, Doppler flow studies and daily fetal activity charts.

THE ANAEMIAS

Anaemia may be caused by a decrease in red blood cell (RBC) production, or a reduction in haemoglobin (Hb) content of the blood, or a combination of these. Signs and symptoms are listed in Box 13.5. A low Hb concentration only indicates that anaemia is present; it does not reveal the cause.

Physiological anaemia of pregnancy

During pregnancy, the maternal plasma volume gradually expands by 50%, an increase of approximately 1200 ml by term. The total increase in RBCs is 25%, or approximately 300 ml. This relative haemodilution produces a fall in Hb concentration, which reaches a nadir during the second trimester of pregnancy and then rises again in the third trimester.

Box 13.5 **Common signs and symptoms of anaemia**

- Pallor of the mucous membranes
- Fatigue
- Dizziness and fainting
- Headache
- Exertional shortness of breath
- Tachycardia
- Palpitations

Iron deficiency anaemia

Iron deficiency anaemia in women is usually due to:

- reduced intake or absorption of iron; this includes dietary deficiency and gastrointestinal disturbances such as diarrhoea or hyperemesis
- excess demand, such as frequent, numerous or multiple pregnancies
- chronic infection, particularly of the urinary tract
- acute or chronic blood loss: e.g. menorrhagia, bleeding haemorrhoids, or antepartum or postpartum haemorrhage.

Investigation

- Mean cell volume (MCV): normal value 80–95 femtolitres.
- Mean cell haemoglobin concentration (MCHC): normal value 32–36 g/dl.
- Serum iron levels: normal value 10–30 µmol/L.
- Total iron-binding capacity (TIBC): normal range 40–70 µmol/L.
- Serum ferritin: normal range 10–300 µg/L.

Management

- Identify the woman at risk through clinical observation and by taking an accurate medical, obstetric and social history.
- Give advice regarding the dietary intake of iron, taking account of how the intake of iron may be affected by social, religious and cultural preferences.
- Iron supplements may be prescribed where the Hb level is outside the range (11 g/dl at first contact, 10.5 g/dl at 28 weeks) and iron deficiency anaemia has been diagnosed.
- Oral iron supplementation should continue postnatally, particularly if the woman is breastfeeding.
- In women who are unable to take, tolerate or absorb oral preparations, iron can also be given intramuscularly or intravenously.

Folic acid deficiency anaemia

Folic acid is needed for the increased cell growth of both the woman and fetus but there is a physiological decrease in serum folate levels in pregnancy. There is a positive correlation between folate deficiency and the development of neural tube defects in the fetus.

Causes

- A reduced dietary intake or reduced absorption, or a combination of these.
- An excessive demand and loss of folic acid, e.g. haemolytic anaemia, multiple pregnancy.
- Interference of some drugs with the utilization of folic acid, e.g. anticonvulsants, sulphonamides and alcohol.

Investigation

Examination of the red cell indices will reveal that the red cells are reduced in number but enlarged in size.

Management

- Advise on the correct selection and preparation of foods that are high in folic acid.
- Recommend supplements of folic acid 400 µg/day for all pregnant women, and those planning a pregnancy.
- Additional supplements may be prescribed for women considered at risk.

HAEMOGLOBINOPATHIES

- This term describes inherited conditions where the haemoglobin is abnormal.
- Defective genes lead to the formation of abnormal Hb; this may be because of impaired globin synthesis (thalassaemia syndromes) or from structural abnormality of globin (Hb variants such as sickle cell anaemia).
- These conditions are found mainly in people whose families come from Africa, the West Indies, the Middle East, the eastern Mediterranean and Asia.
- As these conditions are inherited and in the homozygous form can be fatal, screening of the population at risk should be carried out.
- If both parents are carriers (i.e. heterozygous), there is a 1 in 4 chance that the fetus will be homozygous for the condition.

Thalassaemia

- Thalassaemia is most common in people of Mediterranean, African, Middle and Far Eastern origin.

- The basic defect is a reduced rate of globin chain synthesis in adult Hb. This leads to ineffective erythropoiesis and increased haemolysis with a resultant inadequate Hb content.
- The red cell indices show a low Hb and MCHC level, but raised serum iron level.
- Definitive diagnosis is obtained by electrophoresis.
- The severity of the condition depends on whether the abnormal genes are inherited from one parent or from both.
- There are also different types of thalassaemia, depending on whether the alpha or beta globin chain synthesis is affected:
  - alpha thalassaemia major
  - beta thalassaemia major
  - alpha and beta thalassaemia minor.

Sickle-cell disorders

- Sickle-cell disorders are found most commonly in people of African or West Indian origin.
- In these conditions, defective genes produce abnormal Hb beta chains; the resulting Hb is called HbS.
- In sickle-cell anaemia (HbSS, or SCA) abnormal genes have been inherited from both parents.
- In sickle-cell trait (HbAS) only one abnormal gene has been inherited.

Maternal and fetal/neonatal risks are listed in Box 13.6.

- All women in the at-risk population are screened in early pregnancy, and where possible their partners are screened too.
- Those who are diagnosed as having SCA should be referred to a specialist sickle-cell centre with trained haemoglobinopathy and genetic counsellors.

Sickle-cell trait

This is usually asymptomatic. The blood appears normal, although the sickle screening test is positive. There is no anaemia, even under the additional stress of pregnancy.

DIABETES MELLITUS

The term 'diabetes mellitus' (DM) describes a metabolic disorder of multiple aetiology that affects the normal metabolism of carbohydrates, fats and protein.

> Box 13.6 **Common risks and complications of sickle-cell disorders**
>
> **Maternal risks**
> - Antenatal and postnatal pain crisis
> - Infections
> - Pulmonary complications
> - Anaemia
> - Pre-eclampsia
> - Caesarean section
>
> **Fetal and neonatal complications**
> - Preterm birth
> - Smallness for gestational age
> - Neonatal jaundice

Classification

See Box 13.7.

Diagnosis

- Routine screening for all women in pregnancy is not recommended.
- Women with an increased thirst, increased urine volume, excessive tiredness, unexplained weight loss and a family history require further investigations.
- Similarly, obese women, some ethnicities (Asian, Indian subcontinent, Aboriginal, Torres Strait Islander, Pacific Islander, Maori, Middle Eastern, non-white African), those with polycystic ovarian syndrome, previous perinatal loss or macrosomic babies may need earlier screening.

Monitoring diabetes

The main objectives of diabetic therapy are:
- to maintain blood glucose levels as near to normal as possible
- to reduce the risk of long-term complications.

Long-term blood glucose control can be determined by undertaking a laboratory test to measure glycosylated haemoglobin (HbA1c).

Box 13.7 **Classification of diabetes mellitus (DM)**

Type 1 DM

- Occurs when beta cells in the islets of Langerhans in the pancreas are destroyed, stopping insulin production
- Insulin therapy is required in order to prevent the development of ketoacidosis, coma and death

Type 2 DM

- Results from a defect or defects in insulin action and insulin secretion
- Insulin therapy is not needed to survive
- The risk of developing this type of DM increases with age, obesity and lack of physical activity

Gestational diabetes mellitus (GDM)

- Carbohydrate intolerance resulting in hyperglycaemia of variable severity
- Onset or first recognition is during pregnancy

Impaired glucose regulation

- Includes *impaired glucose tolerance* (IGT) and *impaired fasting glycaemia* (IFG), metabolic states intermediate between normal glucose homeostasis and diabetes

- The HbA1c test counts the number of RBCs that are glycosylated (attached to sugar). For example, if 6 out of every 100 RBCs are attached to sugar, the HbA1c result will be 6%.
- This is different from blood glucose level (BGL) tests. BGL tests measure the amount of sugar that is freely circulating in the blood.
- The degree of Hb glycosylation is dependent on the amount of glucose the RBCs have been exposed to during their 120-day life.
- The higher the HbA1c, the poorer is the blood sugar control.
- Good diabetic control is defined as an HbA1c of < 6.5%.

Carbohydrate metabolism in pregnancy

- Pregnancy is characterized by several factors that produce a diabetogenetic state so that insulin and carbohydrate metabolism is altered in order to make glucose more readily available to the fetus.

- Women with DM do not have the capacity to increase insulin secretion in response to the altered carbohydrate metabolism in pregnancy and therefore glucose accumulates in the maternal and fetal system, leading to significant morbidity and mortality.

Pre-pregnancy care

- Assessment is made of current diabetic control, aiming for premeal glucose levels of < 7 mmol/L and HbA1c of ≤ 6.5%.
- Insulin dosage is reviewed.
- Women on oral hypoglycaemics will need to discuss transfer to insulin to prevent the possibility of teratogenesis.
- Higher-dose folic acid supplementation is given.
- Smoking cessation support is arranged.
- Assessment and management are provided for diabetes complications.

Antenatal care

- Women and their partners should ideally be seen in a combined clinic by a team that includes an endocrinologist, an obstetrician, a specialist diabetes nurse, a specialist midwife and a dietitian.
- They will be seen as often as required in order to maintain good diabetic control and undertake relevant screening, e.g. retinal examination.
- Blood glucose levels should be monitored frequently (four times a day using an approved glucometer) and insulin levels adjusted to achieve premeal blood sugar levels of < 5.3 mmol/L and 1-hour post-meal levels of < 7.8 mmol/L. Additional estimations of blood glucose control, such as monthly HbA1c measurements, are also recommended.
- A diet that is high in fibre is beneficial, as carbohydrates are released slowly and therefore a more constant blood glucose level can be achieved.
- Advise women on early recognition of the signs and symptoms of urinary and vaginal infections.
- Anomaly ultrasound screening should be offered at 20 weeks' gestation and fetal echocardiography at 20–22 weeks if there are clinical signs associated with congenital heart disease or cardiomyopathy, including heart murmur.
- Serum screening for Down syndrome is altered with maternal diabetes and care should be taken when interpreting the results.

- There is an increased risk of growth restriction due to maternal vascular disease, pre-eclampsia or a combination of both. A baseline measurement of the fetal abdominal circumference is taken at 20 weeks. This is followed by serial measurements every 2–4 weeks, commencing at 24 weeks.
- Serial ultrasound should also detect fetal macrosomia and whether polyhydramnios is present.

Intrapartum care

- Ideally, labour should be allowed to commence spontaneously at term for women with uncomplicated DM during pregnancy.
- Poor diabetic control or a deterioration in the maternal or fetal condition may necessitate earlier, planned birth.
- Induction of labour may also be considered where the fetus is judged to be macrosomic.
- Corticosteriods may be used to aid lung maturation and surfactant production, but these will increase insulin requirements.
- The aim of intrapartum care is to maintain normoglycaemia in labour (i.e. < 7.0 mmol/L).
- Continuous electronic fetal monitoring is recommended and fetal blood sampling should be utilized if acidosis is suspected.
- Adequate pain relief, such as epidural analgesia, assists in regulating the blood sugar levels and preventing the development of metabolic acidosis. It is also useful if difficulties should arise with the birth of the shoulders or an operative birth is required.

Postpartum care

- Immediately after the third stage of labour the insulin requirements will fall rapidly to pre-pregnancy levels.
- The insulin infusion rate should be reduced by at least 50%.
- Women with type 2 DM who were previously on oral hypoglycaemics or dietary control need to be reviewed prior to recommencing therapy.
- Breastfeeding should be encouraged in all women with diabetes. An additional carbohydrate intake of 40–50 g is recommended and insulin therapy may need to be adjusted accordingly.
- All women should be offered contraceptive advice so that optimum metabolic control is achieved prior to planning the next pregnancy.

Neonatal care

The development of complications in the neonate is related to maternal hyperglycaemia during pregnancy leading to fetal hyperinsulinaemia. This will result in the following conditions: macrosomia, hypoglycaemia, polycythaemia and respiratory distress syndrome.

Macrosomia

- This is defined as a fetal birth weight > 4500 g.
- The increased fetal size may cause prolonged labour and predisposes the infant to shoulder dystocia and birth injuries.
- Consequently, asphyxia is common and these infants are more likely than babies of normal weight to die from an intrapartum-related event.

Hypoglycaemia.

- Beta-cell hyperplasia causes the baby to continue to produce more insulin than required for up to 24 hours following birth.
- To prevent hypoglycaemia the neonatal blood glucose needs to be assessed 1–2 hours after birth and then every 4–6 hours for the first 24–48 hours.
- Regular feeding is encouraged to maintain a blood glucose of at least 2.6 mmol/L.

Polycythaemia

- Fetal hyperinsulinaemia during pregnancy also leads to an increase in red cell production resulting in polycythaemia (venous haematocrit > 65%).
- The rapid breakdown of the excess RBCs, combined with the relative immaturity of the liver in the newborn, predisposes the baby to jaundice. This will be exacerbated if there is bruising as a result of birth trauma.

Respiratory distress syndrome

- Hyperinsulinaemia is thought to impair the production of surfactant and delay lung maturation. Hence, babies born at term may display symptomatology of respiratory distress.
- Observations of temperature, apex beat and respirations and monitoring of blood sugar levels are important in the first 24–48 hours.

- Clinical signs, together with symptomatology such as respiratory distress, apnoea or tachypnoea, cyanosis, jitteriness, irritability, seizures, feeding intolerance and temperature instability may all be indicative of respiratory distress syndrome.
- Polycythaemia and hypoglycaemia require further investigation and treatment in a neonatal unit.

Gestational diabetes

- There is no agreement among current guidelines on whether screening for gestational diabetes mellitus (GDM) should be universal or focused on women with risk factors.
- Diagnosis of GDM is based solely upon an oral glucose tolerance test (OGTT) (75 g carbohydrate load)
- The International Association of Diabetes in Pregnancy Study Groups (IADPSG) and the World Health Organization (WHO) state that diagnosis of GDM is based on:
  - Fasting glucose greater than or equal to 5.1 mmol/L and/or
  - 1-hour glucose greater than or equal to 10.0 mmol/L and/or
  - 2-hour glucose greater than or equal to 8.5 mmol/L
- Treatment will depend on the blood glucose levels.
- HbA1c levels are useful in women with pre-existing DM, but should not be routinely used to assess women's blood glucose levels in the second and third trimesters.
- Grossly abnormal results are likely to require insulin therapy, which will be discontinued immediately after the birth of the baby.
- It is recommended that a postnatal OGTT is performed at 6 weeks; if the results are abnormal, then appropriate referral should be made.
- Those with normal glucose levels require advice regarding the implications for future pregnancies and the development of type 1 or type 2 DM.

EPILEPSY

- The prevalence of epilepsy in the general population is 1 in 200 and it affects 0.3–0.5% of pregnant women.
- An epileptic seizure results from abnormal electrical activity in the brain, which is manifest by brief sensory, motor and autonomic dysfunction. These disturbances recur spontaneously and are classified according to the parts of the brain affected. Seizures may be described as shown in Box 13.8.

> **Box 13.8 Classification of epilepsy**
>
> **Partial**
> - Usually arising from the temporal or frontal lobe of the brain
>
> **Generalized**
> - Resulting from disturbances involving both halves of the brain: absence seizures (petit mal)
> - Myoclonic seizures
> - Tonic–clonic seizures (grand mal)
> - Atonic seizures
> - Status epilepticus

- Identification of the type of epilepsy is important in its treatment. The aim of treatment is to identify the cause of the seizure and provide appropriate therapy to prevent recurrence.
- The control of seizures can be achieved for most people through the use of antiepileptic drugs (AEDs).

Pre-pregnancy care

- Women on AEDs become folic acid deficient and may develop macrocytic anaemia.
- Folic acid deficiency has also been associated with neural tube defects and other congenital malformations.
- There is a 1–2% risk of neural tube defects if a woman is taking sodium valproate (Epilim) or carbamazepine (Tegretol) in pregnancy.
- Of the other older AEDs, phenytoin gives rise to a combination of malformations termed *fetal hydantoin syndrome,* which comprises craniofacial dysmorphic features, digital defects, microcephaly and growth retardation.
- Preconception advice is therefore essential for women with epilepsy.
- AED therapy may be withdrawn gradually prior to pregnancy to reduce the risk of teratogenicity when women suffer from seizures that are unlikely to harm the fetus, such as absence, partial or myoclonic seizures, or have been seizure free for over 2 years.
- Some medications for epilepsy interfere with folic acid absorption hence higher doses (5 mg/day) should be commenced before pregnancy and continued throughout the first trimester.

Antenatal care

- Antenatal care should include a detailed anomaly scan at 18–22 weeks.
- Abnormalities are more common if AEDs are prescribed in high concentration and particularly if more than one is used.
- Some women may experience an increase in seizures; this is often due to noncompliance with the drug regimen, sleep deprivation during pregnancy and the decline in plasma concentrations of the AED as the pregnancy progresses.
- Particular emphasis should also be placed on the first-aid measures that should be adopted following an epileptic seizure in order to prevent aspiration, and the dangers of hot baths inducing fainting and consequent drowning.

Intrapartum care

Care during labour and childbirth is not likely to be different from that of other women.

Seizures are more likely to occur in conditions such as sleep deprivation, hypoglycaemia, anaemia, stress or hyperventilation – all of which may arise during labour. AEDs should therefore be maintained throughout labour.

Postnatal care

Safety precautions in the home are important. The woman is given advice about how to minimize risks when feeding, bathing, changing and transporting the baby. AED therapy should be reviewed 6 weeks postnatally and the dosage adjusted to pre-pregnancy levels.

Effect of epilepsy on the fetus and neonate

- The majority of women with epilepsy will have uncomplicated pregnancies with normal births and healthy children.
- When status epilepticus occurs, one-third of women and half of the fetuses do not survive. Convulsive status epilepticus is a medical emergency.
- AEDs cross the placenta freely and decrease production of vitamin K, leading to the risk of haemorrhagic disease of the newborn. This can be prevented by routine administration of vitamin K to the woman from 36 weeks' gestation and to the baby shortly after birth.
- The rate of clearance of AEDs varies according to the drug. Newborn infants may therefore suffer harmful effects from the AED level

and, as a group, tend to be less efficient at feeding and gain weight more slowly. A minority will suffer withdrawal symptoms such as tremor, excitability and convulsions.

- AEDs pass into the breast milk in relatively small quantities and therefore breastfeeding is recommended.
- Some AEDs, such as phenobarbital, primidone or benzodiazepines, may have a sedative effect, in which case bottle feeding or mixed feeding may be advised.

AUTOIMMUNE DISEASE

- Autoimmune disease arises from a disruption in the function of the immune system of the body, resulting in the production of antibodies against the body's own cells.
- Antigens normally present on the body's cells stimulate the development of autoantibodies, which, unable to distinguish the self antigens from non-self or foreign antigens, act against the body's cells to cause localized and systemic reactions.
- The cause of this condition is unknown but it is thought to be multifactorial with genetic, environmental, hormonal and viral influences.
- Many autoimmune diseases are more prevalent in women, particularly between puberty and the menopause, which suggests that female hormonal factors may play a role. They broadly fall into two groups:
  - multisystem disease, such as systemic lupus erythematosus (SLE)
  - tissue- or organ-specific disorders, such as autoimmune thyroid disease.
- These disorders are characterized by periods of remission interrupted by periods of crisis, which may require hospitalization.
- Treatment is aimed at lessening the severity of the symptoms rather than effecting a cure. Mild cases usually respond to anti-inflammatory drugs.
- More severe illnesses may require steroids or immunosuppressant therapy.

SYSTEMIC LUPUS ERYTHEMATOSUS

- SLE, or lupus, is an inflammatory disorder of the connective tissue, which forms the fibrous, elastic, fatty or cartilaginous matrix that connects and supports other tissues.

- The initial manifestation of SLE is often arthritis accompanied by fever, fatigue, malaise, weight loss, photosensitivity and anaemia.
- A wide range of skin lesions are seen and an erythematous facial 'butterfly' rash is characteristic of the disorder.
- Depending on the organs involved, inflammatory conditions such as pleuritis, pericarditis, glomerulonephritis, neuritis and gastritis may arise.
- Renal disease and neurological abnormalities are the most serious manifestations of the disease.
- Most people with SLE have a normal life expectancy and serious complications are rare. Infection is the major cause of mortality.

Diagnosis

- The diagnosis of SLE is based on a collection of the signs and symptoms, particularly when joint pain, skin conditions and fatigue occur in combination or evolve over time.
- Blood tests are used to confirm the diagnosis and comprise:
  - full blood count
  - erythrocyte sedimentation rate (ESR)
  - testing for antinuclear antibody (ANA).
- There is often normochromic normocytic anaemia, the ESR is elevated even when the disease is in remission and more than 95% of people with SLE will have ANA.
- Antiphospholipid syndrome (APS) is found in conjunction with SLE in 30% of cases.
- A blood test will detect antiphospholipid antibodies (APL), lupus anticoagulant and anticardiolipin antibodies (anti-Ro and anti-La) if APS is present. This will identify a group of people with SLE at particular risk of thromboembolic disorders and a high rate of fetal loss.

Effects of SLE on pregnancy

- The effects of SLE on pregnancy is variable, although worsening of SLE symptoms is common and may occur at any trimester of pregnancy and in the postpartum period.
- The frequency of the 'flares' is, however, lower in women with mild and well controlled disease.
- Women with SLE should be counselled about planning a pregnancy and the importance of being in remission for at least 6 months before conception.

- Neonatal lupus syndrome is rare but may occur as a result of the transplacental passage of maternal anti-Ro/La antibodies.
- Overall, women with SLE who are pregnant have an increased incidence of adverse outcomes:
  - Approximately one-third of pregnancies will result in spontaneous abortion, therapeutic abortion, intrauterine death or stillbirth.
  - The rate of preterm birth and intrauterine growth restriction is closely related to the incidence of pre-eclampsia.

Antenatal care

- Women should have collaborative care from an obstetrician and a rheumatologist.
- Baseline haematological and immunological blood tests are performed at the first antenatal visit.
- Ongoing blood tests for women with SLE and APS are highly individual and would be coordinated by their obstetrician and rheumatologist.
- An early first trimester scan is undertaken to confirm fetal viability and an anomaly scan is performed at 18–20 weeks.
- Women with SLE and APS are offered a fetal cardiac anomaly scan at 24 weeks' gestation and echocardiography to detect congenital heart block.
- Serial ultrasound examinations for fetal growth, placental size and quality, and amniotic fluid volume should begin at 28–32 weeks.
- Doppler flow studies are performed at 20 and 24 weeks and thereafter according to fetal growth and wellbeing.
- The aim is to control disease activity and achieve clinical remission while keeping drug therapy to a minimum.
- Women who have a mild form of the disease or are in remission require minimal to no medication.
- Avoidance of emotional stress and the promotion of a healthy lifestyle may play a part in reducing the likelihood of flares or exacerbations of SLE arising during pregnancy.
- If treatment is required, simple analgesics such as paracetamol and co-dydramol are used for symptomatic relief.
- Mild flares with joint pain, skin lesions and fatigue respond well to low-dose steroid therapy such as prednisone or prednisolone.
- Antimalarial drugs are effective as maintenance therapy in women with frequent flares and hydroxychloroquine is considered safe to use in pregnancy.

- Advanced renal disease requires immunosuppressants.
- Women with SLE and APS have associated recurrent miscarriage, thrombosis and thrombocytopenia and it is recommended that treatment with low-dose aspirin (75 mg daily) and heparin (5000 IU every 12 hours given subcutaneously) is commenced as soon as these women have a positive pregnancy test. Calcium supplementation is also recommended.

Intrapartum care

- The timing of birth depends on current activity of the disease and whether there are any complications.
- Women with SLE are particularly prone to infection, hypertension, thrombocytopenia and thromboembolic disorders.
- Close monitoring of the maternal condition is required to evaluate cardiac, pulmonary and renal function.
- Blood tests should be undertaken to screen for haematological conditions, which may lead to clotting disorders.
- Comfort measures and thromboembolitic D (TED) stockings can reduce pressure sores and the development of deep vein thrombosis.
- Women who have been on long-term steroid therapy will require parenteral steroid cover during labour.
- As SLE may compromise the uteroplacental circulation, continuous fetal monitoring in conjunction with fetal blood gas estimation is recommended.

Postpartum care

- During the immediate postpartum period the midwife should observe closely for signs of SLE flares and signs and symptoms of infection, pre-eclampsia, renal disease, thrombosis and neurological changes.
- Careful consideration needs to be given to breastfeeding, as most of the drugs used to treat SLE are excreted in breast milk.
- Large doses of aspirin should be avoided and non-steroidal anti-inflammatory drugs (NSAIDs) are contraindicated when breastfeeding jaundiced neonates; paracetamol is the drug of choice for postpartum analgesia.
- Low-dose steroids such as prednisone and prednisolone and the antimalarial hydroxychloroquine are considered safe to use when breastfeeding. Immunosuppressive therapy is contraindicated and should be avoided.

- The choice of contraceptives for a woman with SLE may be limited.

THYROID DISEASE

- In pregnancy, thyroid function is affected by three factors that increase the basal metabolic rate by 20%:
  - Oestrogen stimulates the production of thyroid-binding globulin (TBG), which binds more of the thyroid hormones resulting in a doubling of the total serum levels of *thyroxine* (T_4) and *tri-iodothyronine* (T_3).
  - Human chorionic gonadotrophin (HCG) secreted by the placenta appears to stimulate the thyroid gland directly as *thyroid-stimulating hormone* (TSH) levels fall in early pregnancy and then increase in the second and third trimesters, with a corresponding rise and then fall in the level of HCG.
  - A rise in the glomerular filtration rate in pregnancy leads to increased renal clearance of iodine, resulting in an increase in dietary iodine requirement.
- Clinical assessment of thyroid dysfunction is difficult, as pregnancy-related symptoms are similar to hyperthyroidism and hypothyroidism.
- Thyroid function can be assessed by biochemical tests that measure total T_4, free thyroxine (FT_4), total T_3 and TSH.
- It is important to remember that thyroid function tests may appear abnormal in pregnancy despite normal activity of the thyroid gland.

Hyperthyroidism

- The most common cause of hyperthyroidism in pregnancy is *Graves disease*, which is an autoimmune disorder that results in antibody activation of the thyroid gland.
- The gland becomes enlarged and secretes an increased amount of thyroid hormone. The metabolic processes of the body are accelerated, resulting in fatigue, heat intolerance, palpitations, diarrhoea and mood lability.
- Clinical diagnosis may be difficult, as the physiological signs and symptoms that pregnant women normally exhibit may mask this condition.
- The disease should be suspected in any woman who loses weight despite a good appetite.

- Other symptoms include an enlarged thyroid gland (goitre), exophthalmos, eyelid lag and persistent tachycardia.
- A serious complication of untreated or poorly controlled hyperthyroidism is *thyroid storm*. This may occur spontaneously or be precipitated by infection or stress. It is characterized by signs and symptoms associated with a high metabolic rate:
  - hyperthermia (temperature > 41°C), leading to:
    - dehydration
    - tachycardia
    - acute respiratory distress
    - cardiovascular collapse.
- This is a medical emergency requiring oxygen, cooling, hydration, antibiotics and drug therapy to stop the production and reduce the effect of thyroid hormone.
- Hyperthyroidism in pregnancy is associated with an increase in the incidence of pre-eclampsia, preterm birth, low birth weight and fetal death.

Management

- Treatment of hyperthyroidism is achieved through the use of antithyroid drugs.
- Propylthiouracil and carbimazole may be used in pregnancy. Propylthiouracil is the drug of choice, as less of it crosses the placenta and only small amounts are found in breast milk.
- The aim of management is to use the lowest dose possible, as these drugs may cause goitre and hypothyroidism in the fetus.
- During the antenatal period the pregnant woman should be seen monthly by the endocrinologist for clinical evaluation and monitoring of her thyroid levels.
- Factors that may precipitate thyroid storm include infection, the stress of labour and caesarean section.

Hypothyroidism

- The most common cause of hypothyroidism in pregnancy is *autoimmune thyroiditis* (Hashimoto disease).
- Slowing of the body's metabolic processes may occur, giving rise to mental and physical lethargy, excessive weight gain, constipation, cold intolerance and dryness of the skin.
- However, the symptoms may be non-specific and the condition can be difficult to diagnose.

- Hypothyroidism in pregnancy will result in reduced availability of the hormone for fetal requirements, leading to subsequent poor neurological development.
- Women should be encouraged to increase their dietary iodine intake during pregnancy and hypothyroidism should be treated with daily thyroxine.
- Following birth, the neonate's thyroid status should be checked to identify whether neonatal hypothyroidism is present.
- There is no contraindication to breastfeeding but the dose of thyroxine may need adjustment postpartum because of maternal weight loss following childbirth.

Postpartum thyroiditis

- This is an autoimmune disorder and is a form of Hashimoto thyroiditis, which occurs in 5% of women during the first year following childbirth.
- It is a transient thyroid disorder, characterized by a period of mild hyperthyroidism occurring a few months after birth and followed by a phase of hypothyroidism.
- In both phases the disorder presents with fatigue and a painless goitre; the condition may also mimic postpartum depression.
- Treatment is not required, as recovery is usually spontaneous.

Useful websites

Australian Family Physician. Epilepsy in pregnancy. Available at: http://www.racgp.org.au/afp/2014/march/epilepsy-in-pregnancy/

Khurana, R., Wolf, R.E., 2014. Systemic lupus erythematosus and pregnancy. Available at: http://emedicine.medscape.com/article/335055-overview#a9

NICE Guidelines. Diabetes in pregnancy: management from preconception to the postnatal period. Available at: https://www.nice.org.uk/guidance/ng3/chapter/1-Recommendations#gestational-diabetes-2

Hypertensive Disorders of Pregnancy

Hypertension is the commonest medical condition encountered in pregnancy, complicating approximately 5% of all pregnancies; it is a significant cause of maternal and fetal/neonatal morbidity and mortality. Pregnancy may induce hypertension in women who have been previously normotensive, or may aggravate existing hypertensive conditions.

DEFINITION AND CLASSIFICATION

The definition and classification of the hypertensive disorders are complex (Box 14.1). It is important to recognize the distinction between:
- a woman whose hypertension antedates pregnancy (pre-existing or chronic hypertension)
- a woman who develops an increased blood pressure during pregnancy (new, gestational or pregnancy-induced hypertension).

An incremental rise in blood pressure is not included in this classification system. However, women need close observation if they have a rise in blood pressure of:
- 30 mmHg systolic or
- 15 mmHg diastolic.

Further observation is necessary if proteinuria and hyperuricaemia (raised uric acid level) are also present.

PATHOLOGICAL CHANGES

Blood
- Hypertension, together with endothelial cell damage, affects capillary permeability.
- Plasma proteins leak from the damaged blood vessels, causing a decrease in the plasma colloid pressure and an increase in oedema within the extracellular space.

181

Box 14.1 **Classification and definition of hypertensive disorders in pregnancy**

Chronic hypertension

- Hypertension before pregnancy or a diastolic blood pressure of 90 mmHg or more before 20 weeks' gestation, and persisting 6 weeks after birth

Gestational hypertension (sometimes known as pregnancy-induced hypertension)

- Development of hypertension without other signs of pre-eclampsia
- Diagnosed when, after resting, the woman's blood pressure rises above 140/90 mmHg, on at least two occasions, no more than 1 week apart after the 20th week of pregnancy in a woman known to be normotensive
- Hypertension diagnosed for the first time in pregnancy, which does not resolve postpartum, is also classified as gestational hypertension

Pre-eclampsia

- Diagnosed on the basis of hypertension with proteinuria, when proteinuria is measured as a spot urine protein/creatinine ratio ≥ 30 mg/mmol
- In the absence of proteinuria, pre-eclampsia is suspected when hypertension is accompanied by symptoms including: headache
  - blurred vision
  - abdominal/epigastric pain, *or*
  - altered biochemistry: specifically, low platelet counts, abnormal liver enzyme levels

  These signs and symptoms, together with blood pressure above 160 mmHg systolic or above 110 mmHg diastolic and proteinuria, demonstrate the more severe form of the disease.

Eclampsia

- The new onset of convulsions during pregnancy or postpartum, unrelated to other cerebral pathological conditions, in a woman with pre-eclampsia

Pre-eclampsia superimposed on chronic hypertension

- This may occur in women with pre-existing hypertension (under 20 weeks' gestation) who develop: new proteinuria (> 30 mg/mmol)
  - sudden increases in pre-existing hypertension and proteinuria
  - thrombocytopenia (platelet count $< 100 \times 10^9$/L)
  - abnormal liver enzymes

- The reduced intravascular plasma volume causes hypovolaemia and haemoconcentration, which is reflected in an elevated haematocrit.
- In severe cases the lungs become congested with fluid and pulmonary oedema develops, oxygenation is impaired and cyanosis occurs.
- With vasoconstriction and disruption of the vascular endothelium the coagulation cascade is activated.

Coagulation system

- Increased platelet consumption produces thrombocytopenia.
- Disseminated intravascular coagulation (DIC) is characterized by low platelets and fibrinogen and prolonged prothrombin time.
- As the process progresses, fibrin and platelets are deposited, which will occlude blood flow to many organs, particularly the kidneys, liver, brain and placenta.

Kidneys

- In the kidney, hypertension leads to vasospasm of the afferent arterioles, resulting in a decreased renal blood flow, which produces hypoxia and oedema of the endothelial cells of the glomerular capillaries.
- Glomeruloendotheliosis (glomerular endothelial damage) allows plasma proteins to filter into the urine, producing proteinuria.
- Renal damage is reflected by reduced creatinine clearance and increased serum creatinine and uric acid levels.
- Oliguria develops as the condition worsens, signifying severe and renal vasoconstriction.

Liver

- Vasoconstriction of the hepatic vascular bed will result in hypoxia and oedema of the liver cells.
- In severe cases oedematous swelling of the liver causes epigastric pain and can lead to intracapsular haemorrhages and, in very rare cases, rupture of the liver.
- Altered liver function is reflected by falling albumin levels and a rise in liver enzyme levels.

Brain

- Hypertension, combined with cerebrovascular endothelial dysfunction, increases the permeability of the blood–brain barrier, resulting in cerebral oedema and microhaemorrhaging characterized by the onset of headaches, visual disturbances and convulsions.

- Where the mean arterial pressure (MAP – i.e. the systolic blood pressure plus twice the diastolic pressure divided by 3) exceeds 125 mmHg, the autoregulation of cerebral flow is disrupted, resulting in cerebral vasospasm, cerebral oedema and blood clot formation.
- This is known as *hypertensive encephalopathy*; if left untreated, it can progress to cerebral haemorrhage and death.

Fetoplacental unit

- In the uterus, vasoconstriction caused by hypertension reduces the uterine blood flow which can result in placental abruption and placental scarring.
- The amount of oxygen that diffuses through the cells of the syncytiotrophoblast and cytotrophoblast into the fetal circulation within the placenta is diminished, the placental tissue becomes ischaemic, the capillaries in the chorionic villi thrombose and infarctions occur, leading to fetal growth restriction.

THE MIDWIFE'S ROLE IN RISK ASSESSMENT AND EARLY IDENTIFICATION

- As the hypertensive disorders are unlikely to be prevented, early detection and appropriate management can minimize the severity of the condition.
- A comprehensive history will identify:
  - adverse social circumstances or poverty, which could prevent the woman from attending for regular antenatal care
  - the woman's age and parity
  - primipaternity (pregnancy with a new partner) and partner-related factors
  - a family history of hypertensive disorders
  - a past history of pre-eclampsia
  - the presence of underlying medical disorders: for example, renal disease, diabetes, systemic lupus erythematosus (SLE) and thromboembolic disorders.
- The two essential features of pre-eclampsia, hypertension and proteinuria, are assessed for at regular intervals throughout pregnancy.
- Diagnosis is usually based on the rise in blood pressure and the presence of proteinuria after 20 weeks' gestation.

Blood pressure measurement

- The woman's blood pressure is taken early in pregnancy to compare with all subsequent recordings, taking into account the normal pattern in pregnancy.
- Blood pressure machines should be calibrated for use in pregnancy and regularly maintained.
- Blood pressure can be overestimated by using a sphygmomanometer cuff of inadequate size relative to the arm circumference. The length of the bladder should be at least 80% of the arm circumference. Two cuffs should be available with inflation bladders of 35 cm for normal use and 42 cm for large arms.
- Rounding off of blood pressure measurements should be avoided and an attempt should be made to record the blood pressure as accurately as possible to the nearest 2 mmHg.
- The use of Korotkoff V (disappearance of sound) as a measure of the diastolic blood pressure should be used as this is easy to obtain, more reproducible and closer to the true intraarterial pressure.

Urinalysis

- Proteinuria in the absence of urinary tract infection is indicative of glomerular endotheliosis.
- The amount of protein in the urine is frequently taken as an index of the severity of pre-eclampsia.
- A significant increase in proteinuria, coupled with diminished urinary output, indicates renal impairment.
- Historically, a 24-hour urine collection has been used for quantifying proteinuria in pregnancy although its accuracy was questionable. Currently a spot urine protein/creatinine cut-off level of 30 mg/mmol equates to a 24-hour urine protein > 300 mg per day. This is the recommended method and cut-off for diagnosing proteinuria in pregnancy.

Oedema and excessive weight gain

- These symptoms are usually considered only when a diagnosis of pre-eclampsia has been made based on other criteria.
- The sudden severe widespread appearance of oedema is suggestive of pre-eclampsia or some underlying pathology and further investigations are necessary.
- This oedema puts on pressure and may be found in non-dependent anatomical areas such as the face, hands, lower abdomen, and vulval and sacral areas.

185

> Box 14.2 **Laboratory findings in pre-eclampsia**
>
> - Increased haemoglobin (Hb) and haematocrit levels
> - Thrombocytopenia
> - Prolonged clotting times
> - Raised serum creatinine and urea levels
> - Raised serum uric acid level
> - Abnormal liver function tests, particularly raised transaminases

Laboratory tests

The alterations in the haematological and biochemical parameters listed in Box 14.2 are suggestive of pre-eclampsia.

CARE AND MANAGEMENT

- The aim of care is to monitor the condition of the woman and her fetus and, if possible, to prevent the hypertensive disorder worsening by using appropriate interventions and treatment.
- The ultimate aim is to prolong the pregnancy until the fetus is sufficiently mature to survive, while safeguarding the woman's life.

Antenatal care

Rest

- It is preferable for the woman to rest at home and to be visited regularly by the midwife or GP or attend a specialized hospital clinic as an outpatient.
- When proteinuria develops in addition to hypertension, the risks to the woman and fetus are considerably increased. This would require admission to hospital to monitor and evaluate the maternal and fetal condition.

Diet

- There is little evidence to support dietary intervention for preventing or restricting the advance of pre-eclampsia.

Weight gain

- Weight gain may be useful for monitoring the progression of pre-eclampsia in conjunction with other parameters.

Blood pressure and urinalysis

- The blood pressure is monitored daily at home or every 4 hours when in hospital.
- Urine should be analysed for protein. If proteinuria is evident on dipstick analysis, a 'spot' urine protein:creatinine ratio should be obtained.
- The level of protein indicates the degree of vascular damage. Reduced kidney perfusion is indicated by:
  - proteinuria
  - reduced creatinine clearance
  - increased serum creatinine and uric acid.

Abdominal examination

- This is carried out daily. Any discomfort or tenderness may be a sign of placental abruption.
- Upper abdominal pain is highly significant and indicative of HELLP syndrome (see later) associated with fulminating (rapid-onset) pre-eclampsia.

Fetal assessment

- It is advisable to undertake a biophysical profile to determine fetal health and wellbeing. This is done by the use of:
  - kick charts
  - cardiotocography (CTG) monitoring
  - assessment of liquor volume and fetal breathing movements or Doppler flow studies, or both, to determine placental blood flow.

Laboratory studies

- These include:
  - a full blood count, platelet count and clotting profile
  - urea and electrolytes
  - creatinine and liver function tests, including albumin levels.
- In severe pre-eclampsia, blood samples should be taken every 12–24 hours.

Antihypertensive therapy

- The use of antihypertensive therapy as prophylaxis is controversial, as it shows no benefit in significantly prolonging pregnancy or improving maternal or fetal outcome.

- Its use is, however, advocated as short-term therapy to prevent an increase in blood pressure and the development of severe hypertension, thereby reducing the risk to the woman of cerebral haemorrhage.
- First-line medications used include methyldopa, labetalol and oxprenolol. Second-line medications are hydralazine, nifedipine and prazosin.
- Atenolol used over the long-term is not recommended as it may cause significant fetal growth restriction.

Antithrombotic agents

- Early activation of the clotting system may contribute to the later pathology of pre-eclampsia.
- As a result, the use of anticoagulants or antiplatelet agents has been considered for the prevention of pre-eclampsia and fetal growth restriction.
- Aspirin, recommended for women at risk from 12 weeks' gestation, is thought to inhibit the production of the platelet-aggregating agent, thromboxane A_2.

Intrapartum care

It is essential to monitor the maternal and fetal condition carefully.

Vital signs

- Blood pressure is measured half-hourly, or every 15–20 minutes in severe pre-eclampsia.
- Because of the potentially rapid haemodynamic changes in pre-eclampsia, several authors recommend the measurement of the MAP.
- MAP reflects the systemic perfusion pressure, and therefore the degree of hypovolaemia, whereas manual measurement of diastolic pressure alone is a better indicator of the degree of hypertension.
- Observation of the respiratory rate (> 14/min) will be complemented with pulse oximetry in severe pre-eclampsia; this gives an indication of the degree of maternal hypoxia.
- Temperature should be recorded as necessary.
- In severe pre-eclampsia, examination of the optic fundi can give an indication of optic vasospasm.
- Cerebral irritability can be assessed by the degree of hyper-reflexia or the presence of clonus (significant if more than 3 beats).

Fluid balance

- The reduced intravascular compartment in pre-eclampsia, together with poorly controlled fluid balance, can result in circulatory overload, pulmonary oedema, acute respiratory distress syndrome and ultimately death.
- In severe pre-eclampsia, a central venous pressure (CVP) line may be considered; measurements are taken hourly.
- If the value is > 10 mmHg, then 20 mg furosemide should be considered.
- Intravenous fluids are administered using infusion pumps; the total recommended fluid intake in severe pre-eclampsia is 85 ml/h.
- Oxytocin should be administered with caution, as it has an antidiuretic effect.
- Urinary output should be monitored and urinalysis undertaken every 4 hours to detect the presence of protein, ketones and glucose.
- In severe pre-eclampsia, a urinary catheter should be in situ and urine output is measured hourly; a level > 30 ml/h reflects adequate renal function.

Plasma volume expansion

- Although women with pre-eclampsia have oedema, they are hypovolaemic.
- The blood volume of women with pre-eclampsia is reduced, as shown by a high haemoglobin (Hb) concentration and a high haematocrit level.
- This results in movement of fluid into the extravascular compartment, causing oedema.
- The oedema initially occurs in dependent tissues, but as the disease progresses oedema occurs in the liver and brain.

Pain relief

- Epidural analgesia may procure the best pain relief, reduce the blood pressure and facilitate rapid caesarean section, should the need arise.
- It is important to ensure a normal clotting screen and a platelet count > 100×10^9/L prior to insertion of the epidural.

Fetal condition

- The fetal heart rate should be monitored closely. Deviations from the normal must be reported and acted upon.

Birth plan

- When the second stage commences, the obstetrician and paediatrician should be notified. A short second stage may be prescribed, depending on the maternal and fetal conditions.
- If the maternal or fetal condition shows significant deterioration during the first stage of labour, a caesarean section will be undertaken.
- Oxytocin is the preferred agent for the management of the third stage of labour.
- Ergometrine and syntometrine will cause peripheral vasoconstriction and increase hypertension; they should therefore not normally be used in the presence of any degree of pre-eclampsia, unless there is severe haemorrhage.

Postpartum care

- The maternal condition should continue to be monitored at least every 4 hours for the next 24 hours or more following childbirth, as there is still a potential danger of the woman developing eclampsia.

Signs of impending eclampsia

See Box 14.3.

- The aim of care at this time is to preclude death of the woman and fetus by controlling hypertension, inhibiting convulsions and preventing coma.

Box 14.3 **Signs of impending eclampsia**

- A sharp rise in blood pressure
- Diminished urinary output
- Increase in proteinuria
- Headache, which is usually severe, persistent and frontal in location
- Drowsiness or confusion
- Visual disturbances, such as blurring of vision or flashing lights
- Epigastric pain
- Nausea and vomiting

HELLP SYNDROME

- The syndrome of haemolysis (H), elevated liver enzymes (EL) and low platelet count (LP) is generally thought to represent a variant of the pre-eclampsia/eclampsia syndrome.
- Pregnancies complicated by this syndrome have been associated with significant maternal and perinatal morbidity and mortality.

Clinical presentation

- HELLP syndrome typically manifests itself between 32 and 34 weeks' gestation and 30% of cases will occur postpartum.
- The woman often complains of malaise, epigastric or right upper quadrant pain, and nausea and vomiting.
- Some will have non-specific viral syndrome-like symptoms.
- Hypertension and proteinuria may be absent or slightly abnormal.

Diagnosis

- Pregnant women presenting with the previously mentioned symptoms should have a full blood count, platelet count and liver function tests, irrespective of maternal blood pressure.
- The diagnosis of HELLP syndrome may be assisted by confirming:
  - haemolysis
  - elevated lactate dehydrogenase (LDH)
  - raised bilirubin levels
  - low ($< 100 \times 10^9$/L) or falling platelets
  - elevated liver transaminases (aspartate aminotransferase, alanine transaminase and gamma-glutamyl transferase – AST, ALT and GGT).

Complications

- Subcapsular haematoma or rupture of the liver, or both together, is a rare but potentially fatal complication of the HELLP syndrome.
- The condition usually presents with severe epigastric pain, which may persist for several hours.
- In addition women may complain of neck and shoulder pain.

Management

- Women with the HELLP syndrome should be admitted to an obstetric led unit with intensive or high-dependency care facilities available.
- In pregnancies of less than 32 weeks' gestation expectant management may be undertaken with appropriate safeguards and consent.
- In term pregnancies, or where there is a deteriorating maternal or fetal condition, immediate birth is recommended.

ECLAMPSIA

- Eclampsia is rarely seen in developed countries today; it has an incidence of 1.5 to 10 cases per 10 000 births.
- Eclampsia is associated with increased risks of maternal and perinatal morbidity and mortality.
- Significant maternal life-threatening complications as a result of eclampsia include:
  - pulmonary oedema
  - renal and hepatic failure
  - placental abruption and haemorrhage
  - DIC
  - HELLP syndrome
  - brain haemorrhage.
- Hypertension is not necessarily a precursor to the onset of eclampsia but will almost always be evident following a seizure.
- Detecting and managing imminent eclampsia is also made more difficult in that, unlike other types of seizure, warning symptoms are not always present before onset of the convulsion.

Care of a woman with eclampsia

- The aims of immediate care are to:
  - summon medical aid
  - clear and maintain the woman's airway – this may be achieved by placing the woman in the recovery (semi-prone) position to facilitate the drainage of saliva and vomit
  - administer oxygen and prevent severe hypoxia
  - prevent the woman from being injured.
- In the first instance, all effort is devoted to the preservation of the woman's life; the wellbeing of the fetus is secondary.

- The woman will require intensive/high-dependency care, as she may remain comatose for a time following the seizure or may be sleepy.
- Recordings should be carried out as for severe pre-eclampsia.
- Periodic restlessness associated with uterine contraction may indicate that labour has commenced.
- It is usual to expedite the birth of the baby when eclampsia occurs. In this instance, caesarean section is the usual mode of birth.

Anticonvulsant therapy

- Magnesium sulphate is now the recommended drug of choice for routine anticonvulsant management of women with eclampsia; it is administered intravenously according to a protocol:
  - A loading dose of 4 g (diluted in normal saline) is given over 15 minutes intravenously.
  - This is followed by an infusion of 5 g/500 ml normal saline at a rate of 1–2 g/h until 24 hours following birth or the last seizure.
  - Recurrent seizures should be treated with a further bolus of 2–4 g given over 10 minutes.
- Magnesium sulphate can be toxic and therefore the deep tendon reflexes should be monitored hourly.
- The respiratory rate and oxygen saturation levels are measured hourly and should remain > 14/min and > 95%, respectively.
- In women with oliguria, serum magnesium levels should be monitored and maintained within the therapeutic range (2–3 mmol/L).
- Calcium gluconate is the antidote for magnesium toxicity and should be readily available.

Treatment of hypertension

- Severe hypertension is defined as > 160/110 mmHg or a MAP > 125 mmHg.
- Intravenous hydralazine is the most useful agent to gain control of the blood pressure quickly;
  - 5 mg should be administered slowly and the blood pressure measured at 5-minute intervals until the diastolic pressure reaches 90 mmHg.
  - The diastolic blood pressure may be maintained at this level by titrating an intravenous infusion of hydralazine against the blood pressure.

- Labetalol may be used in preference to hydralazine, in which case 20 mg is given intravenously followed at 10-minute intervals by 40 mg, 80 mg and 80 mg up to a cumulative dose of 300 mg.

Fluid balance

Care must be taken not to overload the maternal system with intravenous fluids.

Anaesthesia

- Both general and regional (epidural/spinal) anaesthesia carry a degree of risk in the eclamptic woman.
- In general, epidural is preferred in eclamptic women who are conscious, haemodynamically stable and cooperative.

Postnatal care

- As almost half of eclamptic fits occur following childbirth, intensive surveillance of the woman is required in a high-dependency or intensive care unit. Parameters to monitor are:
  - a return to normal blood pressure
  - an increase in urine output and reduction in protein
  - a reduction in oedema
  - a return to normal laboratory indices.
- TED stockings should be worn to prevent deep vein thrombosis.
- All the usual postpartum care is given, and as soon as the woman's condition permits, she should be taken to see her baby.
- Alternatively, if the baby's condition is good, he or she may be returned to the woman.

CHRONIC HYPERTENSION

- Chronic hypertension has the following possible causes:
  - It may be a pre-existing disorder: for example, essential hypertension.
  - It may be secondary to existing medical problems, such as renal disease, SLE, coarctation of the aorta, Cushing syndrome or phaeochromocytoma.

Diagnosis

- Consistent blood pressure recordings of 140/90 mmHg or more, on two occasions more than 24 hours apart during the first 20

weeks of pregnancy, suggest that the hypertension is a chronic problem and unrelated to the pregnancy.
- The diagnosis may be difficult to make because of the changes seen with blood pressure in pregnancy.
- This is a particular problem in women who present late in their pregnancy with no baseline blood pressure measurement.

Investigation

- Women with chronic hypertension tend to be older, parous and have a family or personal history of hypertension.
- Accurate measurement of blood pressure is important. Serial blood pressure recordings should be made to determine the true pattern, as even normotensive women show occasional peaks.
- There may be long-term effects of hypertension, such as retinopathy, ischaemic heart disease and renal damage.
- Renal function tests may be performed; however, it is important to realize the extent to which the alterations in the physiological norms may affect clinical interpretation in pregnancy.
- Blood urate levels may help to differentiate between chronic hypertension and pre-eclampsia; they do not rise in the former as they do in the latter.

Complications

- The perinatal outcome in mild chronic hypertension is good.
- However perinatal morbidity and mortality are increased in those women who develop severe chronic hypertension or superimposed pre-eclampsia.
- Other complications are independent of pregnancy and include renal failure and cerebral haemorrhage.
- Maternal mortality is high if phaeochromocytoma is not diagnosed and left untreated.

Management

Mild chronic hypertension
- This is defined as a systolic blood pressure of < 160 mmHg and a diastolic blood pressure of < 110 mmHg.
- The woman is unlikely to need antenatal admission to hospital and may be cared for in the community.
- The woman's condition should be carefully monitored to identify any pre-eclampsia that develops.

Severe chronic hypertension

- The systolic blood pressure is > 160 mmHg and the diastolic blood pressure is > 110 mmHg.
- Ideally, the woman will be cared for by the obstetric team in conjunction with the renal physician.
- Frequent antenatal visits are recommended to monitor the maternal condition.
- Monitoring includes:
  - blood pressure monitoring
  - urinalysis to detect proteinuria
  - blood tests to measure the haematocrit and renal function.
- Antihypertensive drug therapy is used to prevent maternal complications but has no proven benefit for the fetus, nor in the prognosis of the pre-eclamptic process.
- The most commonly used agent is methyldopa 1–4 g/day in divided doses. It has a sedative effect lasting 2–3 days and is generally considered safe in pregnancy.
- As mentioned previously, other drugs in common usage include labetalol, nifedipine and oral hydralazine.
- Sedative drugs may be given to reduce anxiety and help the woman to rest, but are rarely recommended.
- Monitoring of fetal wellbeing and of placental function should be carried out assiduously because of the risk of fetal compromise.
- This would include using serial growth scans and placental blood flow studies by Doppler ultrasound.
- If the maternal or fetal condition causes concern, the woman will be admitted to hospital.
- The timing of the birth is planned according to the needs of woman and fetus. If early birth is deemed necessary, induction of labour is preferred to caesarean section.
- Renal function should be reassessed postnatally and the woman should be seen by the physician with a view to long-term management of persistent hypertension.
- Antihypertensive therapy may be required.

FURTHER READING

Mangesi, L., Hofmeyr, G.J., Smith, V., Smyth, R., 2015. Fetal movement counting for assessment of fetal wellbeing. Cochrane Database Syst. Rev. (10), CD004909. doi: 10.1002/14651858.pub3.

Warland, J., Glover, P., 2016. Fetal movements: what are we telling women? Women Birth. 30 (1), 23–28.

Useful websites

Lowe, S.A., et al., 2014. The SOMANZ guideline for the management of hypertensive disorders of pregnancy. Available at: https://somanz.org/documents/HTPregnancyGuidelineJuly2014.pdf

NICE Guidelines. Hypertension in pregnancy: diagnosis and management. Available at: https://www.nice.org.uk/guidance/cg107/chapter/introduction

Sexually Transmissible and Reproductive Tract Infections in Pregnancy

TRENDS IN SEXUAL HEALTH

Sexually transmitted infections (STIs) are a significant public health issue. Trends of particular concern are the high rates of and increase in STI diagnoses particularly in women aged 16–24. Most at risk are those who have high numbers of sexual partners, partner change and unprotected sexual intercourse. That said there is a pervasive assumption that more mature adults (i.e. those 50 years and older) are less sexually active. Evidence is emerging that there is also a steady increase in STIs in this age group.

Multidisciplinary team work

Joint management between an obstetrician and a sexual health physician specializing in genito-urinary medicine (GUM) during pregnancy is essential for women with infections that are serious, life-threatening, or both, such as human immunodeficiency virus (HIV); in addition, a paediatrician is required in the care and management of the neonate infected through vertical transmission. The midwife plays a vital role in the provision of individualized care throughout pregnancy, labour and the puerperium.

INFECTIONS OF THE VAGINA AND VULVA

There are three main types of vaginal and vulval infection:
- trichomoniasis
- bacterial vaginosis
- candidiasis.

Trichomoniasis

Trichomoniasis is almost exclusively sexually transmissible. It is caused by infection with the parasite *Trichomonas vaginalis*, a round or oval flagellated protozoan. Whereas 10–50% of women are asymptomatic, common symptoms include:

- vaginal discharge, which is present in up to 70% of cases and may vary in consistency from thin and scanty to profuse and thick. A classic frothy yellow–green discharge occurs in 10–30% of women
- vulval pruritus
- inflammation
- dyspareunia
- mild dysuria and lower abdominal pain may also be experienced.

Trichomoniasis in pregnancy

Trichomoniasis has been linked with a small risk of preterm birth and low birth weight, and an increase in the risk of HIV via sexual intercourse. Trichomoniasis may be acquired perinatally.

Diagnosis

In women:

- 95% of cases can be diagnosed by cultures
- 40–80% of cases by microscopic examination of a wet-film or acridine orange-stained slide from the posterior fornix.

Treatment

- The recommended treatment is metronidazole daily for 5–7 days or in a single dose. Although it is contraindicated, meta-analyses have concluded that there is no evidence of teratogenicity from its use in women during the first trimester of pregnancy.
- Clotrimazole pessaries daily for 7 days can be used in early pregnancy. High single-dose regimens should be avoided during pregnancy and breastfeeding.
- It is usual to treat the partner(s) and advise against sexual intercourse until the treatment is completed.
- In addition, patients should be advised not to drink alcohol during the treatment and for at least 48 hours afterwards, as this may cause nausea and vomiting.

Bacterial vaginosis

- Bacterial vaginosis (BV) is the most common cause of vaginal discharge in women of childbearing age. It can arise and remit spontaneously in sexually active and non-sexually active women.

199

It often coexists with other STIs. It is more common in women who:
- have multiple partners
- have an intrauterine contraceptive device (IUCD)
- smoke
- have pelvic inflammatory disease (PID)
- have unprotected sex.
- In this condition the normal lactobacilli-predominant vaginal flora are replaced with a number of anaerobic bacteria.
- The vaginal epithelium is not inflamed; hence the term 'vaginosis' rather than 'vaginitis'.
- The main symptom is a malodorous and greyish watery vaginal discharge, although most women are asymptomatic.
- The odour is usually more pronounced following sexual intercourse owing to the release of amines by the alkaline semen.
- Vulval irritation may occur in approximately one-third of women.

BV in pregnancy

- BV is present in up to 20% of women during pregnancy, although the majority are asymptomatic.
- BV during pregnancy is associated with preterm birth, low birth weight, preterm premature rupture of membranes, intraamniotic infection and postpartum endometritis.

Diagnosis

- A diagnosis of BV is confirmed if three of the following criteria are present:
  - a thin, white-to-grey, homogeneous discharge
  - 'clue cells' on microscopy (squamous epithelial cells covered with adherent bacteria)
  - a vaginal pH of > 4.7
  - the release of a fishy odour when potassium hydroxide is added to a sample of the discharge.
- A Gram-stained vaginal smear is another diagnostic technique.

Treatment

- Antibiotic therapy is highly effective at eradicating infection and improving the outcome of pregnancy for women with a past history of preterm birth.
- The treatment regimen is the same as for trichomoniasis.

- Alternative treatments include oral clindamycin, intravaginal clindamycin cream or metronidazole gel.
- All these treatments have been shown in controlled trials to achieve cure rates of 70–80% after 4 weeks, but recurrences of infection are common.
- Women should be advised to avoid vaginal douching, use of shower gel and use of antiseptic agents or shampoo in the bath.

Candidiasis

- Candidiasis is a common cause of vulvitis, vaginitis and vaginal discharge. The causative organism is usually *Candida albicans*, a fungal parasite.
- It is a commensal and is found in the flora of the mouth, gastrointestinal tract and vagina.
- Colonization of the vagina and vulva may be introduced from the lower intestinal tract or through sexual intercourse.
- During the reproductive years 10–20% of women may harbour *Candida* species but remain asymptomatic and do not require treatment.
- Predisposing factors that encourage *Candida albicans* to convert from a commensal to a parasitic role are listed in Box 15.1.
- The signs and symptoms of candidiasis include:
  - soreness
  - often, a thick, white curdy discharge (not always present)
  - erythema and oedema of the vulva, vagina and cervix may be erythematous and oedematous
  - white plaques of the vulva, vagina and cervix
  - dyspareunia.

Box 15.1 **Factors that provoke the conversion of *Candida albicans* from a commensal to a parasite**

- Local changes to the vaginal immunity (e.g. vaginal douches)
- Immunosuppressant disease or treatment (e.g. acquired immunodeficiency syndrome [AIDS]), chemotherapy)
- Drug therapy (e.g. antibiotics)
- Endocrine disease (e.g. diabetes mellitus)
- Physiological changes (e.g. pregnancy)
- Miscellaneous disorders (e.g. iron deficiency)

Candidiasis in pregnancy

Vaginal candidiasis is found 2–10 times more frequently in pregnant than in non-pregnant women and it is more difficult to eradicate.

Diagnosis

Vaginal culture is the most sensitive method currently available for detecting *Candida albicans* cells.

Treatment

- Candidiasis is treated primarily with antifungal pessaries or cream inserted high into the vagina at night. Preparations that may be given include:
  - clotrimazole pessaries
  - nystatin pessaries or gel
  - oral fluconazole (Diflucan).

Diflucan is available from chemists without a prescription but this form of treatment has not been tested in pregnancy and it cannot be assumed to be safe. It should also be used with caution whilst breast-feeding owing to toxic effects in high doses.

- Recurrence is common. This may be due to resistant cases or failure to complete the treatment.
- It is usual to treat the partner and advise against sexual intercourse until the treatment is completed.
- Vaginal douches and perfumed products should be avoided and tight-fitting synthetic clothing should be discouraged.

BACTERIAL INFECTIONS

Chlamydia

- *Chlamydia trachomatis* is an intracellular bacterium. It is the most common cause of sexually transmitted bacterial infection and a leading cause of PID.
  - Serotypes D–K are sexually transmitted and are important causes of morbidity in both sexes.
  - Serotypes A, B and C cause trachoma and blindness.
  - Serotypes L1–L3 cause the genital disease lymphogranuloma venereum.
- Chlamydial infection is asymptomatic in approximately 80% of cases.

- Some women may have a purulent vaginal discharge, postcoital or intermenstrual bleeding, lower abdominal pain, mucopurulent cervicitis and/or contact bleeding.
- Chlamydial infection of the cervix is found in 15–30% of women attending sexual health clinics, and concurrently in 35–40% of women with gonorrhoea.
- Specific high-risk groups include:
  - women aged less than 25
  - those with a new sexual partner or more than one sexual partner in recent years
  - those not using barrier contraception
  - those using oral contraception
  - those presenting for termination of pregnancy.
- Chlamydial infection has been estimated to account for 40% of ectopic pregnancies.

Chlamydia in pregnancy

It can cause amnionitis and postpartum endometritis.

Fetal and neonatal infections

- The major risk to the infant is from passing through an infected cervix during birth. Up to 70% of babies born to women with chlamydial infection will become infected, with 30–40% developing conjunctivitis and 10–20% a characteristic pneumonia.
- The incubation period of chlamydial ophthalmia is 6–21 days.
- Chlamydial pneumonia usually occurs between the 4th and 11th weeks of life. It affects approximately half the babies who develop conjunctivitis but is not always preceded by it.
- The pharynx, middle ear, rectum and vagina are also targets for infection, with a delay of up to 7 months before cultures become positive.

Diagnosis

Nucleic acid amplification (NAA) tests should be used to screen women for genital chlamydial infection.

Treatment

- Genital chlamydial infections are sensitive to three classes of antibiotic:

- the tetracyclines
- macrolides (e.g. erythromycin)
- the fluorinated quinolones, especially ofloxacin.
- The tetracyclines and the fluoroquinolones are currently contraindicated in pregnancy.
- Erythromycin has long been the preferred treatment for cervical chlamydial infection despite its gastrointestinal effects.
- Erythromycin is also used for chlamydial infections in infants, young children and pregnant and lactating women.
- Single-dose azithromycin is expensive but gaining favour because of its effectiveness, low incidence of adverse gastrointestinal effects and enhanced compliance.

Gonorrhoea

- Gonorrhoea is caused by *Neisseria gonorrhoeae*, a Gram-negative diplococcus.
- Transmission is by sexual contact.
- This organism adheres to mucous membranes. The primary sites of infection are therefore the mucous membranes of the urethra, endocervix, rectum, pharynx and conjunctiva.
- Gonorrhoea may coexist with other genital mucosal pathogens, notably *T. vaginalis, C. albicans* and *C. trachomatis*. According to some epidemiological and biological studies, it is also associated with increased transmission of and susceptibility to HIV infection.
- Gonorrhoea is a major cause of PID. The sequelae of PID include:
  - infertility
  - ectopic pregnancy
  - chronic pelvic pain.
- Although uncommon, gonorrhoea may also cause disseminated systemic disease and arthritis.
  - The most common symptom is an increased or altered vaginal discharge, although up to 50% of women are asymptomatic.
  - Lower abdominal pain, dysuria, intermenstrual uterine bleeding and menorrhagia may also be experienced, ranging in intensity from minimal to severe.

Gonorrhoea in pregnancy

- The incidence of gonorrhoea in pregnancy is low but its presence has been associated with:

- spontaneous abortion
- very low birth weight
- prelabour rupture of the membranes
- chorioamnionitis
- preterm birth
- postpartum endometritis
- pelvic sepsis.

Fetal and neonatal infections

- *N. gonorrhoeae* can be transmitted during birth, or occasionally in utero when there is prolonged rupture of the membranes.
- The risk of transmission is between 30% and 47%.
- Infection usually manifests as gonococcal ophthalmia neonatorum, a notifiable condition.
  - A profuse, purulent discharge is usually evident within a few days of birth.
  - It can be diagnosed by microscopy and culture of an eye swab.
  - The eyes may be cleaned with saline but systemic antibiotics are required.
  - If left untreated, the condition will eventually lead to blindness, and occasionally the neonate may develop further infection such as gonococcal arthritis.

Diagnosis

Culture on antibiotic-containing medium is used for detecting *N. gonorrhoeae*. The sensitivity is almost 100% in specialized clinics, but isolation rates are lower in non-specialized settings.

Treatment

- Pregnant women infected with *N. gonorrhoeae* should be treated with dual therapy consisting of ceftriaxone 250 mg in a single intramuscular (IM) dose and azithromycin 1 g orally as a single dose.

Syphilis in pregnancy

- Syphilis is caused by the bacterium *Treponema pallidum*, a spiral organism (spirochaete), and is usually acquired by sexual contact.
- It can also be congenitally transmitted. It is a complex systemic disease that can involve virtually any organ in the body.

Box 15.2 **Stages of acquired syphilis**

Early infectious

- *Primary*: 9–90 days after exposure (mean 21 days)
- *Secondary*: 6 weeks to 6 months after exposure (4–8 weeks after primary lesion)
- *Latent (early)*: 2 years after exposure

Late non-infectious

- *Latent (late)*: ≥ 2 years after exposure with no symptoms or signs
- *Neurosyphilis, cardiovascular syphilis, gummatous syphilis*: 3–20 years after exposure

- Acquired syphilis is divided into the stages shown in Box 15.2.
- Although sequelae are dependent on the stage of infection in the woman, untreated syphilis in pregnancy may result in:
  - spontaneous abortion
  - preterm birth
  - stillbirth
  - neonatal death
  - significant infant or later morbidity.
- Vertical transmission may occur at any time during pregnancy, but is more likely if the woman has primary, secondary or early latent syphilis.
- The infection does not usually occur before the 4th month of pregnancy because treponemes from the maternal circulation are unable to pass through the Langhans cell layer of the early placenta.

Congenital syphilis

- Approximately two-thirds of live-born infected infants do not have any signs or symptoms at birth, but they present over the following weeks, months or years.
- Lesions develop only after the 4th month when immunological competence becomes established.
- Serology at birth is unreliable owing to passive transfer from the woman and the treponemal-specific IgM test is prone to false positive and negative results.

> Box 15.3 **Serological tests for syphilis**
>
> - Venereal diseases research laboratory (VDRL)
> - Rapid plasma reagin (RPR) test
> - *Treponema pallidum* haemagglutination assay (TPHA)
> - *Treponema pallidum* particle agglutination (TPPA) assay
> - Fluorescent treponemal antibody absorption (FTA-abs) test
> - Treponemal enzyme immunoassay (EIA)

Diagnosis

- Women are screened for syphilis at antenatal booking and treated if need be.
- However, this does not detect women who acquire the infection during pregnancy, or women who are incubating syphilis at the time of serological testing.
- A range of serological tests is used for screening (Box 15.3).

Treatment

- The preferred treatment is IM penicillin.
- In the case of penicillin allergy, the alternative is erythromycin, as tetracycline is contraindicated in pregnancy.
- The poor placental transfer of erythromycin does not reliably cure the fetus and as a precaution the baby may be given a course of penicillin at birth.

Group B Streptococcus (GBS)

- GBS (also known as *Streptococcus agalactiae*) is a Gram-positive bacterium that naturally colonizes the body.
- It is harboured primarily in the gastrointestinal tract, with approximately 30% of adults asymptomatically carrying the organism at any one time.
- It also colonizes the vagina in up to 25% of women.

GBS in pregnancy

- In pregnant women colonized with GBS, high-risk factors associated with vertical transmission include:
  - preterm birth
  - prolonged rupture of membranes
  - maternal pyrexia during labour

- GBS cultured in a urine sample
- known carriage of GBS
- a history of a GBS infection in a previous pregnancy.
- GBS is able to infiltrate the amniotic cavity, whether or not the membranes are intact, and infects the fetus through the lung epithelium.
- Postpartum endometritis and post-caesarean wound infection may also occur in the woman.

Fetal and neonatal infections

- GBS is the commonest cause of overwhelming sepsis in newborns during the first days of life, occurring at a rate of approximately 0.3 per 1000 live births.
- The respiratory infection rapidly progresses to sepsis and shock and causes significant morbidity and mortality. GBS infection in the neonate may be:
  - early onset, in which case the infection starts in utero
  - late onset, which usually presents between 7 days and 3 months of age.

Diagnosis

- Vaginal and rectal swabs can detect colonization with GBS, although higher rates are detected with a special enrichment culture medium.
- The degree of colonization is extremely variable and the tendency for recolonization after treatment makes control difficult.
- Swabs taken late in pregnancy at approximately 35 weeks are more effective in predicting whether or not GBS will be carried during labour.

Treatment

- Intrapartum antibiotic treatment of women colonized with GBS appears to reduce neonatal infection. These are intravenous benzyl penicillin or ampicillin during labour.

VIRAL INFECTIONS

Genital warts

- Genital warts are caused by human papillomavirus (HPV) types 6 and 11.

- Transmission is most often by sexual contact, although infants and young children may develop laryngeal papillomas after being infected from maternal genital warts at birth.
- In pregnancy, genital warts may dramatically increase in size and appear as cauliflower-like masses, although they usually diminish in size following the birth. Occasionally they can obstruct a vaginal birth; therefore, a caesarean section would be indicated.
- Genital warts are difficult and time-consuming to treat.
- They are usually treated initially with locally applied caustic agents such as podophyllum. However, this is contraindicated in pregnancy because of possible teratogenic effects.
- It is recommended that no treatment be offered during pregnancy, although there are alternatives such as trichloroacetic acid, cryotherapy or electrocautery.
- Caesarean section should not be performed solely to prevent transmission of HPV infection to the newborn. However, this could be considered if women have anogenital warts, if the pelvic outlet is obstructed or if vaginal delivery would result in excessive bleeding.
- Women presenting with genital warts should be fully investigated to exclude other STIs. In addition, colposcopy should be performed to exclude flat warts on the cervix.
- Most genital warts are benign, but cervical intraepithelial neoplasia (CIN) is strongly associated with HPV types 16, 18, 31, 33 and 35; therefore, an annual cervical smear is recommended.

Hepatitis B virus (HBV)

- HBV infection is an important cause of morbidity and mortality from acute infection and chronic sequelae that include chronic active hepatitis, cirrhosis and primary liver cancer.
- HBV can be transmitted sexually or parenterally mainly through infected blood or blood products.
- It can be transmitted by means of unsterilized equipment, such as may be used when injecting drug users share needles and syringes, or in tattooing or acupuncture, or as a consequence of needle-stick injury in healthcare workers.
- Vertical transmission is a major mode of transmission, most frequently occurring perinatally.
- Acute HBV infection during pregnancy is associated with an increased rate of spontaneous abortion and preterm labour. There are usually two phases of symptoms:

- The prodromal phase, characterized by flu-like symptoms.
- The icteric phase, characterized by jaundice, anorexia, nausea and fatigue.
- The infection may be asymptomatic in 10–50% of adults in the acute phase and in virtually all infants and children.
- If chronic infection occurs, there are often no physical signs but there may be signs of chronic liver disease.
- In the acute early phase the hepatitis B surface antigen (HBsAg, formally called Australia antigen) is produced by the infected hepatocytes and appears in the sera of most patients.
- The presence of the hepatitis Be antigen (HBeAg) in the serum indicates viral activity, which can persist over days or weeks. IgM- and IgG-type antibodies to the core antigen develop.
- IgG antibodies may be detectable for many years after recovery. As the infection resolves, HBeAg becomes undetectable; once infection is cleared, the antibody to the surface antigen component, anti-HBs, appears, indicating immunity.
- If HBsAg remains detectable for more than 6 months, the patient is usually referred to as a hepatitis B virus carrier.
- All pregnant women should be offered antenatal screening for HBV and babies born to infected women should be vaccinated.
  - The vaccination should be administered at birth and at 1 and 6 months.
  - In addition, the babies of women who have become infected with HBV during pregnancy and those who do not have anti-HBe antibodies should also receive hepatitis B-specific immunoglobulin (HBIg) at birth.
  - This should be injected at a different site to the vaccine (the anterolateral thigh is the preferred site in infants). This confers immediate immunity and reduces vertical transmission by 90%.
  - Infected women should continue to breastfeed, as there is no additional risk of transmission.

Hepatitis C virus (HCV)

- HCV infection is a type of viral hepatitis that affects between 1% and 8% pregnant women.
- The principal route of transmission is by percutaneous inoculation, blood and blood products.
- The incidence of transmission by sexual contact is low.
- Vertical transmission is also low, occurring at 5% or less, but higher rates are seen if the woman is HIV- and HCV-positive.

- At present, there is no known way of reducing the risk of vertical transmission.
- There is no firm evidence that breastfeeding constitutes an additional risk of transmission unless the woman is symptomatic with a high viral load.

Herpes simplex virus (HSV)

- There are two types of HSV: HSV-1 and HSV-2.
  - HSV-1 causes the majority of orolabial infections, and is often acquired during childhood through direct physical contact with oral secretions.
  - HSV-2 is the most common cause of genital herpes and is sexually transmitted via genital secretions.
- Infections may be primary or non-primary. Once infected, the virus remains in the individual for life, causing recurrent infection.
- Prior infection with HSV-1 modifies the clinical manifestations of first infection by HSV-2.
- The incidence of HSV infection depends on factors such as:
  - age
  - duration of sexual activity
  - number of sexual partners
  - socioeconomic status
  - previous genital infections
  - race.
- In adults, HSV infection may be asymptomatic, but painful, vesicular or ulcerative lesions of the skin and mucous membranes occur frequently.
- Dysuria and vaginal or urethral discharge may also occur.
- There may be systemic symptoms of fever and myalgia.
- Symptoms are more common in primary infection.

Genital herpes infection

This is defined as:

- *First episode primary infection* – first infection with either HSV-1 or HSV-2 in an individual with no pre-existing antibodies to either type. The local symptoms tend to be severe and lesions may last for 2–3 weeks.
- *First episode non-primary infection* – first infection with either HSV-1 or HSV-2 in an individual with pre-existing circulating antibodies to the other type.

- *Recurrent infection* – recurrence of clinical symptoms due to reactivation of pre-existent HSV-1 or HSV-2 infection after a period of latency.

HSV in pregnancy

- The most important complication of HSV infection in pregnancy is neonatal herpes, a rare but potentially very serious condition.
- Congenital infection, a consequence of primary infection early in pregnancy, can cause severe abnormalities that in the absence of vesicles are difficult to distinguish from similar syndromes caused by rubella, toxoplasmosis or cytomegalovirus.
- The risk of neonatal infection is approximately 40% with active primary infection, but less than 1% with recurrent infections at the time of birth, and rare with asymptomatic shedding.

Diagnosis

- Viral cultures from open lesions are one of the best methods of diagnosing infection but they have a significant false negative rate. Culture levels are normally available within 48–96 hours.
- Serological tests that demonstrate rising titres of HSV antibodies can be used for the diagnosis of primary infections only by confirming seroconversion.
- The presence of antibody titre in an initial specimen or the presence of a typical lesion is suggestive of non-primary first episode or recurrent disease.
- These tests cannot reliably distinguish between HSV-1 and HSV-2 except by using HSV-type specific glycoprotein G as the antigen.

Treatment

- The treatment and management in pregnancy include:
  - antiviral therapy
  - saline bathing
  - analgesia
  - topical anaesthetic gels.
- Primary infection acquired during the first or second trimester should be treated with oral or intravenous antiviral therapy, depending on the clinical condition.
- Acyclovir reduces viral shedding, reduces pain and promotes the healing of lesions. Currently it is not licensed for use in pregnancy but has been used extensively without any significant reported adverse events or teratogenity.

- The recommended dose is the same as for non-pregnant adults, but higher doses may be required for immunocompromised women.
- Continuous acyclovir in the last 4 weeks of pregnancy reduces the risk of clinical recurrence at term and birth by caesarean section.
- In the third trimester, women with active genital lesions after 34 weeks should have a caesarean section, as the risk of viral shedding and vertical transmission is high.
- Recurrent HSV infection during pregnancy is also treated with acyclovir.
- Caesarean section is not indicated unless genital lesions or prodromal symptoms of an impending outbreak, such as vulval pain or burning, are present.

Cytomegalovirus (CMV)

- Cytomegalovirus, a member of the herpes virus family, is a common infection.
- Most CMV infections are subclinical.
- However, the clinical manifestations of CMV infection vary with age, route of transmission and the immune competence of the subject.
- Primary infection may cause generally mild mononucleosis-type symptoms such as malaise, myalgia and fever in immunocompetent adults, whereas it is particularly pathogenic among immunosuppressed individuals, recipients of organ transplants, premature infants and people with AIDS.

CMV infection in pregnancy

Several studies have shown that primary infection occurs in all trimesters, with approximately 30% of neonates being born with congenital infection. As most of these do not develop the disease, it is not a sufficient criterion to recommend TOP (termination of pregnancy).

Fetal and neonatal infections

- CMV is the most common intrauterine infection, affecting from 0.6% to 0.7% of all live births.
- Unlike rubella, which has a teratogenic effect, CMV allows fetal organs to develop normally but causes disease by the secondary destruction of the cells.
- Perinatal infections result from exposure to CMV in the maternal genital tract at birth or from breast milk.

- 10–15% of infants born to women with primary infection may be symptomatic at birth. These concerns include:
  - a 5–10% chance of mortality in the first 3 months
  - up to 50% chance of microcephaly, seizures (10%), chorioretinitis (10–20%), and developmental delay (≤ 70%)
  - up to 50% chance of sensory neural hearing loss.
- Infants with asymptomatic congenital CMV have a 5% chance of sensory neural hearing loss and a 2% chance of chorioretinitis.
- Infants who develop normally by 12 months have a higher likelihood of a normal development long term.

Diagnosis

CMV infections can be diagnosed by direct methods such as:
- viral cultures (from urine, saliva, breast milk, cervical secretions, biopsy and autopsy specimens)
- polymerase chain reaction (PCR)
- antigen detection.

Treatment

Ganciclovir and foscarnet have been used with encouraging results in life-threatening CMV infections in immunocompromised hosts. Both drugs are, however, extensively toxic.

Human immunodeficiency virus (HIV)

- There are two types of HIV: HIV-1 and HIV-2.
  - HIV-1 is the cause of the worldwide spread of acquired immune deficiency syndrome (AIDS).
  - HIV-2 is largely confined to West Africa.
- The three principal means of HIV transmission are by:
  - blood or blood products
  - sexual contact
  - mother to child transmission (MTCT).
- Two to 6 weeks after exposure to HIV, 50–70% of those infected develop a transient non-specific illness with fever, myalgia, malaise, lymphadenopathy and pharyngitis. Over 50% develop a rash. Oral and genital ulcers have also been reported.
- The illness begins abruptly and usually lasts for 1–2 weeks, but could be more protracted.
- Seroconversion is usually followed by an asymptomatic period lasting on average 10 years without antiretroviral therapy.

- However, although the infection is latent clinically, there is intense viral and lymphocyte turnover with worsening immunodeficiency.
- Approximately one-third of patients will experience persistent generalized lymphadenopathy.
- The average time for progression from HIV to AIDS is between 5 and 20 years.

HIV in pregnancy

- HIV-1 infection is associated with poor pregnancy outcomes.
- The most serious effect of HIV-1 infection during pregnancy is vertical transmission.
- This can occur during pregnancy, in the intrapartum period or postnatally.
- In non-breastfed infants, up to 75% of transmission is thought to occur in late pregnancy and the period covering labour and birth.
- HIV-1 DNA is present in breast milk and so postnatal transmission can occur during breastfeeding. Avoidance of breastfeeding by HIV-1-infected women is therefore recommended if safe and affordable alternatives are available.
- Other factors associated with an increased risk of transmission are listed in Box 15.4.

Box 15.4 Factors associated with an increased risk of transmission in HIV

- Breastfeeding
- Advanced clinical HIV disease
- Impaired maternal immunocompetence
- Maternal nutritional status
- Resistant viral strains
- Vaginal birth
- Prolonged rupture of membranes
- Invasive obstetric procedures
- Maternal ulcerative genital infection
- Recreational drug use during pregnancy
- Prematurity
- Low birth weight

Diagnosis

- Acute infection is accompanied by the development of serum antibodies in the case of core and surface proteins of the virus in 2–6 weeks.
- Over 90% of seroconversions occur within 3 months of infection.
- In a minority of cases seroconversion may be delayed to more than 6 months; therefore, negative diagnostic tests need to be repeated 3 months after possible exposure and after 6–9 months where there has been a high risk of transmission.
- Following seroconversion, antibodies persist indefinitely in the serum and form a highly specific test for HIV infection.
- One or more enzyme immunoassays (EIAs) directed towards HIV-1 and HIV-2 are used as the initial screening tests.
  - Positive screening tests are confirmed by serum titre tests, a Western blot or immunofluorescence assay.
  - Babies born to infected women may have maternal HIV antibodies. A specific test such as PCR can confirm HIV infection in 95% of infected infants by 1 month of age.

Treatment

- The incidence of MTCT can be significantly reduced as a result of measures that include counselling, testing, antiretroviral treatment and infant formula feeding. If women take antiretroviral therapy (ART) medication, and their babies are also appropriately medicated, the risk of transmitting HIV can be 1% or less.
- ART include zidovudine, lamivudine and nevirapine. Regimens involve different combinations over different time periods.
- ART may be given antenatally, intrapartum, postnatally and prophylactically to babies. Highly active ART (HAART) has significantly reduced vertical transmission rates.
- Elective caesarean section should be recommended and breastfeeding avoided in developed countries.
- In the event of labour, measures can be taken to avoid situations known to predispose to vertical transmission of HIV:
  - Amniotomy is contraindicated.
  - If there is spontaneous rupture of membranes, labour should be augmented if contractions are either weak or absent to avoid a prolonged interval between membrane rupture and birth.

- Invasive techniques, such as electronic fetal monitoring via use of fetal scalp electrode and fetal blood sampling, should be avoided.
- Episiotomy should be avoided.
- Instrumental birth should be avoided to minimize abrasions to both woman and baby.

HIV antibody testing and counselling in pregnancy

- An HIV test is offered to all pregnant women.
- Post-test counselling will involve the giving of positive, negative or indeterminate results.
- Issues for discussion include the natural history of the infection, treatment options and safe sex to avoid transmission to an HIV-negative partner(s) and acquisition of other STIs.
- The diagnosis should be confirmed by a second test and an immediate referral should be made for specialist medical assessment.

FURTHER READING

Allstaff, S., Wilson, J., 2012. The management of sexually transmitted infections in pregnancy. The Obstetrician & Gynaecologist 14 (1), 25–32.

Australasian Society for Infectious Diseases, 2014. Management of perinatal infections. Available at: http://www.asid.net.au/documents/item/368.

Useful websites

Useful guidelines on the diagnosis and generic treatment/management of all STIs can be accessed via any of the following websites:

Australian STI management guidelines. Available at: http://www.sti.guidelines.org.au

British Association for Sexual Health and HIV (BASHH). Available at: http://www.bashh.org

Information specific to pregnancy can be accessed via:

Centers for Disease Control, 2016. Sexually transmitted diseases in pregnancy. Available at: http://www.cdc.gov/std/pregnancy/default.htm

Information on the surveillance, epidemiology, screening and management of UTIs can be accessed from the Public Health England website. Available at: http://www.gov.uk

Multiple Pregnancy

The term 'multiple pregnancy' is used to describe the development of more than one fetus in utero at the same time.

TWIN PREGNANCY

Types of twin pregnancy

Twins will be either monozygotic (MZ) or dizygotic (DZ) (Box 16.1). Of all twins born, two-thirds will be DZ and one-third MZ.

Determination of zygosity and chorionicity

Determination of zygosity means determining whether or not the twins are identical.

- In approximately one-third of all twins born, this will be obvious, as the children will be of a different sex.
- At birth, identical twins tend to have a greater weight variation than non-identical ones.
- In approximately two-thirds of identical twins, a monochorionic placenta will confirm monozygosity. If the babies have a single outer membrane, the chorion, they must be MZ.
- In one-third of identical twins, the placenta will have two chorions and two amnions, and either fused placentae or two separate placentae (dichorionic); this situation is indistinguishable from that in non-identical twins. It occurs when the fertilized oocyte splits within the first 3 or 4 days after fertilization and while it is still in the uterine tube.
- When these entities are seen on an early scan they appear as two separate placentae and are dichorionic and diamniotic, exactly the same as non-identical twins.
- In approximately two-thirds of cases the division occurs up to approximately 10–12 days after fertilization; these will be monochorionic and diamniotic.
- Monoamniotic twins occur in approximately 1% of cases, when the embryo divides after 12 days.

Box 16.1 Monozygosity and dizygosity

Monozygotic or uniovular twins

- Also referred to as 'identical twins'
- Develop from the fusion of one oocyte and one spermatozoon, which after fertilization splits into two
- Are of the same sex and have the same genes, blood groups and physical features such as eye and hair colour, ear shapes and palm creases; may be of different sizes and sometimes have different personalities

Dizygotic or binovular twins

- Also referred to as 'non-identical twins'
- Develop from two separate oocytes that are fertilized by two different spermatozoa
- Are no more alike than any brother or sister and can be of the same or different sex

---

- Monochorionic twin pregnancies have a 3–5 times higher risk of perinatal mortality and morbidity than dichorionic twin pregnancies.

Zygosity determination after birth

The most accurate method of determining zygosity is to compare DNA. DNA can be extracted from cells taken from a cheek swab from inside the mouth. Specific genetic markers extracted from different chromosomes are compared and the results are up to 99.99% accurate.

Zygosity determination should be routinely offered to all same-sex twins for the reasons listed in Box 16.2.

Diagnosis of twin pregnancy

- This is usually through ultrasound examination. Diagnosis can be made as early as 6 weeks into the pregnancy, or later at the routine detailed structural scan between the 18th and 20th weeks.
- A family history of twins should alert the midwife to the possibility of a multiple pregnancy.
- Occasionally (1 in 12 000 live births), one fetus may die in the second trimester and become a fetus papyraceous, which becomes

> ### Box 16.2 **Reasons for determining zygosity**
>
> - Most parents will want to know whether or not their twins are identical
> - If parents are considering further pregnancies, they will want to know the likelihood of having twins again: DZ twins tend to run in families and the increased likelihood is approximately fivefold
> - MZ twins do not run in families and the likelihood does not change
> - It will help the twins in establishing their sense of identity; it will influence their life and family relationships
> - The information is important for genetic reasons: not just the monogenic disorders but with any serious illness later in life
> - Twins are frequently asked to be involved in research where knowledge of zygosity is essential

embedded in the surface of the placenta and expelled with the placenta at birth.

Abdominal examination

See Box 16.3.

The pregnancy

A multiple pregnancy tends to be shorter than a single pregnancy. The average gestation for twins is 37 weeks, for triplets 34 weeks, and for quadruplets 33 weeks. There can be an increase in complications of pregnancy.

Effects of pregnancy

Exacerbation of common disorders

More than one fetus and the higher levels of circulating hormones often exacerbate the common disorders of pregnancy. Sickness, nausea, backache and heartburn may be more persistent and more troublesome than in a singleton pregnancy.

Anaemia

- Iron deficiency and folic acid deficiency anaemias are common.
- Early growth and development of the uterus and its contents make greater demands on the maternal iron stores; in later

---

Box 16.3 **Abdominal examination in the diagnosis of multiple pregnancy**

Inspection

- The size of the uterus may be larger than expected for the period of gestation, particularly after the 20th week. The uterus may look broad or round
- Fetal movements may be seen over a wide area, although the findings are not diagnostic of twins
- Fresh striae gravidarum may be apparent
- Up to twice the amount of amniotic fluid is normal in a twin pregnancy but polyhydramnios is not an uncommon complication of a twin pregnancy, particularly with monochorionic twins

Palpation

- The fundal height may be greater than expected for the period of gestation
- The presence of two fetal poles (head or breech) in the fundus of the uterus may be noted; multiple fetal limbs may also be palpable
- The head may be small in relation to the size of the uterus
- Lateral palpation may reveal two fetal backs or limbs on both sides
- Pelvic palpation may give findings similar to those on fundal palpation, although one fetus may lie behind the other and make detection difficult
- Location of three poles in total is diagnostic of at least two fetuses

Auscultation

- Hearing two fetal hearts is not diagnostic; however, if simultaneous comparison of the heart rates reveals a difference of at least 10 beats per minute, it may be assumed that two hearts are being heard

---

pregnancy (after the 28th week) fetal demands may lead to maternal anaemia.

- Routine prescription of iron and folic acid supplements is not necessary.

Polyhydramnios

This is particularly associated with monochorionic twins and with fetal malformations. Polyhydramnios will add to any discomfort that the woman is already experiencing. Acute polyhydramnios can lead to miscarriage or premature labour.

221

Pressure symptoms

Impaired venous return from the lower limbs increases the tendency to varicose veins and leg oedema. Backache is common and the increased uterine size may also lead to marked dyspnoea and indigestion.

Antenatal screening

- Nuchal translucency for Down syndrome is accurate only if performed between 11 and 13 weeks.
- Serum screening is not usually performed in multiple pregnancy, as results are too complex to interpret, and can lead to false positives.
- In addition, there are not enough data to determine whether the non-invasive prenatal tests (NIPT) is accurate in multiple pregnancies.
- Chorionic villus sampling (CVS) is sometimes performed in multiple pregnancy, but loss rates have been recorded as higher than singleton pregnancies with this procedure.
- Amniocentesis, performed in a specialist fetal medicine unit, can be performed in twin pregnancies, usually between 15 and 20 weeks' gestation. Most obstetricians prefer to do a dual needle insertion so there is no chance of contamination between the two sacs.
- Via ultrasound scan, chorionicity should be determined in the first trimester to prepare and support the parents.
- All MZ twins should have echocardiography performed at approximately 20 weeks' gestation, as there is a much higher risk of cardiac anomalies in these babies.

Ultrasound examination

- Monochorionic twin pregnancies should be scanned every 2 weeks from diagnosis to check for discordant fetal growth and signs of twin-to-twin transfusion syndrome (TTTS).
- Dichorionic twin pregnancies should be scanned at 20 weeks for anomalies, and then usually every 4 weeks.

Preparation for breastfeeding

Women should be advised not only that it is possible to breastfeed two, and in some cases three, babies, but also that, nutritionally, this is the best way for her to feed her babies.

LABOUR AND BIRTH

Onset of labour

- The higher the number of fetuses the woman is carrying, the earlier labour is likely to start.
- Term for twins is usually considered to be 37 weeks rather than 40, and approximately 30% of twins are born preterm.
- In addition to being preterm the babies may be small for gestational age and therefore prone to the associated complications of both conditions.
- If spontaneous labour begins very early the woman may be given drugs to inhibit uterine activity. Known causes of preterm labour, for example urinary tract infection, should be treated with antibiotics.
- If the first twin is in a cephalic presentation, labour usually continues normally to a vaginal birth, but if the first twin is presenting in any other way (Fig. 16.1), an elective caesarean section is often recommended.

Management of labour

- Induction of labour usually occurs at approximately 38 weeks' gestation.
- The presence of complications such as pregnancy-induced hypertension, intrauterine growth restriction or TTTS may be reasons for earlier induction.
- The majority will go into labour spontaneously. There is an increased incidence of dysfunctional labour in twin pregnancies, possibly because of overdistension of the uterus.
- Continuous fetal heart monitoring of both babies is advocated. This can be achieved:
  - with two external transducers, *or*
  - once the membranes are ruptured, with a scalp electrode on the presenting twin and an external transducer on the second.
- If a 'twin monitor' is available, both heartbeats can be monitored simultaneously to give a more reliable reading. Uterine activity will also need to be monitored.
- If cardiotocography (CTG) is not available, use of the Doptone or Sonicaid may be more practical in providing accurate recordings of the fetal heart rates than a fetal stethoscope. If the latter has to

Fig. 16.1 Presentation of twins before birth. (After Bryan 1984, with permission of Edward Arnold.)

be used, two people must auscultate simultaneously so that fetal heart rates are counted over the same minute.

- Mobilization is encouraged or the adoption of whichever position the woman finds most comfortable. When using the birthing bed, a foam rubber wedge under the side of the mattress will help to prevent supine hypotensive syndrome by giving a lateral tilt. A birthing chair or a reclining chair may be more comfortable than a birthing bed.

- Pain relief must be based on the woman's informed decision and every effort must be taken not to medicalize care. However, it is widely acknowledged that regional epidural block provides excellent analgesia and, if necessary, allows easier assisted birth and also manipulation of the second twin. The use of inhalation analgesia may be helpful, either before the epidural is in situ or during the second stage if the epidural is not as effective as the woman wishes.
- If fetal compromise occurs during labour, birth will need to be expedited, usually by caesarean section. Action may also need to be taken if the woman's condition gives cause for concern.
- If uterine activity is poor, the use of intravenous oxytocin may be required once the membranes have been ruptured.
- If the babies are expected to be premature and of low birth weight or known to have any other problems, the neonatal unit must be informed.

Management of the births

- Although every effort must be taken to normalize the care the woman receives, the second stage of labour may be confirmed by a vaginal examination. The obstetrician, paediatric team and anaesthetist should be present for the births because of the risk of complications.
- If epidural analgesia has been used, and all remains well with mother and fetuses it may be 'topped up'. This allows for a passive second stage to allow descent of the fetal head of the first twin.
- The possibility of emergency caesarean section is ever-present and the operating theatre should be ready to receive the woman at short notice.
- Monitoring of both fetal hearts should continue.
- Provided that the first twin is presenting by the vertex, the birth can be expected to proceed normally.
- When the first twin is born, the time of birth and the sex are noted. This baby and cord must be labelled as 'twin one' immediately.
- The baby may be put to the breast to aid the stimulation of uterine contractions, unless active neonatal resuscitation is required.
- After the birth of the first twin, abdominal palpation is carried out to ascertain the lie, presentation and position of the second twin and to auscultate the fetal heart:

- If the lie is not longitudinal, an attempt may be made to correct it by external cephalic version.
- If it is longitudinal, a vaginal examination is made to confirm the presentation.
- If the presenting part is not engaged, it should be guided into the pelvis by fundal pressure before the second sac of membranes is ruptured, if spontaneous rupture has not occurred following the first birth.

- The fetal heart should be auscultated again once the membranes are ruptured.
- If uterine activity does not recommence, intravenous oxytocin may be used to stimulate it.
- When the presenting part becomes visible, the woman should be encouraged to push with contractions to give birth to the second twin.
- Owing to the reduced size of the placental site following the birth of the first twin, the second fetus may be somewhat deprived of oxygen.
- The birth of the second twin should be completed within 30 minutes of the first twin (there are higher rates of fetal acidosis and pathological CTG tracings with birth intervals > 30 minutes).
- A uterotonic drug (usually Syntocinon or Syntometrine) is usually given intramuscularly or intravenously, after the birth of the anterior shoulder, depending on local policy.
- This baby and cord are labelled as 'twin two'. A note of the time of birth and the neonate's sex is documented.
- The risk of asphyxia is greater for the second twin. The baby may need to be transferred to the neonatal unit but must be labelled with identification tags and shown to the woman/parents prior to transfer.
- Once the uterotonic drug has taken effect, controlled cord traction is applied to both cords simultaneously and the placentae should be delivered without delay. Emptying the uterus enables bleeding to be controlled and postpartum haemorrhage (PPH) is prevented. An infusion of 40 IU of Syntocinon usually in 500 ml of normal saline (depends on local policy) should be prepared for PPH prophylaxis.
- The placenta(e) and cords should be examined and the number of amniotic sacs, chorions, placentae, and cord vessels noted. Pathological examination of placentae and membranes may be needed to confirm chorionicity.

Complications associated with multiple pregnancy

The high perinatal mortality associated with twinning is largely due to complications of pregnancy, such as the premature onset of labour, intrauterine growth restriction and complications of birth.

Polyhydramnios

Acute polyhydramnios may occur as early as 18–20 weeks. It may be associated with fetal malformation but it is more likely to be due to TTTS.

Twin-to-twin transfusion syndrome (TTTS)

- Also known as *fetofetal transfusion syndrome* (FFTS), this can be acute or chronic. The acute form usually occurs during labour and is the result of a blood transfusion from one fetus (donor) to the other (recipient) through vascular anastomosis in a monochorionic placenta.
- Both fetuses may die of cardiac failure if not treated immediately.
- Chronic TTTS can occur in up to 20% of monochorionic twin pregnancies and with treatment, accounts for approximately 15–17% of perinatal mortality in these twins.
- The placenta in TTTS transfuses blood from one twin fetus to the other. These cases are characterized by one or more deep unidirectional arteriovenous anastomoses.
- This results in anaemia and growth restriction in the donor twin and polycythaemia with circulatory overload in the recipient twin (hydrops).
- The fetal and neonatal mortality is high but some infants may be saved by early diagnosis and prenatal treatment with either amnioreduction, which may have to be repeated regularly as fluid can reaccumulate rapidly, or laser coagulation of communicating placental vessels. Selective fetocide is sometimes considered.

Fetal malformation

This is particularly associated with MZ twins (see Ch. 34 for congenital malformations).

Conjoined twins

This extremely rare malformation of MZ twinning results from the incomplete division of the fertilized oocyte. Birth has to be by caesarean section. Separation of the babies is sometimes possible and will depend on how they are joined and which internal organs are involved.

Acardiac twins (twin reversed arterial perfusion – TRAP)

One twin presents without a well-defined cardiac structure and is kept alive through placental anastomoses to the circulatory system of the viable fetus.

Fetus-in-fetu (endoparasite)

Parts of one fetus may be lodged within another fetus; this can happen only in MZ twins.

Malpresentations

The fetuses can restrict each other's movements, which may result in malpresentations, particularly of the second twin. After the birth of the first twin, the presentation of the second twin may change.

Preterm prelabour rupture of the membranes

Malpresentations due to polyhydramnios may predispose to preterm prelabour rupture of the membranes.

Prolapse of the cord

This is associated with malpresentations and polyhydramnios and is more likely if there is a poorly fitting presenting part. The second twin is particularly at risk.

Prolonged labour

Malpresentations are a poor stimulus to good uterine action and a distended uterus is likely to lead to poor uterine activity and consequently prolonged labour.

Monoamniotic twins

Monoamniotic twins risk cord entanglement with occlusion of the blood supply to one or both fetuses. Birth is usually at approximately 32–34 weeks and by caesarean section.

Locked twins

This is a rare but serious complication. There are two types: one occurs when the first twin presents by the breech and the second by the vertex, the other when both are vertex presentations (Fig. 16.2). In both instances the head of the second twin prevents the continued descent of the first.

Fig. 16.2 Locked twins. (A) Both fetuses are presenting vertex. (B) The first fetus is presenting breech and the second fetus is vertex.

Delay in the birth of the second twin

After birth of the first twin, uterine activity should recommence within 5 minutes. Birth of the second twin is usually completed within 30 minutes of the first birth. With the introduction of fetal heart rate monitoring the interval time between babies is not so crucial as long as the fetal condition is monitored. Poor uterine action as a result of malpresentation may be the cause of delay. The risks of delay are:

- intrauterine hypoxia
- birth asphyxia following premature separation of the placenta

- sepsis as a result of ascending infection from the first umbilical cord, which lies outside the vulva.

After the birth of the first twin the lower uterine segment begins to reform and the cervical canal may have to dilate fully again. The midwife may need to 'rub up' a contraction and to put the first twin to the woman's breast to stimulate uterine activity.

- If there appears to be an obstruction, a caesarean section may be necessary.
- If there is no obstruction, oxytocin infusion may be commenced or instrumental birth considered.

Premature expulsion of the placenta

The placenta may be expelled before the birth of the second twin.

- In dichorionic twins with separate placentae, one placenta may be delivered separately.
- In monochorionic twins, the shared placenta may be expelled. The risks of severe asphyxia and death of the second twin are then very high.
- Haemorrhage is also likely if one twin is retained in utero, as this prevents adequate retraction of the placental site.

Postpartum haemorrhage

Poor uterine tone as a result of overdistension or hypotonic activity is likely to lead to postpartum haemorrhage.

Undiagnosed twins

The possibility of an unexpected undiagnosed second baby should be considered if the uterus appears larger than expected after the birth of the first baby or if the baby is surprisingly smaller than expected. If a uterotonic drug has been routinely given after the birth of the anterior shoulder of the first baby, the second baby is in great danger and birth should be expedited. He or she will require active resuscitation because of severe asphyxia.

POSTNATAL PERIOD

Care of the babies

Immediate care at birth is the same as for a single baby. Identification of the infants should be clear and the parents should be given the opportunity to check the identity bracelets and have skin-to-skin contact with their babies.

Nutrition

Both babies may be breastfed, either simultaneously or separately.

- If the babies are small for gestational age or preterm, the paediatrician may recommend that the babies be 'topped up' after a breastfeed, ideally with expressed breast milk.
- If the babies are not able to suck adequately at the breast, then the woman should be encouraged to express her milk regularly for her babies.
- If she does not have sufficient breast milk, milk from a human milk bank can be used, which is much better for preterm babies than formula milk.
- The more stimulation the breasts are given, the more plentiful is the milk supply.

Care of the woman

- Involution of the uterus will be slower because of its increased bulk. 'Afterpains' may be troublesome and analgesia should be offered.
- A good diet is essential, and if the woman is breastfeeding, she requires a high-protein, high-calorie diet and plenty of fluids. It is quite common for breastfeeding mothers to feel hungry between meals.
- Once the woman is at home she must be encouraged to rest and eat a well-balanced diet. Psychosocial support and routine are the essence of coping with new babies.
- Isolation can be a real problem for new mothers. The incidence of postnatal depression has been shown to be significantly higher in women with twins.

Triplets and higher-order births

- The rapidly increasing number of surviving triplets and higher-order births will produce many more families needing special advice and support from healthcare workers.
- A woman expecting three or more babies is at risk of all the same complications as one expecting twins, but more so. She is more likely to have a period in hospital resting before the babies are born and they will almost certainly be born prematurely.

- Perinatal mortality rates are higher for triplets than twins and the incidence of cerebral palsy is also increased.
- The mode of birth for triplets or more babies is usually by caesarean section. It is essential that the paediatric team be present. The special dangers associated with these births are:
  - asphyxia
  - intracranial injury
  - perinatal death.
- Organizing extra help for these families must occur before the babies are born.

Disability and bereavement

- Perinatal mortality and long-term morbidity are both more common among multiples than singletons. The perinatal mortality rate for twins is approximately four times that of singletons, and that of triplets 12 times higher.
- The grief of parents following the death of one of a multiple set is often underestimated. Addresses of organizations that offer support should be made available to the parents.
- Where one or more of a multiple set has a disability, it is often the healthy child who needs special attention. He or she may feel guilt about doing something that caused the twin's disability and may be resentful of the attention that the other one needs, or of the loss of twinship.

EMBRYO REDUCTION

- This is the reduction of an apparently healthy higher-order multiple pregnancy down to two or even one embryo so the chances of survival are much higher.
- The procedure may be offered to parents who have conceived triplets or more.
- The procedure is usually carried out between the 10th and 12th weeks of the pregnancy.
- Various techniques may be used, involving the insertion of a needle under ultrasound guidance either via the vagina or, more commonly, through the abdominal wall into the fetal thorax.
- Potassium chloride is usually used, although some doctors prefer saline. All embryos remain in the uterus until birth.

SELECTIVE FETOCIDE

- This may be offered to parents with a multiple pregnancy when one of the babies has a serious abnormality.
- The affected fetus is injected as described in embryo reduction, so allowing the healthy fetus to grow and develop normally.
- The full impact of either of these procedures on the parents and their feelings of bereavement will often not be felt until the birth of their remaining baby (or babies) many weeks later.

SOURCES OF HELP

- The hospital social work team are able to coordinate extra services to support families with multiples. Sources of support include:
  - Home Start (UK based)
  - Twins and Multiple Births Association (UK based)
  - Australian Multiple Birth Association (Australia based).

FURTHER READING

Hofmeyr, G., Barrett, J.F., Crowther, C.A., 2015. Planned caesarean section for women with a twin pregnancy. Cochrane Database Syst. Rev. (12), CD006553. doi: 10.1002/14651858.CD006553.pub3.

Sekar, R., 2013. Managing multiples. Obstet. Gynaecol. Mag. 15 (4), 39–40.

Useful websites

Twins and Multiple Births Association. Available at: https://www.tamba.org.uk/

Australian Multiple Birth Association. Available at: http://www.amba.org.au/

Section | 3 |

Labour

The First Stage of Labour

Normal labour is spontaneous in onset between 37 and 42 weeks' gestation with the fetus presenting by the vertex, culminating in a healthy mother and baby.

Phases of the first stage

These are described in Box 17.1.

THE ONSET OF SPONTANEOUS NORMAL LABOUR

The onset of labour appears to be initiated by a combination of hormonal and mechanical factors.

- Levels of maternal oestrogen rise sharply during the last weeks of pregnancy, resulting in changes that overcome the inhibiting effects of progesterone.
- High levels of oestrogens cause uterine muscle fibres to display oxytocic receptors and form gap junctions with each other.
- Oestrogen also stimulates the placenta to release prostaglandins that induce a production of enzymes that will digest collagen in the cervix, helping it to soften.
- It is thought that both fetal and placental factors are involved in the process. Uterine activity may also result from mechanical stimulation of the uterus and cervix, brought about by overstretching or pressure from a presenting part that is well applied to the cervix.

When the woman is in labour, uterine contractions will often be accompanied or preceded by a blood-stained mucoid 'show'; this results from the operculum, which formed the cervical plug during pregnancy, being lost when the cervix dilates.

Occasionally the membranes will rupture; this should always be reported to the midwife, who will check that the fetal heart rate is within normal limits and that meconium is not present in the liquor.

Spurious labour

Many women experience contractions before the onset of labour; these may be painful and may even be regular for a time, causing a

---

Box 17.1 **Phases of the first stage of labour**

The latent phase

- Precedes the active first stage of labour
- May last up to 12 hours in nulliparous women, but this is highly variable
- The cervix dilates and effaces

The active first stage

- Traditionally this was thought to occur when the cervix is 3–4 cm dilated, however, new research has shown that the active phase of labour may not start until 5 cm of cervical dilation in multiparas and even later in nulliparas
- In the presence of rhythmic contractions, is complete when the cervix is fully dilated (10 cm)
- Usually completed within 6–12 hours

The transitional phase

- The cervix expands from approximately 8 cm dilated until it is fully dilated (or until the expulsive contractions during the second stage are felt by the woman)
- There is often a brief lull in the intensity of uterine activity at this time

---

woman to think that labour has started. The two features of true labour that are absent here are:

- effacement of the cervix
- dilatation of the cervix (see later).

PHYSIOLOGICAL PROCESSES

Uterine action

Fundal dominance (Fig. 17.1)

- Each uterine contraction starts in the fundus near one of the cornua and spreads across and downwards.
- The contraction lasts longest in the fundus where it is also most intense, but the peak is reached simultaneously over the whole uterus and the contraction fades from all parts together and is weakest in the lower segment.

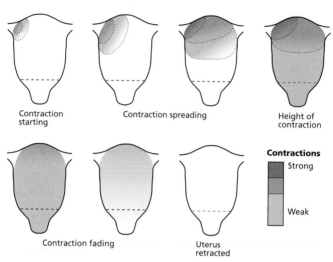

Contraction starting

Contraction spreading

Height of contraction

Contraction fading

Uterus retracted

Contractions

Strong

Weak

Fig. 17.1 Fundal dominance during uterine contractions.

Polarity

- Polarity is the neuromuscular harmony that prevails between the two poles or segments of the uterus throughout labour. During each uterine contraction:
  - the upper pole contracts strongly and retracts to expel the fetus
  - the lower pole contracts slightly and dilates to allow expulsion to take place.
- If polarity is disorganized, then the progress of labour is inhibited.

Contraction and retraction

- Retraction is when the uterine muscle fibres retain some of the shortening of the contraction instead of becoming completely relaxed (Fig. 17.2).
- It assists in the progressive expulsion of the fetus; the upper segment of the uterus becomes gradually shorter and thicker and its cavity diminishes.
- Before labour becomes established, uterine contractions may occur every 15–20 minutes and may last for approximately 30 seconds; they may be imperceptible to the mother.

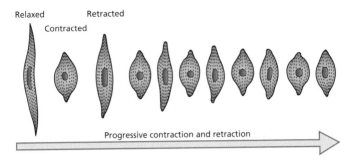

Fig. 17.2 How uterine muscle retains some shortening after each contraction.

- By the end of the first stage they occur at 2- to 3-minute intervals, last for 50–60 seconds and are very powerful.

Formation of upper and lower uterine segments

- By the end of pregnancy, the body of the uterus is described as having divided into two anatomically distinct segments:
  - The upper uterine segment is formed from the body of the uterus.
  - The lower uterine segment is formed from the isthmus and the cervix, and is approximately 8–10 cm in length.
- The muscle content reduces from the fundus to the cervix, where it is thinner.
- When labour begins, the retracted longitudinal fibres in the upper uterine segment pull on the lower uterine segment, causing it to stretch; this is aided by the force applied by the descending presenting part.
- A ridge forms between the upper and lower uterine segments; this is known as the *physiological retraction ring*.

Cervical effacement

'Effacement' refers to the inclusion of the cervical canal into the lower uterine segment (Fig. 17.3). Effacement may occur late in pregnancy, or it may not take place until labour begins.

- In the nulliparous woman, the cervix will not usually dilate until effacement is complete.

Fig. 17.3 (A) The cervix before effacement. (B) The cervix after effacement. The cervical canal is now part of the lower uterine segment.

- In the parous woman, effacement and dilatation may occur simultaneously and a small canal may be felt in early labour. This is often referred to as a 'multips os'.

Cervical dilatation

Dilatation of the cervix is the process of enlargement of the os uteri from a tightly closed aperture to an opening large enough to permit passage of the fetal head.
- Dilatation is measured in centimetres and full dilatation at term equates to approximately 10 cm.
- Dilatation occurs as a result of uterine action and the counterpressure applied by either the intact bag of membranes or the presenting part, or both.
- A well-flexed fetal head closely applied to the cervix favours efficient dilatation.
- Pressure applied evenly to the cervix causes the uterine fundus to respond by contraction and retraction.

Mechanical factors
Formation of the forewaters
- As the lower uterine segment forms and stretches, the chorion becomes detached from it; the increased intrauterine pressure causes this loosened part of the sac of fluid to bulge downwards into the internal os.
- The well-flexed head fits snugly into the cervix and cuts off the fluid in front of the head, the 'forewaters', from that which surrounds the body, the 'hindwaters'.

240

General fluid pressure

- While the membranes remain intact, the pressure of the uterine contractions is exerted on the fluid and, as fluid is not compressible, the pressure is equalized throughout the uterus and over the fetal body; it is known as 'general fluid pressure'.
- Preserving the integrity of the membranes optimizes the oxygen supply to the fetus and helps to prevent intrauterine and fetal infection.

Rupture of the membranes

- The optimum physiological time for the membranes to rupture spontaneously is at the end of the first stage of labour after the cervix becomes fully dilated and no longer supports the bag of forewaters.
- The uterine contractions are also applying increasing force at this time.
- Membranes may sometimes rupture days before labour begins or during the first stage.
- If there are no other signs of labour but the history of ruptured membranes is convincing or obvious liquor is draining, then digital examination should be avoided owing to an increased risk of ascending infection.
- If the diagnosis is not obvious, then one sterile speculum examination should be performed to try to visualize pooling of liquor in the posterior fornix; endocervical swabs may also be taken at this time.
- Most women will labour spontaneously within 24 hours. After 24 hours, an obstetrician may consider augmentation of labour.
- Women with prelabour ruptured membranes should have their temperature recorded and be monitored for signs of fetal compromise associated with infection.
- Occasionally, the membranes do not rupture, even in the second stage, and appear at the vulva as a bulging sac covering the fetal head as it is born; this is known as the 'caul'.

Fetal axis pressure

- During each contraction, the uterus rises forward and the force of the fundal contraction is transmitted to the upper pole of the fetus and down the long axis of the fetus, and applied by the presenting part to the cervix.

- This is known as 'fetal axis pressure' and becomes much more significant after rupture of the membranes and during the second stage of labour.

OBSERVATIONS AND CARE IN LABOUR

Maternal wellbeing

Women must be enabled to be in control throughout labour, with the midwife providing evidence-based information, listening to the woman and ensuring consent is given before any intervention.

Past history and reaction to labour

Factors of particular relevance at the onset of labour are listed in Box 17.2.

Pulse rate

This is recorded every 1–2 hours during early labour and every 30 minutes when labour is more advanced. It is also necessary to record the maternal pulse rate regularly if she has external fetal monitoring in situ. If the rate increases to more than 100 beats per minute, it may be indicative of:

- anxiety
- pain
- infection
- ketosis
- haemorrhage.

Box 17.2 Important factors in the history at the onset of labour

- The birth plan – whatever choices the woman makes, she must be the focus of the care, and should be able to feel she is in control of what is happening to her and able to make decisions about her care
- Parity and age
- Character and outcomes of previous labours
- Weights and condition of previous babies
- Attendance at any specialist clinics
- Any known problems – social or physical
- Blood results, including Rhesus isoimmunization and haemoglobin (Hb)

Temperature

This is recorded at least every 4 hours in normal labour. Pyrexia is indicative of infection or ketosis, or may be associated with epidural analgesia. Be aware that a high maternal temperature can increase the fetal heart rate.

Blood pressure

This is measured every 2–4 hours, unless it is abnormal. The blood pressure must be monitored very closely following epidural or spinal anaesthetic. Hypotension may be caused by:
- the supine position
- shock
- epidural anaesthesia.

Urinalysis and bladder care

The woman should be encouraged to empty her bladder every 1–2 hours during labour. The urine passed should be tested for glucose, ketones and protein.
- A low level of ketones is very common during labour and is not thought to be significant.
- A trace of protein may be a contaminant following rupture of the membranes or a sign of a urinary infection, but more significant proteinuria, accompanied by hypertension, may indicate pre-eclampsia.

A full bladder may prevent the fetal head from entering the pelvic brim and can increase the risk of postpartum haemorrhage. If the bladder is incompletely emptied or the woman is unable to void for some hours, it may become necessary to pass a catheter.

Fluid balance

A record should be kept of all urine passed and fluids administered.

Abdominal examination

- This is undertaken at the initial assessment and then repeated at intervals throughout labour, in particular before a vaginal examination, to assess the length, strength and frequency of contractions and the descent of the presenting part.
- Contractions that are unduly long or very strong and coming in quick succession should give cause for concern (i.e. more than 5 in 10 minutes or exceeding 2 minutes in duration).

243

- Hypervigilance is necessary to prevent hyperstimulation if augmentation of labour with oxytocin is implemented.
- Descent of the presenting part is usually described in terms of fifths of the head palpable, i.e. the amount palpated above the pelvic brim.

Vaginal examination (VE) and progress in labour

- Although it is not essential to examine the woman vaginally at frequent intervals, it may be useful to do so when progress is in doubt or another indication arises. The features that are indicative of progress on VE are:
  - effacement and dilatation of the cervix
  - descent, flexion and rotation of the fetal head.
- Progressive dilatation is monitored as labour continues and charted on the partogram.
- The level or station of the presenting part is estimated in relation to the ischial spines; during normal labour the head descends progressively (Fig. 17.4).

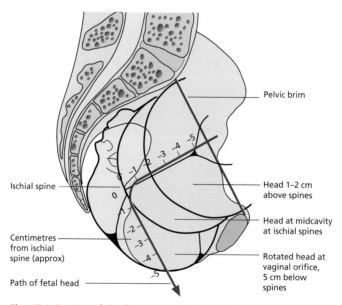

Pelvic brim

Ischial spine

Head 1–2 cm above spines

Head at midcavity at ischial spines

Centimetres from ischial spine (approx)

Rotated head at vaginal orifice, 5 cm below spines

Path of fetal head

Fig. 17.4 Stations of the fetal head in relation to the pelvic canal.

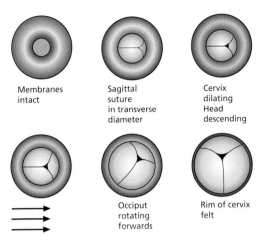

Fig. 17.5 Dilatation of the cervix and rotation of the fetal head, as felt on vaginal examination.

- Moulding or a large caput will give a false impression of the level of the fetal head.
- In vertex presentations, progress depends partly on increased flexion. Flexion is assessed by the position of the sutures and fontanelles:
  - If the head is fully flexed, the posterior fontanelle becomes almost central (Fig. 17.5).
  - If the head is deflexed, both anterior and posterior fontanelles may be palpable.
- Rotation is assessed by noting changes in the position of the presenting part between one examination and the next.
- The sutures and fontanelles are palpated to determine position.

Under no circumstances should a midwife make a vaginal examination if there is any frank bleeding.

Nutrition

- In normal labour women may take a low-fat, low-residue diet according to appetite.
- The vigorous muscle contractions of the uterus during labour demand a continuous supply of glucose. If this is not obtained from the diet, the body will start to metabolize protein and fat

245

stores in an effort to provide glucose (gluconeogenesis). This relatively inefficient method of producing glucose results in the occurrence of ketoacidosis.

Prevention of infection

- Invasive procedures should be kept to a minimum.
- Personal hygiene is important for both the woman and her attendants.
- The fetal membranes should be preserved intact unless there is a positive indication for their rupture that would outweigh the advantage of their protective functions.
- Women whose labour is prolonged are at particular risk of infection and are often subjected to a number of invasive procedures.
- Some women will need specialized care, especially women with any transmissible infection such as gastroenteritis, hepatitis or HIV infection.

Bowel preparation

If there has been no bowel action for 24 hours or the rectum feels loaded on vaginal examination, the woman should be offered an enema or suppositories. This is never done as a routine procedure.

Position and mobility

Mobility in labour should be encouraged, as it lessens the need for pharmacological analgesia, and aids optimal fetal position, and descent of the presenting part, as well as overall progress. Furthermore, the woman is more likely to feel less confined, more in in control and an active participant in her care.

Pain management

The biological, psychological, social, spiritual, cultural and educational dimensions of each woman have an impact on how she expresses herself and how she perceives pain during labour.

Midwives should work with women to encourage them to maintain control and be as mobile as possible throughout labour.

Non-pharmacological methods of pain control

These are listed in Box 17.3.

> Box 17.3 **Non-pharmacological methods of pain control**
>
> - Breathing and relaxation techniques
> - Massage
> - Hydrotherapy
> - Aromatherapy
> - Transcutaneous electrical nerve stimulation (TENS)
> - Reflexology
> - Homoeopathy
> - Music therapy
> - Acupuncture
> - Herbal medicine

Pharmacological methods of pain control

Opiate drugs

Three systemic opioids are commonly used for pain relief in labour:

Pethidine: usually administered intramuscularly in doses of 50–150 mg; takes approximately 20 minutes to have an effect.

Diamorphine (or morphine in some countries): usual dosage 5–10 mg given via intramuscular injection.

Meptazinol: usually given in doses of 100–150 mg intramuscularly.

Remifentanil: used in a patient controlled intravenous analgesia (PCIA) apparatus (for those women who have poorly controlled pain/ contraindications to epidural analgesia). However, there must be safeguards against respiratory depression in place (i.e. regular assessment and documentation of respiratory rate and oxygen saturation levels). The continuous presence of a midwife when remifentanyl is in use is also imperative.

Inhalation analgesia

The most commonly used inhalation analgesia in labour is a premixed gas made up of 50% nitrous oxide and 50% oxygen administered through a piped system or via the Entonox apparatus. It takes effect within 20 seconds, maximum efficacy occurring after approximately 45–50 seconds.

Regional (epidural) analgesia

- A local anaesthetic is administered via a catheter into the epidural space of the lumbar region, usually between vertebrae L1 and L2, or between L2 and L3, or between L3 and L4.

- Bolus injections of bupivacaine (Marcain) or continuous infusion of dilute bupivacaine and opioids (usually fentanyl) may be used.
- An intravenous infusion of crystalloid fluids is commenced prior to siting the epidural.
- After the administration of the first dose of bupivacaine and any subsequent top-up doses of local anaesthetic, the blood pressure and pulse should be measured and recorded every 5 minutes for 20–30 minutes, and then every 30 minutes. The fetal heart is usually monitored electronically.
- The mother may sit up in bed once it has been established that her blood pressure is stable, but should be tilted to one side to prevent aortocaval compression.
- The spread of the block (by assessing dermatomes) is checked regularly by the midwife (see Fig. 17.6).

Fig. 17.6 Dermatomes of the body.

Table 17.1 Contraindications to regional analgesia, with associated risks

Contraindication	Risk
Uncorrected anticoagulation or coagulopathy	Vertebral canal haematoma
Local or systemic sepsis (pyrexia above 38°C not treated with antibiotics)	Vertebral canal abscess
Hypovolaemia or active haemorrhage	Cardiovascular collapse secondary to sympathetic blockade
Patient refusal	Legal action
Lack of sufficient trained midwives for continuous care and monitoring of mother and fetus for the duration of the epidural blockade	Maternal collapse, convulsion, respiratory arrest; fetal compromise

Table 17.2 Advantages and disadvantages of epidural analgesia

Disadvantages	Advantages
Ineffective blocks	Effective pain relief
More frequent monitoring of vital signs	Tendency to lower blood pressure can be advantageous in cases of pregnancy-induced hypertension
Lengthens first stage of labour	
Mother less able to adopt different birth positions	If labour is prolonged, gives effective pain relief, allowing mother to rest
Less sensation of expulsive efforts and lengthens second stage of labour	Does not depress respiratory centre of fetus
Increase in instrumental vaginal delivery	

Table 17.1 shows contraindications to regional analgesia and Table 17.2 lists the advantages and disadvantages of epidural analgesia.

Fetal wellbeing

Fetal condition during labour can be assessed by obtaining information about:

- the fetal heart rate and patterns
- the pH of the fetal blood (if electronic fetal monitoring [EFM] is in use)
- the amniotic fluid.

The fetal heart

- Women with an uncomplicated pregnancy should have intermittent auscultation with a Pinard stethoscope or hand-held Doppler device.
- There is no evidence to support an admission cardiotocography (CTG); it should therefore not be routinely performed.
- For women with problems in their pregnancy or other risk factors, including the use of oxytocin or epidural analgesia, or EFM is appropriate.
- The use of a CTG will limit women's choice of position in labour.

Intermittent fetal monitoring

Women with no medical or obstetric risk factors should be offered intermittent fetal monitoring. The fetal heart rate should be counted over a complete minute.

- The baseline rate should be between 110 and 160 beats per minute (bpm).
- Variability should be between 5 bpm and 25 bpm.

If slowing of the fetal heart is heard in the first stage of labour with a Pinard or Doppler instrument, then EFM may be indicated.

It is important to monitor maternal pulse as well especially when a Doppler device is in use.

Continuous EFM

This combines a fetal cardiograph and a maternal tocograph in a CTG apparatus. It presents a graphic record of the response of the fetal heart to uterine activity, as well as information about its rate and variability. It is used as a tool to indicate fetal welfare, but is not diagnostic.

Findings

The CTG provides information on:

- baseline fetal heart rate
- baseline variability
- accelerations from baseline rate
- decelerations from baseline rate
- uterine activity.

It is important for midwives to remember that EFM is only an adjunct to care it cannot replace skills of clinical judgement and decision making To ensure accuracy, the CTG machines should be regularly checked to ensure they are in good working order.

Response of the fetal heart to uterine contractions

- The fetal heart rate will normally remain stable or accelerate during uterine contractions during the first stage of labour.
- Compression of the umbilical cord or fetal head will result in some decelerations, particularly if the membranes are not intact. These would be early or type 1 variable decelerations lasting less than 3 minutes, with good recovery to the baseline.
- A late or type 11 variable deceleration lasting longer than 3 minutes begins during or after a contraction, reaches its nadir (lowest point) after the peak of the contraction and has not recovered when the contraction has ended. The *time lag* between the peak of the contraction and the nadir of the deceleration is more significant in terms of severity than the drop in the fetal heart rate.

Interpretation of CTG

DR C BRAVADO is a useful mnemonic for evaluating a CTG (see Box 17.4). Two midwives or a midwife and doctor should work collaboratively to monitor and review CTG traces. Best practice is to review and sign the CTG trace hourly. This can help to identify early deviations from normal, which ultimately prevent adverse outcomes and litigation. In the UK, this is ubiquitously referred to as a buddying system or

---

Box 17.4 **The DR C BRAVADO mnemonic**

- **DR** – Determine Risk
- **C** – Contractions
- **BR** – Baseline Rate
- **A** – Accelerations
- **V** – Variability
- **A** – Accelerations
- **D** – Decelerations
- **O** – Overall evaluation

'fresh eyes approach'. The key areas that can result in misinterpretation of CTGs are identified as:

- familiarity
- fatigue
- limited knowledge.

See Fig. 17.7 for information on how to interpret fetal heart rate features and classify CTG tracings.

All areas that use EFM should have ready 24-hour access to fetal blood sampling (FBS) facilities. All CTG traces should be secured in the notes.

Fetal blood sampling

When the fetal heart rate pattern is suspicious or pathological and fetal acidosis is suspected, then FBS should be carried out unless the birth is imminent.

- An FBS result of 7.25 or below should be repeated usually within 30 minutes to an hour.
- An FBS below 7.20 indicates that birth should be expedited.

Amniotic fluid

- If the fetus becomes hypoxic, meconium may be passed, causing the amniotic fluid to be stained green.
- Amniotic fluid that is a muddy yellow colour or is only slightly green may signify a previous event from which the fetus has recovered; it is also common and of no significance in postdates babies.
- If the breech is presenting, the fetus may pass meconium because of the compression of the abdomen or as a result of hypoxia.
- Bleeding of sudden onset at the time of rupture of the membranes may be the result of ruptured vasa praevia and is an acute emergency.

Fetal compromise

Signs of fetal compromise resulting from oxygen deprivation are:

- fetal tachycardia
- a pathological CTG and corresponding poor FBS result
- fetal bradycardia or a severe change in fetal heart rate or decelerations related to uterine contractions, or both
- passage of meconium-stained amniotic fluid.

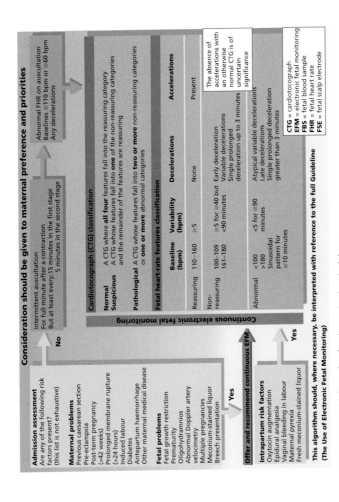

Consideration should be given to maternal preference and priorities

Admission assessment
Are any of the following risk factors present?
(this list is not exhaustive)

Maternal problems
Previous caesarean section
Pre-eclampsia
Post-term pregnancy
(>42 weeks)
Induced labour
Prolonged membrane rupture
(>24 hours)
Diabetes
Antepartum haemorrhage
Other maternal medical disease

Fetal problems
Fetal growth restriction
Prematurity
Oligohydramnios
Abnormal Doppler artery
velocimetry
Multiple pregnancies
Meconium-stained liquor
Breech presentation

↑ Yes

Offer and recommend continuous EFM

Intrapartum risk factors
Oxytocin augmentation
Epidural analgesia
Vaginal bleeding in labour
Maternal pyrexia
Fresh meconium-stained liquor

↑ Yes

No →

Intermittent auscultation
For full minute after a contraction
But at least every: 15 minutes in the first stage
5 minutes in the second stage

↑

Abnormal FHR on auscultation
Baselines ≤110 bpm or ≥60 bpm
Any decelerations

Continuous electronic fetal monitoring

Cardiotocograph (CTG) classification

Normal	A CTG where **all four** features fall into the reassuring category
Suspicious	A CTG whose features fall into **one** of the non-reassuring categories and the remainder of the features are reassuring
Pathological	A CTG whose features fall into **two or more** non-reassuring categories or **one or more** abnormal categories

Fetal heart-rate features classification

	Baseline (bpm)	Variability (bpm)	Decelerations	Accelerations
Reassuring	110–160	≥5	None	Present
Non-reassuring	100–109 161–180	<5 for ≥40 but <90 minutes	Early deceleration Variable decelerations Single prolonged deceleration up to 3 minutes	
Abnormal	<100 >180 Sinusoidal pattern for ≥10 minutes	<5 for ≥90 minutes	Atypical variable decelerations Late decelerations Single prolonged deceleration greater than 3 minutes	

The absence of accelerations with an otherwise normal CTG is of uncertain significance

CTG = cardiotocograph
EFM = electronic fetal monitoring
FBS = fetal blood sample
FHR = fetal heart rate
FSE = fetal scalp electrode

This algorithm should, where necessary, be interpreted with reference to the full Guideline
(The Use of Electronic Fetal Monitoring)

Fig. 17.7 Guidelines for fetal monitoring in labour.

Midwife's management of fetal compromise

- Identify any causes of the abnormality and initiate appropriate action (e.g. turn woman onto her left side, correct maternal hypotension, rehydrate with intravenous fluid, reduce or cease oxytocin and inform obstetrician who will initiate tocolysis if there is uterine hyperstimulation)
- Summon medical assistance. Oxygen therapy is not used to manage fetal compromise per se and is only administered if the maternal condition warrants it.
- Assist with arrangements to expedite the birth.

Preterm labour

- Preterm labour is defined as labour commencing before the 37th completed week of pregnancy.
- A woman who is at risk of giving birth preterm should be transferred to a unit with intensive neonatal facilities, preferably with the fetus in utero.
- If there are no contraindications tocolytic drugs may be used in very early labour to try to delay the birth.
- Antenatal administration of steroids has been shown to reduce the incidence of hyaline membrane disease, intraventricular haemorrhage and necrotizing enterocolitis in fetuses of 26–34 weeks' gestation. Two doses given over 24 hours last for at least 7 days.

Records

- The record of labour is a legal document and must be kept meticulously. It provides current, comprehensive and concise information regarding:
  - the woman's physical, psychological and sociological state
  - any problems that arose
  - the midwife's response to that problem, including any interventions.
- An accurate record during labour provides the basis on which clinical improvements, progress or deterioration of the mother or fetus can be judged. For this reason, the notes should be kept in chronological order.
- Key points for practice are summarized in Box 17.5.

Box 17.5 **Key points for practice**

- Women should be well informed and offered choice founded on evidence-based information where possible
- A competent woman can give or withhold consent for any procedure
- Another adult cannot consent or withhold consent on behalf of a competent woman
- Good communication between women and midwives and between professionals is a fundamental component of maternity services
- The latent phase of labour should be more widely acknowledged in hospital settings
- The use of strict time limits for first and second stages of labour should be reviewed in problem-free pregnancies
- Good record keeping and care plans are an essential aspect of care

FURTHER READING

Lutomski, J.E., Meaney, S., Greene, R.A., et al., 2015. Expert systems for fetal assessment in labour. Cochrane Database Syst. Rev. (4), CD010708. doi: 10.1002/14651858.pub2.

Zhang, J., Landy, H.J., Branch, D.W., et al., 2010. Contemporary patterns of spontaneous labor with normal neonatal outcomes. Consortium on Safe Labor. Obstet. Gynecol. 116, 1281–1287.

Useful websites

Advanced Life Support in Obstetrics. Available at: http://www.also-uk.com and http://www.also.net.au

NICE. Intrapartum care for healthy women and babies. Available at: https://www.nice.org.uk/guidance/cg190/chapter/1-recommendations#first-stage-of-labour

The Second Stage of Labour

THE NATURE OF TRANSITION AND SECOND-STAGE PHASES OF LABOUR

- The second stage of labour is the phase between full dilatation of the cervical os and the birth of the baby.
- However, most midwives and labouring women are aware of a transitional period between the dilatation, or first stage of labour, and the time when active maternal pushing efforts begin.
- This period is typically characterized by maternal restlessness, discomfort, desire for pain relief, a sense that the process is never-ending and demands to attendants to get the birth over with as quickly as possible.
- Some women may experience the urge to push before the cervix is fully dilated, and others may have a lull in activity before the full expulsive nature of the second-stage contractions becomes evident. This latter phenomenon is termed the *resting phase* of the second stage of labour.
- The onset of the second stage of labour is traditionally confirmed with a vaginal examination, however it may not be necessary unless there are signs that the labour is not progressing as anticipated.

Uterine action

- Contractions become stronger and longer but may be less frequent.
- The membranes often rupture spontaneously towards the end of the first stage or during transition to the second stage.
- The contractions become expulsive as the fetus descends further into the vagina.
- Pressure from the presenting part stimulates nerve receptors in the pelvic floor (this is termed the 'Ferguson reflex') and the woman experiences the need to push.
- This reflex may initially be controlled to a limited extent but becomes increasingly compulsive, overwhelming and involuntary during each contraction. The woman's response is to employ her secondary

powers of expulsion by contracting her abdominal muscles and diaphragm.

Soft tissue displacement

- With descent of the head, the soft tissues of the pelvis become displaced.
  - Anteriorly, the bladder is pushed upwards; this results in the stretching and thinning of the urethra so that its lumen is reduced.
  - Posteriorly, the rectum becomes flattened into the sacral curve and the pressure of the advancing head expels any residual faecal matter.
  - The levator ani muscles dilate, thin out and are displaced laterally, and the perineal body is flattened, stretched and thinned.
- The fetal head becomes visible at the vulva, advancing with each contraction and receding between contractions until crowning takes place.
- The head is then born. The shoulders and body follow with the next contraction, accompanied by a gush of amniotic fluid and sometimes of blood.
- The second stage culminates in the birth of the baby.

Duration of the second stage

The time taken to complete the second stage will vary considerably. Although many maternity units do currently impose routine limits on the duration of the second stage, beyond which medical help should be called, these are not based on good evidence.

MATERNAL RESPONSE TO TRANSITION AND THE SECOND STAGE

Pushing

- The urge to push may come before the vertex is visible.
- Traditionally, in order to conserve maternal effort and allow the vaginal tissues to stretch passively, the woman is encouraged to avoid active pushing at this stage.
- It is now accepted that managed active pushing accompanied by breath holding (the *Valsalva manœuvre*) has adverse consequences.

257

- Whenever active pushing commences, the woman should be encouraged to follow her own inclinations in relation to expulsive effort. Few women need instruction on how to push unless they are using epidural analgesia. Some women vocalize loudly as they push.

Position

- If the woman lies flat on her back, then vena caval compression is increased, resulting in hypotension. This can lead to reduced placental perfusion, diminished fetal oxygenation and the efficiency of uterine contractions may be reduced.
- The woman's instinctive preference is the primary consideration:
  - *Semirecumbent or supported sitting position, with the thighs abducted.*
  - *Squatting, kneeling, all fours or standing.* Radiological evidence demonstrates an average increase of 1 cm in the transverse diameter and 2 cm in the anteroposterior diameter of the pelvic outlet when the squatting position is adopted.
  - *Left lateral position.* An assistant may be required to support the right thigh, which may not be ergonomic. It is an alternative position for women who find it difficult to abduct their hips.

THE MECHANISM OF NORMAL LABOUR

- As the fetus descends, soft tissue and bony structures exert pressures that lead to descent through the birth canal by a series of movements, called *mechanism of labour*.
- During vaginal birth, the fetal presentation, position and size will govern the exact mechanism, as the fetus responds to external pressures. Principles common to all mechanisms are:
  - Descent takes place.
  - Whichever part leads and first meets the resistance of the pelvic floor will rotate forwards until it comes under the symphysis pubis.
  - Whichever part emerges from the pelvis will pivot around the pubic bone.
- During the mechanism of normal labour the fetus turns slightly to take advantage of the widest available space in each plane of the pelvis.
- The widest diameter of the pelvic brim is the transverse; at the pelvic outlet, the greatest space lies in the anteroposterior diameter.

- At the onset of labour, the most common presentation is the vertex and the most common position either left or right occipitoanterior.
- When these conditions are met, the way that the fetus is normally situated can be described as follows:
  - the lie is longitudinal
  - the presentation is cephalic
  - the position is right or left occipitoanterior
  - the attitude is one of good flexion
  - the denominator is the occiput
  - the presenting part is the posterior part of the anterior parietal bone.

Main movements

Descent

Throughout the first stage of labour the contraction and retraction of the uterine muscles allow less room in the uterus, exerting pressure on the fetus to descend. Following rupture of the forewaters and the exertion of maternal effort, progress speeds up.

Flexion

Pressure exerted down the fetal axis will increase flexion, resulting in smaller presenting diameters that will negotiate the pelvis more easily.
- At the onset of labour the suboccipitofrontal diameter (10 cm) is presenting.
- With flexion, the suboccipitobregmatic diameter (9.5 cm) presents.
- The occiput becomes the leading part.

Internal rotation of the head

During a uterine contraction, the leading part is pushed downwards onto the pelvic floor. The resistance of this muscular diaphragm brings about internal rotation of the fetal head.
- In a well-flexed vertex presentation, the occiput leads and meets the pelvic floor first and rotates anteriorly through one-eighth of a circle.
- This causes a slight twist in the neck of the fetus, as the head is no longer in direct alignment with the shoulders.
- The anteroposterior diameter of the fetal head now lies in the widest (anteroposterior) diameter of the pelvic outlet.

- The occiput slips beneath the subpubic arch and crowning occurs when the fetal head no longer recedes between uterine contractions and the widest transverse diameter (biparietal) is born.
- While flexion is maintained, the suboccipitobregmatic diameter (9.5 cm) distends the vaginal orifice.

Extension of the head

Once crowning has occurred, the fetal head can extend, pivoting on the suboccipital region around the pubic bone. The sinciput, face and chin sweep the perineum and are born.

Restitution

The twist in the neck of the fetus that resulted from internal rotation is corrected by a slight untwisting movement. The occiput moves one-eighth of a circle towards the side from which it started (Fig. 18.1A and B).

Internal rotation of the shoulders

The anterior shoulder is the first to reach the levator ani muscle and it therefore rotates anteriorly to lie under the symphysis pubis. This movement can be clearly seen as the head turns at the same time (external rotation of the head) (Fig. 18.1C).

Lateral flexion

The anterior shoulder is usually born first, although it has been noted by midwives who commonly use upright or kneeling positions that the posterior shoulder is commonly seen first. In the former case the anterior shoulder slips beneath the subpubic arch and the posterior shoulder passes over the perineum. The remainder of the body is born by lateral flexion as the spine bends sideways through the curved birth canal.

OBSERVATIONS AND CARE DURING THE SECOND STAGE OF LABOUR

Principles of care

See Box 18.1.

- Surgical gloves should be worn during the birth for the protection of both the woman and midwife from infection. In some

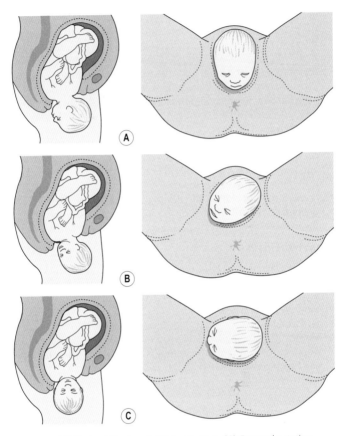

Fig. 18.1 (A) Birth of the head. (B) Restitution. (C) External rotation.

Box 18.1 **Principles of care during the second stage of labour**

- Observation of progress
- Prevention of infection
- Emotional and physical comfort of the woman
- Anticipation of normal events
- Recognition of abnormal developments

261

units, goggles or plain glasses are also advised to minimize the risk of transmission of infection through blood splashes to the eyes.

- If the woman has not requested physiological management of the third stage of labour, and there are no risk factors for a post-partum haemorrhage, a uterotonic agent is prepared, commonly oxytocin 5 or 10 units. Syntometrine 1 ml is used if there is a high risk of haemorrhage post-birth but there is no history of hypertension.
- Whether birth is taking place at home or in the hospital setting, neonatal resuscitation equipment should be thoroughly checked and readily accessible and blood bottles prepared if, for example, the woman is rhesus negative.
- A warm cot and clothes should be prepared for the baby.
- Encourage and involve the birth support partner/s in the care of the woman, as appropriate.

Observations

At least five factors determine whether the second stage is continuing optimally, and these must be carefully observed:
- uterine contractions
- descent, rotation and flexion
- fetal condition
- suspicious/pathological changes in the fetal heart (these terms are only applicable if cardiotocography [CTG] is in use where the trace can be objectively viewed and quantified)
- maternal condition.

Uterine contractions

The strength, length and frequency of contractions should be assessed continuously by observation of maternal responses, and regularly by uterine palpation.

Descent, rotation and flexion

If there is a delay in progress despite regular strong uterine contractions and active maternal pushing, a vaginal examination may be performed:
- to confirm whether internal rotation of the head has taken place
- to assess the position, attitude and station of the presenting part

- to assess degree of any moulding and determine whether a caput succedaneum has formed.

In the absence of good rotation and flexion, or a weakening of uterine contractions, or both, then a change of position, nutrition and hydration or use of optimal fetal positioning techniques may be considered. If there is evidence that either the fetal or maternal condition is compromised, an experienced obstetrician must be consulted. A full bladder impedes progress.

Fetal condition

- If the membranes are ruptured, the liquor amnii is observed to ensure that it is clear.
  - Thick, fresh meconium is always ominous.
  - Thin, old meconium staining is not always regarded as a sign of fetal compromise.
- As the fetus descends, fetal oxygenation may be less efficient owing either to cord or head compression or to reduced perfusion at the placental site. A well-grown healthy fetus will not be compromised by this transitory hypoxia.
- This will tend to be manifest in early decelerations of the fetal heart, with a swift return to the normal baseline after a contraction.
- During the second stage the fetal heart is usually auscultated immediately after a contraction, with some readings being taken through a contraction if the woman can tolerate this.

Suspicious/pathological changes in the fetal heart when CTG in use

- Signs for concern include:
  - late or prolonged decelerations
  - type 2 variable decelerations with biphasic feature, reduced variability and no acceleration preceding and following a contraction (i.e. no reassuring features)
  - lack of return to the normal baseline
  - a rising/tachycardic baseline
  - a lack of variability (< 5 beats per minute).
- If decelerations are heard for the first time in second stage, they may be due to cord or head compression, which may be helped by a change in maternal position.
- If they persist following such a change, then medical advice must be sought.

263

- If the labour is taking place in a unit that is distant from an obstetric unit, an episiotomy may be considered but only if the birth is imminent and the woman consents.
- Midwives who are trained and experienced in ventouse birth may consider expediting the birth at this point. Otherwise, transfer to an obstetric unit should be arranged.

Maternal condition

Monitoring includes an appraisal of the woman's ability to cope emotionally, as well as an assessment of her physical wellbeing. Maternal pulse rate is usually recorded every half hour and blood pressure every hour, provided that these remain within normal limits. The woman should be encouraged to pass urine at the beginning of the second stage, unless she has recently done so.

Birth of the head

- With each contraction, the head descends. As it does so, the superficial muscles of the pelvic floor can be seen to stretch.
- The head recedes between contractions, which allows these muscles to thin gradually.
- The skill of the midwife in ensuring that the active phase is unhurried helps to safeguard the perineum from trauma. She must either watch the advance of the fetal head or control it with light support from her hand, or both.
- Once the head has crowned, the woman can achieve control by gently blowing or 'sighing' out each breath to minimize active pushing.
- The head is born by extension as the face appears.
- During the resting phase before the next uterine contraction, the midwife may check that the cord is not around the baby's neck.
- If it is, then the usual practice is to slacken it to form a loop through which the shoulders may pass.
- If the cord is very tightly wound around the neck, it is common practice to apply two artery forceps approximately 3 cm apart and to sever the cord between the two clamps. However, this is rarely necessary.
- Once severed, the cord may be unwound from around the neck.
- The woman may now be able to see and touch her baby's head and assist in the birth of the trunk while welcoming her baby into the world.

Birth of the shoulders

- Restitution and external rotation of the head usually occurs, maximizing the smooth birth of the shoulders and minimizing the risk of perineal laceration.
- If the woman is in an upright position, the shoulders may be left to birth spontaneously with the help of gravity.
- During a water birth, it is important not to touch the emerging baby to avoid stimulating it to gasp underwater. It is for this reason why it is important for the head to emerge first from the water.
- Once restitution has occurred fully; a hand is placed on each side of the baby's head, over the ears, and gentle downward traction is applied. The anterior shoulder escapes under the symphysis pubis. When the axillary crease is seen, the head and trunk are guided in an upward curve to allow the posterior shoulder to pass over the perineum. (These manoeuvres are reversed if the woman is, for example, on 'all fours'.) The midwife/woman, or woman's partner, may now grasp the baby around the chest to aid the birth of the trunk and lift the baby towards the woman's abdomen.
- Alternatively, midwives may use the 'hands poised' technique whereby the perineum is not supported, the baby's head is not touched and the shoulders are born spontaneously.
- The time of birth is noted.
- Once the cord has finished pulsating (generally between 1 and 3 minutes) it is severed between two clamps and a cord clamp is applied close to the umbilicus.
- If the woman has opted for a physiological third stage the umbilical cord can be clamped and cut once the placenta has been expelled by maternal effort.
- Record the time of placental expulsion.
- The baby is dried and placed in the skin-to-skin position with the woman, unless she requests otherwise.
- A warm cover is placed over the exposed areas of the baby to prevent cooling.
- The mother and baby should be left together undisturbed to facilitate the first breastfeed.

Episiotomy

- This is an incision through the perineal tissues to enlarge the vulval outlet during the birth (Fig. 18.2).
- The evidence does not support liberal use of episiotomy.

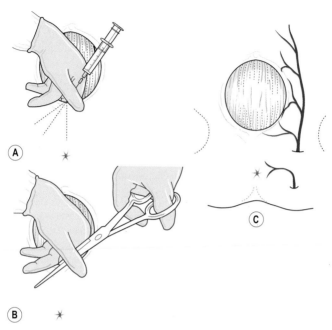

Fig. 18.2 (A) Infiltrating the perineum. (B) Performing an episiotomy. (C) Innervation of the vulval area and perineum.

- As the perineum distends, a decision to undertake an episiotomy may very occasionally be necessary, for example, in women who have been infibulated (i.e. type 3 female genital mutilation) The rationale for its use depends largely on the need to minimize the risk of severe, spontaneous, maternal trauma and to expedite the birth when there is evidence of fetal compromise.
- The woman needs to give consent prior to the procedure.
  - The perineum should be adequately anaesthetized prior to the incision. Lidocaine is commonly used, either 0.5% 10 ml or 1% 5 ml.
  - The incision is made during a contraction when the tissues are stretched so that there is a clear view of the area and bleeding is less likely to be severe.

> **Box 18.2 Classification of perineal trauma**
>
> **Classification of perineal trauma**
> - **First degree** – Injury to perineal skin **ONLY**
> - **Second degree** – Injury to the perineum involving perineal muscles but not involving the anal sphincter
> - **Third degree** – Injury involves the anal sphincter complex
>   - 3a: less than 50% of external anal sphincter thickness torn
>   - 3b: more than 50% of external anal sphincter thickness torn
>   - 3c: internal anal sphincter torn
> - **Fourth degree** – Injury to perineum involving the anal sphincter complex (internal and external anal sphincters) and anal epithelium.

Source: National Institute for Care Excellence, 2014. Intrapartum care for healthy mothers and babies, CG190. Available at: https://www.nice.org.uk (accessed 6 Sept 2016)

- Birth of the head should follow immediately and its advance must be controlled to avoid extension of the episiotomy.

Types of incision

- *Mediolateral.* Begins at the midpoint of the fourchette and is directed at a 40–60° angle to the midline towards a point midway between the ischial tuberosity and the anus (Box 18.2). There is evidence that when this angle is employed to effect the episiotomy, there are fewer obstetric anal sphincter injuries [OASIS] (i.e. 3rd and 4th degree tears) than episiotomies performed at a more acute angle.
- *Median.* A midline incision that follows the natural line of insertion of the perineal muscles. It is associated with reduced blood loss but a higher incidence of damage to the anal sphincter.

Perineal trauma

Spontaneous trauma may be of the labia anteriorly, the perineum posteriorly or both. A gentle, thorough examination must be carried out to assess the extent of the trauma accurately and to determine who should carry out the repair.

- *Anterior labial tears.* A suture may be necessary to secure haemostasis.

> Box 18.3 **Key points for practice**
>
> - The transitional and second-stage phases of labour are emotionally intense and physically hard
> - The vast majority of labours will progress physiologically
> - Maternal behaviour is usually a good indication of progress during this time
> - The core midwifery skill is to support the woman in the context of a sound knowledge of the physiology and the mechanisms of this phase of labour
> - Support should be unobtrusive
> - Midwifery care should be evidence-based and tailored to the woman's needs
> - Clear, comprehensive and contemporaneous documentation is essential

- *Posterior perineal trauma.* Spontaneous tears are usually classified in degrees (see Box 18.2). Third- and fourth-degree tears should be repaired by an experienced obstetrician. A general anaesthetic or effective epidural or spinal anaesthetic is necessary. A multidisciplinary approach to care is essential when caring for women with OASIS with input from a urogynecologist and physiotherapist.

Records

Documentation during labour and birth should be detailed, contemporaneous, and in line with the midwife's statutory professional responsibilities.

See Box 18.3 for key points relating to the second stage of labour.

FURTHER READING

Gupta, J.K., Hofmeyr, G.J., Shehmar, M., 2012. Position in the second stage of labour for women without epidural anaesthesia. Cochrane Database Syst. Rev. (5), CD002006. doi: 10.1002/14651858.CD002006.pub3.

McDonald, S.J., Middleton, P., Dowswell, T., Morris, P.S., 2013. Effect of timing of umbilical cord clamping of term infants on maternal and neonatal outcomes. Cochrane Database Syst. Rev. (7), CD004074, doi: 10.1002/14651858.CD004074.pub3.

Petrocnik, P., Marshall, J.E., 2015. Hands-poised technique: the future technique for perineal management of second stage of labour? A modified systematic literature review. Midwifery 31 (2), 274–279.

Useful website

NICE Guidelines. Available at: https://www.nice.org.uk/guidance/cg190/chapter/1-recommendations. These guidelines also address the evidence base relating to perineal trauma.

The Third Stage of Labour

PHYSIOLOGICAL PROCESSES

Labour should be seen as one continuous process. Factors affecting the first and second stage of labour will also impact on the third stage, which is concerned with separation and expulsion of the placenta and membranes alongside the achievement of haemostasis following the birth of the baby.

- Physiologically the third stage of labour is the result of an interplay of mechanical and haemostatic factors.
- The time at which the placenta actually separates from the uterine wall can vary; it may occur during the final expulsive contractions accompanying the birth of the baby or remain adherent to the uterine wall for some considerable time.
- The third stage usually lasts between 5 and 15 minutes, but any period up to 1 hour may be considered within normal limits.

Separation and descent of the placenta

Mechanical factors (Fig. 19.1)

- The majority of placentae are situated on the anterior or posterior aspect of the uterine wall.
- Separation usually begins from the lower pole of the placenta and gradually moves upwards.
- Placentae that are situated at the fundus of the uterus tend to separate first at both poles, followed by the fundal aspect.
- When separation begins centrally a retroplacental clot is formed (Fig. 19.2). Two methods of separation are described:
  - Schultze (Fig. 19.3A) and Matthews Duncan (Fig. 19.3B).

Once separation has occurred, the uterus contracts strongly, forcing the placenta and membranes to fall into the lower uterine segment and finally into the vagina.

Haemostasis

The four factors that are critical to control of bleeding and prevention of maternal morbidity and mortality are the following:

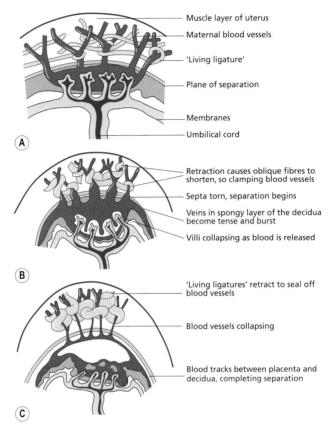

Fig. 19.1 The placental site during separation. (A) Uterus and placenta before separation. (B) Separation begins. (C) Separation is almost complete.

- *Retraction* of the oblique uterine muscle fibres in the upper uterine segment through which the tortuous blood vessels intertwine.
- The presence of vigorous uterine *contraction* following separation – this brings the walls into apposition so that further pressure is exerted on the placental site.
- The achievement of *haemostasis* – following separation, the placental site is rapidly covered by a fibrin mesh utilizing 5–10% of the circulating fibrinogen.

271

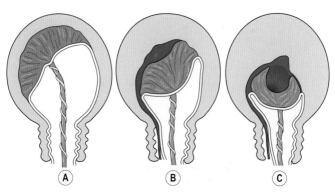

Fig. 19.2 The mechanism of placental separation. (A) Uterine wall is partially retracted, but not sufficiently to cause placental separation. (B) Further contraction and retraction thicken the uterine wall, reduce the placental site and aid placental separation. (C) Complete separation and formation of the retroplacental clot. *Note*: the thin lower segment has collapsed like a concertina following the birth of the baby.

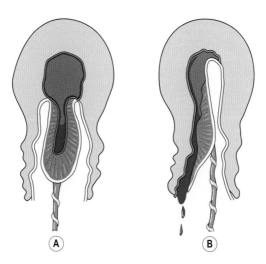

Fig. 19.3 Expulsion of the placenta. (A) Schultze method. (B) Matthews Duncan method.

- Breastfeeding – oxytocin released from the posterior lobe of the pituitary gland stimulates uterine contraction.

MANAGEMENT OF THE THIRD STAGE

Expectant or physiological management: This management policy allows the physiological changes within the uterus that occur at the time of birth to take their natural course with minimal intervention; it excludes the administration of uterotonic drugs. The processes of placental separation and expulsion are quite distinct from one another and the signs of separation and descent must be evident before maternal effort can be used to expedite expulsion.

- The normal physiological mechanisms involved in labour are supported.
- Routine administration of the uterotonic drug is withheld.
- The umbilical cord is best left unclamped until after the birth of the placenta.
- If the baby needs to be separated from the placenta or the mother requests the cord to be clamped and cut it is best to await cessation of cord pulsation.
- In any event, any mild resuscitation of the baby can be undertaken at the site of the birth, with the benefit of continued oxygen flow to the baby through the umbilical cord.
- Maintaining a calm, warm and stress free environment where the mother is comfortable and in an optimal position to facilitate gravity and placental descent is necessary. If sitting or squatting, gravity will aid expulsion.
- If good uterine contractions are sustained, maternal effort will usually bring about expulsion. The mother simply pushes, as during the second stage of labour.
- Watchful waiting, breast-feeding and enabling mother-baby dynamic interaction are encouraged.
- Early attachment of the baby to the breast may enhance these physiological changes by stimulating the release of oxytocin from the posterior lobe of the pituitary gland.
- The placenta is expelled by use of gravity and maternal effort – not through traction on the cord.
- Encouragement is important, as by now the mother may be exhausted and the contractions will feel weaker and less expulsive than those during the second stage of labour.

- Providing that fresh blood loss is not excessive, the mother's condition remains stable and her pulse and respiratory rate are within normal parameters, there need be no anxiety. This spontaneous process can take from 20 minutes to an hour to complete.
- It is important that the midwife monitors uterine action by placing a hand lightly on the fundus. She can thus palpate the contraction while checking that relaxation does not result in the uterus filling with blood.
- Vigilance is crucial, as it should be remembered that the longer the placenta remains undelivered, the greater the risk of bleeding because the uterus cannot contract down fully while the bulk of the placenta is in situ.

With this approach, *therapeutic* uterotonic administration would ONLY be administered either to stop bleeding once it has occurred or to maintain the uterus in a contracted state when there are indications that excessive bleeding is likely to occur.

- Active management: this is a policy whereby *prophylactic* administration of an uterotonic is applied, regardless of the assessed obstetric risk status of the woman. This is undertaken in conjunction with clamping of the umbilical cord shortly after birth of the baby and delivery of the placenta by the use of controlled cord traction.

Uterotonics agents

These are drugs (also known as *oxytocics* or *ecbolics*), for example:
- Syntometrine
- Syntocinon
- ergometrine
- prostaglandins

that stimulate the smooth muscle of the uterus to contract. They may be administered with crowning of the baby's head, at the time of birth of the anterior shoulder of the baby, at the end of the second stage of labour or following the delivery of the placenta and membranes.

Information related to the best available research information on the use of uterotonic drugs during the third stage of labour should be provided in an objective manner.

Intravenous ergometrine 0.25–0.5 mg
- This drug acts within 45 seconds; therefore, it is particularly useful in securing a rapid contraction where hypotonic uterine action results in haemorrhage.

- If a doctor is not present in such an emergency, a midwife may give the injection, if it is within her scope of practice.

Combined ergometrine and oxytocin

(A commonly used brand is Syntometrine)
- A 1 ml ampoule contains 5 IU of oxytocin and 0.5 mg ergometrine and is administered by intramuscular injection.
- The oxytocin acts within 2.5 minutes, and the ergometrine within 6–7 minutes.
- Their combined action results in a rapid uterine contraction enhanced by a stronger, more sustained contraction lasting several hours.
- Administered, normally, at birth of the anterior shoulder.
- *Caution.* No more than two doses of ergometrine 0.5 mg should be given, as it can cause headache, nausea and an increase in blood pressure; it is normally contraindicated where there is a history of hypertensive or cardiac disease.

Oxytocin

(A commonly used brand is Syntocinon)
- Oxytocin can be administered as both an intravenous and an intramuscular injection. However, an intravenous bolus of oxytocin can cause profound, fatal hypotension, especially in the presence of cardiovascular compromise.
- No more than 5 IU should be given by slow intravenous injection.

Prostaglandins

In recent years, a great deal of time and resource has been invested in seeking alternative ways to reduce the risk of postpartum haemorrhage (PPH), especially in resource poor countries.
- Misoprostol (a prostaglandin E1 analogue) is cheap, not prone to the loss of potency, does not need to be sterile or refrigerated and has the advantage of being licensed to be administered vaginally, orally and rectally.
- Although systematic reviews from the Cochrane Database suggests that it should be replaced by tried and tested uterotonic agents such as those previously identified, it may be useful in circumstances where nothing else is available.

Clamping of the umbilical cord

Traditionally, this may have been carried out during birth of the baby if the cord was tightly around the neck.

- Preferred practice is to loosen the loop of cord and slip it over the baby's head or emerging shoulder. The baby's body is born beside the loop.
- Previously, early clamping of the cord was carried out in the first 1–3 minutes immediately after birth, regardless of whether cord pulsation has ceased.

The evidence base is that early clamping of the umbilical cord denies the baby his/her full quota of placental blood, which may constitute as much as 30–40% of the circulating blood volume.

Proponents of late clamping suggest that:

- No action be taken until cord pulsation ceases or the placenta has been completely delivered, thus allowing the physiological processes to take place without intervention.
- Delayed cord clamping may decrease the risk of feto-maternal transfusion when caring for women with a rhesus negative blood group.

DELIVERY OF THE PLACENTA AND MEMBRANES

Controlled cord traction (CCT)

This manoeuvre according to the evidence base has no effect on major PPH (> 1000 ml) and little, if no effect on mild PPH (> 500 ml). It does however shorten the third stage of labour by 6 minutes. Before starting CCT check that the conditions listed in Box 19.1 have been met.

- At the beginning of the third stage, a strong uterine contraction results in the fundus being palpable below the umbilicus. It feels broad, as the placenta is still in the upper segment.

Box 19.1 **Conditions for starting controlled cord traction**

- A uterotonic drug has been administered
- It has been given time to act
- The uterus is well contracted
- Countertraction is applied
- Signs of placental separation and descent are present

- As the placenta separates and falls into the lower uterine segment there is a small fresh blood loss, the cord lengthens and the fundus becomes rounder, smaller and more mobile as it rises in the abdomen.
- (*Note*: there is a school of thought that does not believe it is necessary to wait for signs of separation and descent *but* the uterus must be well contracted and care exerted with cord traction.)

It is good practice throughout labour to ensure the woman does not have a full bladder.

- It is important not to manipulate the uterus in any way, as this may precipitate incoordinate action.
- No further step should be taken until a strong contraction is palpable. If tension is applied to the umbilical cord without this contraction, uterine inversion may occur (see Ch. 23).

When CCT is the preferred method of management, the following sequence of actions is usually undertaken:

- Once the uterus is found on palpation to be contracted, one hand is placed above the level of the symphysis pubis with the palm facing towards the umbilicus and exerting pressure in an upwards direction. This is countertraction.
- Grasping the cord, traction is applied in a downward and backward direction following the line of the birth canal.
- Some resistance may be felt but it is important to apply steady tension by pulling the cord firmly and maintaining the pressure. Jerky movements and force should be avoided.
- The aim is to complete the action as one continuous, smooth, controlled movement. However, it is only possible to exert this tension for 1 or 2 minutes, as it may be an uncomfortable procedure for the mother and the midwife's hand will tire.
- Downward traction on the cord must be released *before* uterine countertraction is relaxed, as sudden withdrawal of countertraction while tension is still being applied to the cord may also cause uterine inversion.
- If the manoeuvre is not immediately successful, there should be a pause before uterine contraction is again checked and a further attempt is made.
- Should the uterus relax, tension is temporarily released until a good contraction is again palpable.
- Once the placenta is visible, it may be cupped in the hands to ease pressure on the friable membranes.

- A gentle upward and downward movement or twisting action will help to coax out the membranes and increase the chances of delivering them intact. Great care should be taken to avoid tearing the membranes.

Asepsis

The need for asepsis is even greater now than in the preceding stages of labour.
- Laceration and bruising of the cervix, vagina, perineum and vulva provide a route for the entry of micro-organisms.
- The placental site, a raw wound, provides an ideal medium for infection.
- Strict attention to the prevention of sepsis is therefore vital.

Cord blood sampling

This may be required:
- when the mother's blood group is rhesus negative or her rhesus type is unknown
- when atypical maternal antibodies have been found during an antenatal screening test
- where a haemoglobinopathy is suspected (e.g. sickle cell disease).

The sample should be taken from the fetal surface of the placenta where the blood vessels are congested and easily visible.

In the event of paired cord blood sampling for reasons outlined by local and national guidelines, blood will be taken from the umbilical cord. To achieve this an additional clamp will need to be applied resulting in double-clamping of the cord.

COMPLETION OF THE THIRD STAGE

- Once the placenta is delivered, the uterus should be well contracted and fresh blood loss minimal.
- Perineum and lower vagina should be checked for trauma.
- Blood loss is estimated, including blood that has soaked into linen and swabs, as well as measurable fluid loss and clot formation.
- A thorough inspection of the placenta and membranes must be carried out to make sure that no part has been retained.
- If there is any suspicion that the placenta or membranes are incomplete, they must be kept for inspection and a doctor informed immediately.

Immediate care

It is advisable for mother and infant to remain in the midwife's care for at least an hour after birth, regardless of the birth setting.

- The woman should be encouraged to pass urine because a full bladder may impede uterine contraction.
- Uterine contraction and blood loss should be checked on several occasions during this first hour.
- Throughout this same period the midwife should pay regard to the baby's general wellbeing. She should check the security of the cord clamp and observe general skin colour, respirations and temperature.
- The warmest place for a baby to be placed is in a direct skin-to-skin contact position with the mother or wrapped and cuddled, whichever she prefers.
- Most women intending to breastfeed will wish to put their baby to the breast during these early moments of contact.

COMPLICATIONS OF THE THIRD STAGE OF LABOUR

Postpartum haemorrhage (PPH)

PPH is defined as excessive bleeding from the genital tract at any time following the baby's birth up to 12 weeks after birth.

- If it occurs during the third stage of labour or within 24 hours of birth, it is termed *primary postpartum haemorrhage*.
- If it occurs subsequent to the first 24 hours following birth up until the 12th week postpartum, it is termed *secondary postpartum haemorrhage*.

Primary postpartum haemorrhage

A measured loss that reaches 500 ml or any loss that adversely affects the mother's condition constitutes a PPH.

There are several reasons why a PPH may occur, best summarized as the four T's:

1. Tone of uterus – atonic uterus
2. Tissue – retained placenta/membranes
3. Trauma – genital tract trauma (cervix, vagina, perineum, ruptured vulval or perineal varicosities)
4. Thrombin – blood coagulation disorder.

Atonic uterus

This is a failure of the myometrium at the placental site to contract and retract, and to compress torn blood vessels and control blood loss by a living ligature action.

- Causes of atonic uterine action resulting in PPH are listed in Box 19.2.
- There are, in addition, a number of factors that do not directly *cause* a PPH, but do increase the likelihood of excessive bleeding (Box 19.3).

Signs of PPH

These may be obvious, such as:
- visible bleeding
- maternal collapse.

However, more subtle signs may present, such as:
- pallor
- rising pulse rate
- falling blood pressure
- altered level of consciousness; the mother may become restless or drowsy
- an enlarged uterus that feels 'boggy' on palpation (i.e. soft, distended and lacking tone), even if little visible blood loss.

Box 19.2 **Causes of atonic uterine action**

- Incomplete separation of the placenta
- Retained cotyledon, placental fragment or membranes
- Precipitate labour
- Prolonged labour resulting in uterine inertia
- Polyhydramnios or multiple pregnancy causing overdistension of uterine muscle
- Placenta praevia
- Placental abruption
- General anaesthesia, especially halothane or cyclopropane
- Mismanagement of the third stage of labour
- A full bladder
- Ruptured varicosities, perineal or genital tract trauma
- Aetiology unknown

> **Box 19.3 Predisposing factors which might increase the risks of postpartum haemorrhage**
>
> - Previous history of postpartum haemorrhage or retained placenta
> - High parity, resulting in uterine scar tissue
> - Presence of fibroids
> - Maternal anaemia
> - Ketoacidosis
> - Multiple pregnancy
> - Caesarean section
> - Infection – HIV/AIDS

Prophylaxis
- During the antenatal period, identify risk factors, e.g. previous obstetric history, anaemia.
- During labour, prevent prolonged labour and ketoacidosis.
- Ensure the mother does not have a full bladder at any stage.
- Give prophylactic administration of an uterotonic agent.
- If a woman is known to have a placenta praevia, keep 2 units of cross-matched blood available.
- Attend to repair of all perineal trauma in a timely manner to arrest early any associated bleeding.

Management of PPH
Three basic principles of care:
- call for medical aid
- stop the bleeding:
  - rub up a contraction
  - give a uterotonic
  - empty the bladder
  - empty the uterus
  - apply pressure if there is trauma
- resuscitate the mother.

See Fig. 19.4 for a summary of management; at the same time as taking these measures, check the blood is clotting.

Secondary postpartum haemorrhage

See Chapter 25.

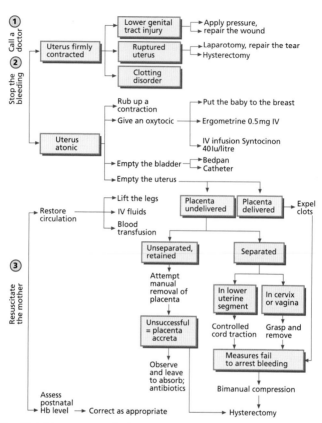

Fig. 19.4 Management of primary postpartum haemorrhage.

SUGGESTED READING

Andersson, O., Hellström-Westas, L., Andersson, D., et al., 2011. Effect of delayed versus early umbilical cord clamping on neonatal outcomes and iron status at 4 months: a randomised controlled trial. BMJ 343, d7157. doi: 10.1136/bmj.d7157. Available at: http://www.bmj.com (accessed 10 April 2016).

Fahy, K., Hastie, C., Bisits, A., et al., 2010. Holistic physiological care compared with active management of the third stage of labour for

women at low risk of postpartum haemorrhage: a cohort study. Women
Birth 23 (4), 146–152.

Useful website

The Cochrane Library. Available from: http://www.cochranelibrary.com.
Provides helpful systematic reviews to inform practice such as the
management of the third stage of labour.

Prolonged Pregnancy and Disorders of Uterine Action

POST-TERM, POST-DATES OR PROLONGED PREGNANCY

- Post-dates is defined as $40+^0$ to $40+^6$ weeks.
- Post-term pregnancy is one where the gestation exceeds 42 completed weeks (294 days).
- Prolonged pregnancy is a pregnancy equal to or beyond 42 completed weeks. The term is often used interchangeably with 'post-term' and 'post-dates', thus creating some confusion and ambiguity in the literature.
- There is a growing body of evidence that prolonged pregnancy might be a normal variation on human gestation, especially in some ethnicities/racial groups.
- Accurate dating of a pregnancy is essential, as incorrect diagnosis that a pregnancy has gone beyond term may lead to inappropriate or unnecessary intervention.
- Ostensibly, prolonged pregnancy it could be argued, is the largest single indication for induction of labour.
- If prolonged pregnancy is to be construed as a 'complication' the possible perceived 'risks' in terms of morbidity and mortality need to be considered from the perspective of the mother, fetus and neonate (Fig. 20.1).

Plan of care for prolonged pregnancy

Two approaches to care are offered:
- Expectant management with fetal surveillance.
- Cervical membrane sweep at 41 weeks/elective induction of labour after 41 weeks of gestation.

Key points in the management of prolonged pregnancy:
- Accurate estimation of date of birth (EDB) based on last menstrual period (LMP) and early ultrasound scan (USS) reduces the incidence of pregnancies diagnosed as prolonged.

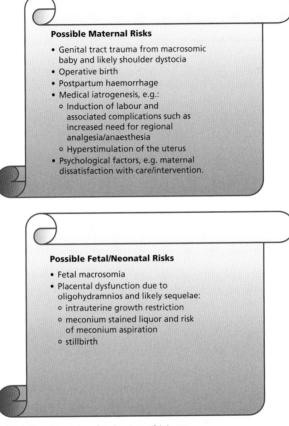

Possible Maternal Risks

- Genital tract trauma from macrosomic baby and likely shoulder dystocia
- Operative birth
- Postpartum haemorrhage
- Medical iatrogenesis, e.g.:
  - Induction of labour and associated complications such as increased need for regional analgesia/anaesthesia
  - Hyperstimulation of the uterus
- Psychological factors, e.g. maternal dissatisfaction with care/intervention.

Possible Fetal/Neonatal Risks

- Fetal macrosomia
- Placental dysfunction due to oligohydramnios and likely sequelae:
  - intrauterine growth restriction
  - meconium stained liquor and risk of meconium aspiration
  - stillbirth

Fig. 20.1 Possible risks of induction of labour.

- The evidence base points to the fact that genetic factors create disparity; therefore, the gestation in some ethnicities/racial groups must be considered with regards to the definition of prolonged pregnancy in these racial groups to improve perinatal outcomes.
- A membrane sweep can be offered to women from 40 weeks' gestation to increase the chances of the initiation of labour.

Box 20.1 **Indications for induction of labour**

Maternal
- Prolonged or post-term pregnancy
- Hypertension, including pre-eclampsia
- Diabetes
- Medical problems, e.g. renal, respiratory or cardiac disease
- Placental abruption
- Obstetric history, such as previous stillbirth or previous caesarean section
- Prelabour rupture of membranes
- Maternal request

Fetal
- Suspected fetal compromise
- Intrauterine death
- Fetal anomaly incompatible with life

- If there are underlying pregnancy complications approaching or beyond term, then care needs to be prioritized in terms of how best to manage the specific complication.
- Where the woman makes an informed choice for expectant management, she must be informed that any deviations highlighted in antenatal surveillance will necessitate a reevaluation and review of the agreed plan of care and options available to her.

Indications for induction

Induction is indicated when the benefits to the mother or the fetus outweigh those of continuing the pregnancy. It is associated with the maternal and fetal factors described in Box 20.1.

Some contraindications to induction

These include:
- placenta praevia
- transverse or compound fetal presentation
- cord presentation or cord prolapse when vaginal birth is not imminent
- known cephalo-pelvic disproportion

- HIV-positive women not receiving any antiretroviral therapy or women on any antiviral therapy with a viral load of 400 copies/ml or more
- severe acute fetal compromise
- active genital herpes.

If birth of the baby is imperative, it should be effected by caesarean section.

Cervical ripening

Structural changes in ripening

- Successful induction occurs when the cervix is favourable or so-called 'ripe'.
- The cervix is then more compliant, offering less soft tissue resistance to the actions of the myometrium and the presenting part.

Prostaglandins (PGE₂)

- Pre-induction PGE_2 can be used to prime or mature the cervix for induction.
- A low-dose PGE_2 is administered to bring about effacement and dilatation without stimulating contractions.

Methods of inducing labour

Prostaglandins and induction

- Prior to prescribing PGE_2, the cervix is assessed using the Bishop score (Table 20.1).
- PGE_2 preparations are available in gels, tablets or controlled-release pessary form; they are inserted close to the cervix within the posterior fornix of the vagina.

Table 20.1 Modified Bishop pre-induction pelvic scoring system				
Inducibility features	0	1	2	3
Dilatation of cervix (cm)	< 1	1–2	2–4	> 4
Consistency of cervix	Firm	Firm	Medium	Soft
Cervical canal length (cm)	> 4	2–4	1–2	< 1
Position of cervix	Posterior	Mid	Anterior	–
Position/station of presenting part (cm above or below ischial spine)	–3	–2	–1	+1, +2

- Fetal heart rate and uterine contractions should be monitored continuously for 30–60 minutes thereafter.
- The mother remains recumbent or resting for 1 hour, but tilted with a wedge/pillow to avoid aorta-caval compression.
- Changes in the cervix can be assessed by an increase in the Bishop score.

Recommended prescribed doses of PGE_2 are dependent on local and national guidelines and it is for this reason that it is recommended that the reader consults the evidence base alongside the guidelines currently used in practice.

Associated risks of PGE_2 preparations

- Uterine hyperstimulation
- Placental abruption
- Fetal hypoxia
- Pulmonary embolism
- Amniotic fluid embolism
- Uterine rupture (rare)

Sweeping or stripping of cervical membranes

- Sweeping the cervical membranes is an adjunct to rather than a method of inducing labour per se.
- During a vaginal examination, the clinician inserts a finger into the cervical os, and using a sweeping or circular movement releases the fetal membranes from the lower uterine segment.
- Detaching the membranes from the decidua results in an increase in the concentration of circulating PGE_2 that may contribute to the initiation of the onset of labour in some women.
- The woman should be made aware that it may cause some discomfort and bleeding.
- Additional membrane sweeping may be offered if labour does not start spontaneously.

Amniotomy

- Amniotomy is the artificial rupture of the fetal membranes (ARM), resulting in drainage of liquor.
- It is performed to induce labour when the cervix is favourable or during labour to augment contractions.
- ARM may also be carried out to visualize the colour of the liquor or to attach a fetal scalp electrode for the purposes of continuous

---

Box 20.2 **Amniotomy procedures**

Prior to intervention

- Informed maternal consent is obtained
- The reason for the amniotomy is clearly stated in the records
- Presentation and degree of engagement of the presenting part are confirmed by abdominal palpation
- The fetal heart rate is auscultated
- The presence of a low-lying placenta or cord is excluded (check USS record)

Following intervention

- Note the colour and quantity of liquor
- Check the presentation, position and station of the fetus
- Ensure no cord has prolapsed
- Auscultate the fetal heart rate
- Document findings and communicate them to the woman

---

electronic monitoring of the fetal heart rate when the external transducer is ineffective or produces an unsatisfactory trace.
- A well-fitting presenting part is essential to prevent cord prolapse.

The fetal heart rate should be auscultated before and after an ARM in conjunction with maternal pulse and documented contemporaneously.

ARM is carried out using an amnihook or an amnicot. Procedures are shown in Box 20.2.

Hazards of ARM

These include:
- intrauterine infection
- early decelerations of the fetal heart
- cord prolapse
- bleeding from fetal vessels in the membranes (vasa praevia); friable vessels in the cervix; or placenta praevia.

Oxytocin

Synthetic oxytocin (Syntocinon) is a powerful uterotonic agent used in conjunction with amniotomy and may be commenced at the same time as ARM or after a delay of several hours, especially where PGE_2 has been employed. Current evidence concludes that amniotomy alone

289

or with oxytocin, should not be used as a primary method of induction of labour unless there are specific clinical reasons for not using vaginal PGE$_2$, in particular the risk of uterine hyperstimulation.

Administration of oxytocin to induce labour

- Oxytocin is used intravenously, diluted in an isotonic solution such as normal saline.
- The infusion should be controlled through an infusion pump or syringe driver with non-return valve to enable accurate assessment of volume and rate.
- The dosage or infusion rate should follow local protocol based on evidence based national guidelines. The midwife should aim to administer the lowest dose required to maintain effective, well-spaced uterine contractions, with a maximum of 3–4 contractions every 10 minutes.
- To prevent overstimulation of the uterus and its associated deleterious effects, oxytocin should not be started within 6 hours of the administration of prostaglandins.

Risks associated with oxytocin infusion

- Hyperstimulation of the uterus, which could cause fetal hypoxia and uterine rupture.
- Fluid retention (oxytocin has an antidiuretic effect).
- Amniotic fluid embolism.
- Prolonged use may contribute to uterine atony and primary postpartum haemorrhage.

Alternative approaches to inducing labour include:
- ingestion of castor oil
- nipple stimulation
- sexual intercourse
- acupuncture
- homoeopathy.

The Cochrane Database systematic reviews provide evidence regarding the efficacy of the above methods.

Responsibilities of the midwife in the care of a mother where labour is induced

The role of the midwife is to monitor the wellbeing of the mother and fetus throughout the process of induction, assess progress in labour and observe for signs of side effects of oxytocin. The parameters listed in Box 20.3 should be monitored.

Box 20.3 **The midwife's responsibilities in induction of labour**

Baseline observations

- Maternal pulse rate, blood pressure, respiratory rate and temperature are recorded

Uterine contractions

- Frequency, duration and strength are monitored every 15–30 minutes during the first stage of labour
- Continuous tocography is recommended when oxytocin is in use and for an hour following insertion of prostaglandins

Fetal wellbeing

- Fetal heart rate is recorded every 15 minutes during the first stage of labour
- There should be continuous monitoring in conjunction with oxytocin, using an abdominal ultrasound transducer or a fetal scalp electrode if external monitoring is difficult to achieve

Assessment of pain

- The rapid build-up of contractions can be difficult to cope with

Assessment of progress

- Position and station of the presenting part are noted
- Length, consistency, position and dilatation of the cervix are monitored
- Vaginal examinations are usually carried out every 4 hours

The midwife should be aware of the risk of uterine rupture associated with excessive use of oxytocin, particularly if there is a previous history of caesarean section.

PROLONGED LABOUR

- Prolonged labour is associated with the medical model of management of childbirth and for many women – and midwives – the attempts to place time limits on the physiological process of labour is problematic.
- Prolonged labour is associated with increasing risks to mother and fetus.

Prolonged labour is most common in primigravidae and may be caused by:

- ineffective uterine contractions
- cephalopelvic disproportion
- an occipitoposterior position.

Dystocia literally means 'difficult labour' and is associated with slowness or lack of progress in labour. Possible problems include:

- contractions being ineffective in dilating and effacing the cervix
- uncoordinated contractions, where the two segments of the uterus fail to work in harmony
- contractions giving inadequate involuntary expulsion.

Other causes of dystocia are:

- fetal malpresentations and malposition
- the pelvis
- the birth canal and congenital malformations.

Delay in the latent phase

The latent phase of labour is still poorly understood and its duration difficult to define; therefore, a diagnosis of a prolonged latent phase may be arbitrary and result in inappropriate intervention.

Delay in the active phase

- Slow progress may be defined either as total duration of hours in labour or as failure of the cervix to dilate at a fixed rate per hour.
- A rate of 1 cm per hour is still widely applied to both nulliparous and multiparous women and most commonly taken as normal, but use of a standardized progress rate is now being questioned.
- A prolonged active phase is caused by a combination of factors such as:
  - maternal age
  - maternal size and nutritional status
  - parity
  - the cervix
  - the uterus
  - the fetus
  - the mother's pelvis.

Such variables as detailed previously mean that labour does not conform to a pre-determined time limit.

Inefficient uterine action

In the absence of effective contractions, descent of the presenting part and dilatation of the cervix may be delayed.

Factors that may affect uterine action

- Restricting food and fluids to mothers in labour may have a detrimental effect.
- Ambulation may promote more effective uterine activity.
- An upright position improves the application of the presenting part on to the cervix, and may trigger the neuroendocrine Ferguson reflex.
- Stress and psychosocial factors can adversely affect contractions due to the release of stress hormones cortisol and catecholamines as a 'fight or flight' response.

Augmentation of labour

Augmentation of labour refers to intervention to correct slow progress in labour. Correction of ineffective uterine contractions includes:
- amniotomy
- administration of oxytocin and amniotomy or administration of oxytocin in the presence of the previously ruptured membranes.

Cephalopelvic disproportion should be excluded before any method of augmenting labour is introduced.

Incoordinate uterine activity

This may be hypertonic and also inefficient. Possible signs include the following:
- fundal dominance is lacking
- polarity is reversed
- resting tone of the uterus is raised
- pain is intense and out of proportion to the effect of the contraction on the dilatation of the cervix
- where coordination of the contractions is completely lacking, different areas of the uterus contract independently, causing a 'colicky' uterus
- the mother suffers severe generalized pain
- fetal compromise may occur due to diminished placental perfusion.

Constriction ring dystocia

This is a localized spasm of a ring of muscle fibres that occurs at the junction of the upper and lower segments of the uterus. It is associated with the use of oxytocin.

Management of prolonged labour

Determining the cause is necessary before deciding on management.

- Hypotonic uterine activity may be corrected with amniotomy or oxytocin infusion, or both.
- If, however, there have been strong contractions and slow progress, a caesarean section is likely.
- Obvious disproportion or malpresentation is an indication for caesarean section.

Principles of care are summarized in Box 20.4.

Box 20.4 Principles of care in prolonged labour

Comfort and analgesia
- Adequate analgesia should be offered
- Regional analgesia (i.e. epidural) may be beneficial

Observations
- Temperature is recorded every 4 hours
- Vaginal swabs may be taken and broad-spectrum antibiotics commenced if infection is suspected
- Pulse, respiratory rate and blood pressure recorded hourly, or more frequently if the woman's condition dictates this

Fluid balance
- Input and output should be recorded
- The mother should be encouraged to empty her bladder every 2 hours; a full bladder may affect the uterine action in labour
- Reduced urinary output and ketones may indicate dehydration

Assessment of progress
- Vaginal examination is usually carried out 4 hourly

Fetal wellbeing
- Fetal heart is monitored continuously
- The presence of meconium-stained liquor and an abnormal fetal heart tracing are suggestive of fetal hypoxia; fetal blood sampling may be carried out
- A paediatrician may be required, and if the mother is in labour at home it may be necessary for her to be transferred into hospital

---

Prolonged second stage of labour

Provided that there is evidence of descent of the fetus and in the absence of fetal or maternal compromise, there is no basis for placing a time limit on the duration of the second stage of labour.

Causes of delay in the second stage

These are listed in Box 20.5.

Management of a prolonged second stage of labour

- Perform a thorough abdominal examination.
- Confirm the position, attitude and station of the presenting part by vaginal examination.
- Auscultate the fetal heart after every contraction or use electronic monitoring.
- In the presence of inefficient uterine contractions where labour is protracted the woman should be referred to the obstetric team who might consider implementing an infusion of oxytocin after careful and through assessment.
- Where the mother is in labour at home, arrange for transfer to hospital after discussion with the mother and consent has been obtained.
- Birth may be expedited where the conditions alter and maternal or fetal wellbeing become compromised.
- Ventouse or forceps will be utilized where the pelvic outlet is adequate and vaginal birth can be safely carried out.
- Caesarean section may be necessary where there is evidence of cephalopelvic disproportion.

Box 20.5 **Causes of delay in the second stage of labour**

- Ineffective contractions
- Poor maternal effort
- Loss or absence of a desire to push caused by epidural analgesia
- Fetal macrosomia, malpresentation or malposition
- A full bladder or a full rectum
- A reduced pelvic outlet, in association with an occipitoposterior position may result in deep transverse arrest

Cervical dystocia

- This occurs rarely and is often acquired as a consequence of scarring of the cervix or a congenital structural abnormality.
- Despite effective contractions the cervix fails to dilate, although it may efface.
- Caesarean section is necessary to birth the baby.

PRECIPITATE LABOUR

- Defined as expulsion of the fetus within three hours of the onset of uterine contractions.
- The contractions are strong and frequent from the onset of labour.
- Resistance from the soft tissue is low, resulting in rapid completion of the first and second stages.
- The mother may be distressed by the intensity of the contractions and the unexpected speed of the birth, both physically and psychologically.
- Soft tissue damage to the cervix or perineum may complicate the birth.
- The uterus may fail to retract during the third stage, leading to retained placenta or postpartum haemorrhage.
- Fetal hypoxia and rapid moulding can occur.
- The speed of the birth may result in the baby being born in an inappropriate place and sustaining injury.

Precipitate labour tends to recur, but there is no evidence to support induction of labour as a prophylactic measure.

TRIAL OF LABOUR

- A trial of labour is offered to mothers when there is a minor degree of cephalopelvic disproportion.
- Review of place of birth may be necessary.
- If, despite good uterine contractions, cervical dilatation is slow and the head fails to descend, the outlook for vaginal birth is poor and the decision must be made whether to allow labour to continue.
- If at any stage during this labour the mother or fetus is under stress, then a caesarean section will be performed.
- A trial of labour (also referred to as a trial of scar) for vaginal birth may also be considered following previous caesarean section (VBAC).

OBSTRUCTED LABOUR

Labour is obstructed when there is no advance of the presenting part despite strong uterine contractions. The obstruction usually occurs at the pelvic brim but may occur at the outlet.

Causes of obstructed labour

- Cephalopelvic disproportion.
- Deep transverse arrest.
- Malpresentation, e.g. shoulder or brow presentation, or in persistent mentoposterior position.
- Pelvic mass, e.g. fibroids, ovarian or pelvic tumours.
- Fetal malformations, e.g. hydrocephalus, conjoined twins.

Signs of obstructed labour

These are listed in Box 20.6.

On examination, the vagina feels hot and dry; the presenting part is high and feels wedged and immovable. It may be difficult to assess the station of the presenting part accurately due to excessive moulding of the fetal skull and a large caput succedaneum.

Management of obstructed labour

- An intravenous infusion to correct dehydration.
- Blood is taken for cross-matching in case a transfusion is needed.
- Antibiotics should be given to overcome any infection or if mother develops pyrexia.
- If obstructed labour is recognized in the first stage of labour, birth should be expedited by caesarean section.
- In the second stage of labour, failure to progress and descent may be due to deep transverse arrest. If rotation and assisted birth fail, caesarean section should be performed.
- If the mother is in labour at home, arrangements should be made to transfer her to the nearest maternity unit with facilities for an immediate caesarean section. Blood is taken for cross-matching and an intravenous infusion is sited prior to transfer.
- The paediatrician should be present at the birth.

Complications of obstructed labour

Complications are listed in Box 20.7.

Box 20.6 Signs of obstructed labour

Early signs

- The presenting part does not enter the pelvic brim despite good contractions (exclude full bladder, loaded rectum or excessive liquor)
- Cervical dilatation is slow; the cervix hangs loosely like 'an empty sleeve'
- Pressure may result in early rupture or formation of a large elongated sac of forewaters

Late signs

- The mother is dehydrated, ketotic and in constant pain
- The mother is pyrexial
- Urinary output is poor and haematuria may be present
- There is evidence of fetal compromise
- The uterus becomes moulded round the fetus and fails to relax properly between contractions
- Contractions continue to build in strength and frequency until the uterus is in a continuous state of tonic contraction
- A visible retraction ring (Bandl ring), similar in appearance to a full bladder, appears at an oblique angle across the abdomen
- In a primigravida, uterine contractions may cease for a while before recommencing with renewed vigour

Box 20.7 Complications of obstructed labour

Maternal

- There is trauma to the bladder, e.g. vesicovaginal fistula
- There is intrauterine infection due to prolonged rupture of membranes
- Neglected obstruction will result in rupture of the uterus, leading to haemorrhage and possible death of the mother and the fetus

Fetal

- Intrauterine asphyxia may result in a fresh stillbirth or, if the baby is born alive, permanent brain damage
- Ascending infection can cause neonatal pneumonia; this may also develop as a consequence of meconium aspiration

SUGGESTED READING

Galal, M., Symonds, I., Murray, H., et al., 2012. Postterm pregnancy. Facts Views Vis. Obgyn. 4 (3), 175–187.

Papoutsis, D., Antonakou, A., Tzavara, C., 2016. The effect of ethnic variation on the success of induced labour in nulliparous women with postdates pregnancies. Scientifica (Cairo) 2016, 9569725. doi: 10.1155/2016/9569725. Available at: http://www.hindawi.com/journals/scientifica/2016/9569725 (accessed 10 April 2016).

Useful website

World Health Organization. Available at: http://www.who.int. Provides useful health bulletins on statistical information on a global perspective on issues such as obstructed labour.

Malpositions of the Occiput and Malpresentations

- Malposition is any position other than occipitoanterior in a fetus with a vertex presentation.
- Malpresentation is any presentation of the fetus other than the vertex.
- Both malpositions and malpresentations are associated with a difficult labour and an increased risk of operative birth.

OCCIPITOPOSTERIOR POSITIONS

- Occipitoposterior positions are the most common type of malposition of the occiput and occur in approximately 10–30% of labours but only approximately 5% of births.
- A persistent occipitoposterior position results from a failure of internal rotation prior to birth.
- The vertex is presenting, but the occiput lies in the posterior rather than the anterior part of the pelvis. As a consequence, the fetal head is deflexed and larger diameters of the fetal skull present.

Causes

The direct cause is often unknown, but it may be associated with an android- or anthropoid-shaped pelvis.

Antenatal diagnosis

History

- Listen to the woman as she may complain of persistent backache and be specific where she feels fetal movements, often across both sides of her abdomen.

Abdominal examination

Inspection

- There is a saucer-shaped depression at or just below the umbilicus.

Palpation
- The back is difficult to palpate; it is well out to the maternal side, sometimes almost adjacent to the maternal spine.
- Limbs can be felt on both sides of the midline.
- The head is usually high.
- The occiput and sinciput are on the same level.

Auscultation
- The fetal heart can be heard in the midline or at the flank.

Diagnosis during labour

- The woman may complain of continuous and severe backache worsening with contractions.
- Spontaneous rupture of the membranes may occur at an early stage of labour.
- Contractions may be incoordinate.
- There is slow descent of the head, even with good contractions.
- The woman may have a strong desire to push early in labour.

Vaginal examination

The findings will depend upon the degree of flexion of the head; locating the anterior fontanelle in the anterior part of the pelvis is diagnostic. The direction of the sagittal suture and location of the posterior fontanelle will help to confirm the diagnosis.

Management of labour

Labour with a fetus in an occipitoposterior position can be long and painful. The deflexed head does not fit well onto the cervix and therefore does not produce optimal stimulation.

Management is described in Box 21.1.

Mechanism of the right occipitoposterior position (Long rotation)

See Figs 21.1–21.4 and Table 21.1.
- *Flexion.* Descent takes place with increasing flexion. The occiput becomes the leading part.
- *Internal rotation of the head.* The occiput reaches the pelvic floor first and rotates forwards three-eighths of a circle along the right side of the pelvis to lie under the symphysis pubis. The shoulders follow, turning two-eighths of a circle from the left to the right oblique diameter.

Box 21.1 Management of labour: occipitoposterior positions

First stage of labour

- Assist with pain management techniques, such as massage, changes of posture and optimal positions to aid flexion and rotation of the fetal head. Pharmacological pain control methods as appropriate are provided if this is the mother's request
- Prevent dehydration and ketosis
- Correct any incoordinate uterine action or ineffective contractions with an oxytocin infusion
- The urge to push long before the cervix has become fully dilated may be eased by a change in position, use of water (bath, birthing pool) and the use of breathing techniques or nitrous oxide and oxygen to enhance relaxation

Second stage of labour

- Full dilatation of the cervix may need to be confirmed by a vaginal examination
- Encourage the woman to remain upright
- If contractions are weak and ineffective, an oxytocin infusion may be necessary
- The length of the second stage of labour is increased when the occiput is posterior, and there is an increased likelihood of assisted/operative birth

Fig. 21.1 Head descending with increased flexion. Sagittal suture in right oblique diameter of the pelvis.

Fig. 21.2 Occiput and shoulders have rotated one-eighth of a circle forwards. Sagittal suture in transverse diameter of the pelvis.

Fig. 21.3 Occiput and shoulders have rotated two-eighths of a circle forwards. Sagittal suture in the left oblique diameter of the pelvis. The position is right occipitoanterior.

Fig. 21.4 Occiput has rotated three-eighths of a circle forwards. Note the twist in the neck. Sagittal suture in the anteroposterior diameter of the pelvis.

- *Crowning.* The occiput escapes under the symphysis pubis and the head is crowned.
- *Extension.* The sinciput, face and chin sweep the perineum and the head is born by a movement of extension.
- *Restitution.* The occiput turns one-eighth of a circle to the right and the head realigns itself with the shoulders.

Table 21.1 Terminology for mechanisms of the right occipitoposterior, left mentoanterior and left sacroanterior positions

	Right occipitoposterior	**Left mentoanterior**	**Left sacroanterior**
Lie	Longitudinal	Longitudinal	Longitudinal
Attitude	Deflexion of head	Extension of head and back	Complete flexion
Presentation	Vertex	Face	Breech
Denominator	Occiput	Mentum	Sacrum
Presenting part	Middle or anterior area of left parietal bone	Left malar bone	Anterior (left) buttock
Diameter	Occipitofrontal diameter (11.5 cm) lies in right oblique diameter of pelvic brim		Bitrochanteric diameter (10 cm) enters pelvis in the oblique diameter of brim
	Occiput points to right sacroiliac joint and sinciput to left iliopectineal eminence		Sacrum points to left iliopectineal eminence

- *Internal rotation of the shoulders.* The shoulders enter the pelvis in the right oblique diameter; the anterior shoulder reaches the pelvic floor first and rotates forwards one-eighth of a circle to lie under the symphysis pubis.
- *External rotation of the head.* At the same time the occiput turns a further one-eighth of a circle to the right.
- *Lateral flexion.* The anterior shoulder escapes under the symphysis pubis, the posterior shoulder sweeps the perineum and the body is born by a movement of lateral flexion.

Possible course and outcomes of labour

Long internal rotation

This is the most common outcome, with good uterine contractions producing flexion and descent of the head so that the occiput rotates forward three-eighths of a circle, as described previously.

Short internal rotation (persistent occipitoposterior position)

This results from failure of flexion.
- The sinciput reaches the pelvic floor first and rotates forwards.
- The occiput goes into the hollow of the sacrum.
- The baby is born facing the pubic bone (face to pubis).

Diagnosis

In the first stage of labour:
- there is slow descent with a deflexed head and fetal heart audible in the flank or in the midline.

In the second stage of labour:
- delay is common
- on vaginal examination, the anterior fontanelle is felt behind the symphysis pubis
- dilatation of the anus and gaping of the vagina may occur while the fetal head is barely visible; there may also be excessive bulging of the perineum.

The birth

- The sinciput will first emerge from under the symphysis pubis; the midwife maintains flexion to prevent it from escaping further than the glabella.
- The occiput sweeps the perineum and is born.
- The head is then extended to bring the face down from under the symphysis pubis. An episiotomy may be considered in some cases.

Deep transverse arrest

- This occurs when the occiput begins to rotate forwards but flexion is not maintained; the occipitofrontal diameter becomes caught at the narrow bispinous diameter of the outlet.
- Arrest may be due to weak contractions, a straight sacrum or a narrowed outlet.

Diagnosis

On vaginal examination:
- The sagittal suture is in the transverse diameter of the pelvis and both fontanelles are palpable.
- The head is at the level of the ischial spines and there is no advance.

Management

Pushing may not resolve the problem, though a change of position and sighing out slowly (SOS) breathing may help to overcome the urge to bear down.

An assisted vaginal birth may be required to rotate the head to an occipitoanterior position before birth. Adequate analgesia or regional anaesthesia should be given.

Conversion to face or brow presentation

- This occurs when the head is deflexed at the onset of labour and extension occurs instead of flexion.
- Complete extension results in a face presentation; incomplete extension leads to a brow.

Complications

- Prolonged labour with increased likelihood of instrumental vaginal birth
- Obstructed labour
- Maternal perineal trauma
- Neonatal trauma/cerebral haemorrhage
- Cord prolapse

FACE PRESENTATION

The attitude of the head is one of complete extension. It may be primary (presents before labour) or secondary (develops during labour). The denominator is the mentum and the presenting diameters are the submentobregmatic (9.5 cm) and the bitemporal (8.2 cm) (Figs 21.5–21.10).

Causes

- Anterior obliquity of the uterus
- Contracted pelvis
- Polyhydramnios
- Congenital malformation, e.g. anencephaly

Diagnosis during labour

Abdominal palpation

Face presentation may be difficult to diagnose.
- The occiput feels prominent, with a groove between head and back.

Fig. 21.5 Right mentoposterior. **Fig. 21.6** Left mentoposterior.

Fig. 21.7 Right mentolateral. **Fig. 21.8** Left mentolateral.

- The limbs may be palpated on the side opposite to the occiput.
- The fetal heart is best heard through the fetal chest on the same side as the limbs. It is difficult in a mentoposterior position.

Vaginal examination

- The presenting part is high, soft and irregular.
- The orbital ridges, eyes, nose and mouth may be felt.

Fig. 21.9 Right mentoanterior.

Fig. 21.10 Left mentoanterior.

- As labour progresses the face becomes oedematous, making it more difficult to distinguish from a breech presentation.
- Care must be taken not to injure or infect the eyes.

Mechanism of the left mentoanterior position

See Table 21.1.

- *Extension*. Descent takes place with increasing extension. The mentum becomes the leading part.
- *Internal rotation of the head*. This occurs when the chin reaches the pelvic floor and rotates forwards one-eighth of a circle. The chin escapes under the symphysis pubis.
- *Flexion*. Flexion takes place when the sinciput, vertex and occiput sweep the perineum; the head is born.
- *Restitution*. This occurs when the chin turns one-eighth of a circle to the woman's left.
- *Internal rotation of the shoulders*. The shoulders enter the pelvis in the left oblique diameter, and the anterior shoulder reaches the pelvic floor first and rotates forwards one-eighth of a circle along the right side of the pelvis.
- *External rotation of the head*. This occurs simultaneously. The chin moves a further one-eighth of a circle to the left.
- *Lateral flexion*. The anterior shoulder escapes under the symphysis pubis, the posterior shoulder sweeps the perineum and the body is born by a movement of lateral flexion.

Possible course and outcomes of labour

Prolonged labour

This is due to an ill-fitting presenting part and facial bones that do not mould. The fetal axis pressure is directed to the chin and the head is extended almost at right angles to the spine, increasing the diameters to be accommodated in the pelvis.

Mentoanterior positions

With good uterine contractions, descent and rotation of the head occur and labour progresses to a spontaneous birth.

Mentoposterior positions

If the head is completely extended and the contractions are effective, the mentum will rotate forwards and the position becomes anterior.

Persistent mentoposterior position

If the head is incompletely extended and the sinciput reaches the pelvic floor first and rotates forwards one-eighth of a circle, bringing the chin into the hollow of the sacrum, no further mechanism is possible and labour becomes obstructed.

Management of labour

See Box 21.2.

Complications

- Obstructed labour
- Cord prolapse
- Facial bruising/oedema
- Cerebral haemorrhage
- Maternal perineal and vaginal trauma

BROW PRESENTATION

The fetal head is partially extended with the frontal bone (bounded by the anterior fontanelle and the orbital ridges) lying at the pelvic brim. The presenting diameter is the mentovertical (13.5 cm).

Box 21.2 **Management of labour: face presentations**

First stage of labour
- Inform the obstetrician
- Do not apply a fetal scalp electrode and take care not to infect or injure the eyes during vaginal examinations
- Following rupture of the membranes, exclude cord prolapse
- Observe descent of the head by abdominal palpation
- Assess cervical dilatation and descent of the head by vaginal examination every 2–4 hours. In mentoposterior positions, note whether the mentum is lower than the sinciput. If the head remains high in spite of good contractions, caesarean section is likely.

Birth of the head
- When the face appears at the vulva, maintain extension by holding back the sinciput and permitting the mentum to escape under the symphysis pubis before the occiput is allowed to sweep the perineum. In this way, the submentovertical diameter (11.5 cm), instead of the mentovertical diameter (13.5 cm), distends the vaginal orifice
- Because the perineum is also distended by the biparietal diameter (9.5 cm), an elective episiotomy may be considered, but will need the mother to consent to the intervention.
- If the head does not descend in the second stage and is in a mentoanterior position, it may be possible for the obstetrician to assist the baby's birth with forceps; when rotation is incomplete, or the position remains mentoposterior, a rotational forceps may be feasible
- If the head has become impacted, or there is any suspicion of disproportion, a caesarean section will be necessary

Causes

These are the same as for a secondary face presentation; during extension from a vertex presentation to a face presentation, the brow will present temporarily and in a few cases this will persist.

Diagnosis

Brow presentation is not usually detected before the onset of labour.

Abdominal palpation

- The head is high, appears unduly large and does not descend into the pelvis despite good uterine contractions.

Box 21.3 **Management of labour: brow presentations**

- Inform the obstetrician immediately this presentation is suspected; vaginal birth is extremely rare unless the woman has a large pelvis and a small baby
- If there is no evidence of fetal compromise, the woman may be allowed to labour for a short while in case further extension of the head converts the brow presentation to a face presentation
- Occasionally, spontaneous flexion may occur, resulting in a vertex presentation

Vaginal examination

- The presenting part is high.
- The anterior fontanelle may be felt on one side of the pelvis and the orbital ridges, and possibly the root of the nose, at the other.
- A large caput succedaneum may mask these landmarks if the woman has been in labour for some hours.

Management

Management of brow presentations is summarized in Box 21.3.

Complications

These are the same as in a face presentation, except that obstructed labour requiring caesarean section is the probable outcome.

BREECH PRESENTATION

Here the fetus lies longitudinally with the buttocks in the lower pole of the uterus. There are six positions (Figs 21.11–21.16).

Types of breech presentation position

- Breech with extended legs (frank breech) (Fig. 21.17)
- Complete breech (Fig. 21.18)
- Footling breech (Fig. 21.19)
- Knee presentation (Fig. 21.20)

Fig. 21.11 Right sacroposterior.

Fig. 21.12 Left sacroposterior.

Fig. 21.13 Right sacrolateral.

Fig. 21.14 Left sacrolateral.

Causes

Often no cause is identified, but the following circumstances favour breech presentation:

- extended legs
- preterm labour

Fig. 21.15 Right sacroanterior.

Fig. 21.16 Left sacroanterior.

Fig. 21.17 Frank breech.

Fig. 21.18 Complete breech.

- multiple pregnancy
- polyhydramnios
- hydrocephaly
- uterine malformations
- placenta praevia.

Fig. 21.20 Knee presentation.

Fig. 21.19 Footling presentation.

Antenatal diagnosis

Abdominal examination

Palpation

The lie is longitudinal with a soft presentation, which is more easily felt using Pawlik's grip. However, this is usually uncomfortable for the mother. It is important that she has an empty bladder to minimize discomfort.

- The head can usually be felt in the fundus as a round hard mass, which may be made to move independently of the back by ballottement with one or both hands.
- If the legs are extended, the feet may prevent such nodding.
- When the breech is anterior and the fetus well flexed, it may be difficult to locate the head, but use of the combined grip, in which the upper and lower poles are grasped simultaneously, may aid diagnosis.
- The woman may complain of discomfort under her ribs, especially at night, owing to pressure of the head on the diaphragm.

Auscultation

- When the breech has not passed through the pelvic brim, the fetal heart is heard most clearly above the umbilicus.
- When the legs are extended, the breech descends into the pelvis easily. The fetal heart is then heard at a lower level.

Ultrasound examination

- This may be used to demonstrate a breech presentation.

X-ray examination

This has now been superseded by ultrasound in resource rich countries.

Diagnosis during labour

Abdominal examination

- Breech presentation is sometimes missed antenatally and is diagnosed when the woman is in labour.

Vaginal examination

- The breech feels soft and irregular with no sutures palpable.
- The anus may be felt and fresh meconium on the examining finger is usually diagnostic.
- If the legs are extended (Fig. 21.21), the external genitalia are very evident but it must be remembered that these become oedematous.
- The heel of a foot must be differentiated from a hand (Fig. 21.22).

Presentation may be confirmed by ultrasound scan.

Antenatal management

If the midwife suspects or detects a breech presentation at 36 weeks' gestation or later, she should refer the woman to an obstetrician.

Fig. 21.21 No feet felt; the legs are extended.

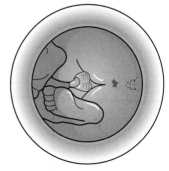

Fig. 21.22 Feet felt; complete breech presentation.

There are differing opinions among obstetricians as to the management of breech presentation during pregnancy and a decision on management is usually deferred until near term.

External cephalic version

External cephalic version (ECV) involves external manipulation on the mother's abdomen to convert a breech to a cephalic presentation. ECV may be offered at term and should only be undertaken in a unit where there are facilities for emergency caesarean section. Contraindications include:

- pre-eclampsia or hypertension
- multiple pregnancy
- oligohydramnios
- ruptured membranes
- a hydrocephalic fetus
- any condition that would require birth by caesarean section.

Persistent breech presentation

At 37 weeks' gestation, a discussion of the available options should take place between the mother and an experienced practitioner, and a decision made as to whether to perform an elective caesarean section or to attempt a vaginal birth.

Assessment for vaginal birth

Any doubt as to the capacity of the pelvis to accommodate the fetal head must be resolved before the buttocks are born and the head attempts to enter the pelvic brim.

Fetal size

This, especially in relation to maternal size, can be assessed on abdominal palpation but is more accurately judged in association with an ultrasound examination.

Pelvic capacity

- Can be judged on vaginal assessment.
- Provides information on the shape of the sacrum, as well as a clinical judgement of the anteroposterior diameters of the pelvic brim, cavity and outlet.
- In a multigravida, information about the type of birth and the size of previous babies when compared with the size of the present fetus can be helpful.

Mechanism of the left sacroanterior position

This is described in Table 21.1.

- *Compaction*. Descent takes place with increasing compaction, owing to increased flexion of the limbs.
- *Internal rotation of the buttocks*. The anterior buttock reaches the pelvic floor first and rotates forwards one-eighth of a circle along the right side of the pelvis to lie underneath the symphysis pubis. The bitrochanteric diameter is now in the anteroposterior diameter of the outlet.
- *Lateral flexion of the body*. The anterior buttock escapes under the symphysis pubis, the posterior buttock sweeps the perineum and the buttocks are born by a movement of lateral flexion.
- *Restitution of the buttocks*. The anterior buttock turns slightly to the mother's right side.
- *Internal rotation of the shoulders*. The shoulders enter the pelvis in the same oblique diameter as the buttocks, the left oblique. The anterior shoulder rotates forwards one-eighth of a circle along the right side of the pelvis and escapes under the symphysis pubis, the posterior shoulder sweeps the perineum and the shoulders are born.
- *Internal rotation of the head*. The head enters the pelvis with the sagittal suture in the transverse diameter of the brim. The occiput rotates forwards along the left side and the suboccipital region (the nape) impinges on the undersurface of the symphysis pubis.
- *External rotation of the body*. At the same time the body turns so that the back is uppermost.
- *Birth of the head*. The chin, face and sinciput sweep the perineum and the head is born in a flexed attitude.

Fig. 21.23A–H summarizes the spontaneous manoeuvres for a vaginal breech (with extended legs) birth.

Management of labour

Careful assessment should be made at the start of labour and anticipated labour management should be reviewed (Box 21.4). A consultant obstetrician should be informed of a breech presentation in labour, even if the woman is birthing at home in case transfer to hospital is necessary.

- Breech births follow the same physiological process as any other spontaneous vaginal birth. It is therefore important not to interfere unnecessarily with the process of labour.

317

Breech Birth

Fig. 21.23 Spontaneous vaginal breech birth with extended legs. (A) Breech with extended legs engaging in left sacrum anterior (LSA) position. (B) Descent of the breech with the left sacrum transverse (LST) position. Note the anterior buttock is the leading part. (C) Birth of the anterior buttock (this emerges first) as it follows the curve of carus. Note that the body of the baby should rotate to sacro-anterior. (D) Spontaneous birth of the extended fetal legs; occurs in the presence of effective uterine contractions followed by progressive descent. It is important not to rush the process. Watchful waiting should be the norm if all is progressing well. (E) Birth of the legs and visualization of the umbilicus. Avoid touching the umbilicus but do observe the baby for: tone, colour, movement or flexion. If full rotation has not occurred and there is no sign of progress, assistance with birth of the arms will be required. A second midwife/scribe is advisable to document the timing/sequence of events as they unfold. (F) Note spontaneous rotation to bring the anterior arm below the pubic arch. (G) Complete birth of the fetal arms. Note baby's abdomen is facing maternal buttocks/(back is uppermost) 'tum to bum'. (H) Birth of the head (attitude is that of flexion).

> Box 21.4 **Management of labour: breech presentations**
>
> **First stage of labour**
>
> - Basic care during this stage is the same as in normal labour
> - Meconium-stained liquor is sometimes found owing to compression of the fetal abdomen and is not always a sign of fetal compromise
> - A vaginal examination should be performed to exclude cord prolapse as soon as the membranes rupture. If they do not rupture spontaneously at an early stage, it is considered safer to leave them intact until labour is well established and the breech is at the level of the ischial spines.
>
> **Second stage of labour**
>
> - Full dilatation of the cervix should always be confirmed by vaginal examination before the woman commences active pushing
> - In hospital, inform the obstetrician of the onset of the second stage
> - A paediatrician should be present for the birth
> - Inform the anaesthetist too in case a general anaesthetic is required
> - Active pushing is commenced when the buttocks are distending the vulva. Failure of the breech to descend onto the perineum in the second stage despite good contractions may indicate a need for caesarean section.

Types of vaginal birth

- *Spontaneous breech birth.* The birth occurs with little or no assistance from the midwife or obstetrician, whose hands are kept poised to receive the baby.
- *Assisted breech birth.* The buttocks are born spontaneously, but some assistance is necessary for birth of extended legs or arms and the head.
- *Breech extraction.* This is a manipulative procedure carried out by an obstetrician and is employed to hasten birth in an emergency situation such as fetal compromise.

Management of breech birth

- *When the buttocks are distending the perineum,* the woman is upright (i.e. kneeling or 'all fours' position). This is especially the case if the woman is at home or in a midwifery-led unit following her own instinct. The lithotomy position is commonly employed if birth is in the hospital setting.
- The bladder must be empty and it is usually catheterized at this stage. In the hospital setting, if epidural analgesia is not being used, the perineum is infiltrated with local anaesthesia in line with local protocol if an episiotomy is to be performed (pudendal block is sometimes used by an obstetrician).
- The buttocks are born spontaneously.
- If the legs are flexed, the feet disengage at the vulva and the baby is born as far as the umbilicus.
- It is best not to handle the umbilical cord unless absolutely necessary; it is more prudent to observe the baby's colour, tone, flexion or movement and fullness of the cord.
- In a flexed breech the arms are usually flexed and tend to be born spontaneously providing there is good descent with the next uterine contraction, and there is no unnecessary interference from the midwife. However, if they do not emerge spontaneously, the midwife should feel for the elbows, if the arms are not felt on the chest of the fetus, they are extended.

Birth of the shoulders

- The shoulders should rotate into the anteroposterior diameter of the pelvic outlet.
- When the anterior shoulder has escaped, the buttocks are lifted towards the mother's abdomen to enable the posterior shoulder and arm to pass over the perineum.

- The head enters the pelvic brim and descends through the pelvis with the sagittal suture in the transverse diameter.

Birth of the head

- The baby's abdomen should be in the direction of the mother's buttocks ('tum to bum') once the arms have been born via the physiological process of internal rotation.
- Once external rotation of the back has been observed, the baby's body should be allowed to hang unsupported.
- The baby's weight brings the head onto the pelvic floor on which the occiput rotates forwards.
- The sagittal suture is now in the anteroposterior diameter of the outlet.
- A well-flexed head should pass through the pelvis unimpeded.
- However, if descent of the head is not realized with the next uterine contraction and progress appears to be arrested, especially if baby's colour and tone are not reassuring, assisting the birth of the head will be required. This can be realized in a number of ways:
  - If rotation of the head fails to take place, two fingers should be placed on the malar bones and the head rotated.
  - The baby can be allowed to hang unimpeded by his/her own weight for 1 or 2 minutes.
- Gradually the neck elongates, the hairline appears and the suboccipital region can be felt.

Controlled birth of the head is vital to avoid any sudden change in intracranial pressure and subsequent cerebral haemorrhage.

There are three methods:
- forceps birth
- Burns Marshall method (if the head is flexed – mainly employed by the obstetrician)
- Mauriceau–Smellie–Veit manoeuvre (jaw flexion and shoulder traction).

Forceps birth

Most breech births are performed by an obstetrician, who will apply forceps to the after-coming head for better control.

Burns Marshall method (least favoured by midwives)

- With the left hand, grasp the baby's ankles from behind with forefinger between the two (Fig. 21.24A).

Ⓐ   Ⓑ

Fig. 21.24 Burns Marshall method of facilitating birth of the after-coming head of a breech presentation. (A) The baby is grasped by the feet and held on the stretch. (B) The mouth and nose are free. The vault of the head is delivered slowly.

- The baby is kept on the stretch with sufficient traction to prevent the neck from bending backwards and being fractured.
- The suboccipital region, and not the neck, should pivot under the apex of the pubic arch or the spinal cord may be crushed.
- The feet are taken up through an arc of 180° until the mouth and nose are free at the vulva.
- The right hand may support perineum to prevent sudden escape of the head. The mother should be asked to take deliberate, regular breaths that allow the vault of the skull to escape gradually (Fig. 21.24B).

Mauriceau–Smellie–Veit manoeuvre (more suitable for midwives)
- This is mainly used when there is delay in descent of the head because of extension.
- The baby is laid astride the right arm with the palm supporting the chest. Two fingers are placed on the malar bones.
- Two fingers of the left hand are hooked over the shoulders, with the middle finger pushing on the occiput to aid flexion.
- Traction is applied to help birth the head from the vagina.
- When the suboccipital region appears, the body is lifted to assist the head to pivot around the symphysis pubis.
- The speed of delivery of the head must be controlled so that it does not emerge suddenly.

Use of uterotonics for third stage
- These are withheld until the head is born.

Birth of extended legs
- Delay may occur at the outlet because the legs splint the body and impede lateral flexion of the spine.
- When the popliteal fossae appear at the vulva, two fingers are placed along the length of one thigh with the fingertips in the fossa.
- The leg is swept to the side of the abdomen (abducting the hip) and the knee is flexed by the pressure on its undersurface. As this movement is continued, the lower part of the leg will emerge from the vagina (Fig. 21.25).
- Repeat to release the second leg. The knee is a hinge joint, which bends in one direction only. If the knee is pulled forwards from the abdomen, severe injury to the joint can result.

Birth of extended arms
Extended arms are diagnosed when the elbows are not felt on the chest after the umbilicus is born. This may be dealt with by using the Løvset manoeuvre (Figs 21.26 and 21.27). This is a combination of rotation and downward traction to free the arms, whatever position they are in. The direction of rotation must always bring the back uppermost and the arms emerge from under the pubic arch.
- When the umbilicus is born and the shoulders are in the anteroposterior diameter, the baby is grasped by the iliac crests with the thumbs over the sacrum.

Fig. 21.25 Assisting birth of extended leg by pressure on the popliteal fossa.

Fig. 21.26 Correct grasp for Løvset manoeuvre.

Fig. 21.27 Løvset manoeuvre for birth of extended arms (see text).

- Downward traction is applied until the axilla is visible.
- Maintaining downward traction throughout, the body is rotated through a half-circle, 180°, starting by turning the back uppermost.
- The friction of the posterior arm against the pubic bone as the shoulder becomes anterior sweeps the arm in front of the face. The movement allows the shoulders to enter the pelvis in the transverse diameter.
- The first two fingers of the hand that is on the same side as the baby's back are used to splint the humerus and draw it down over the chest as the elbow is flexed.
- The body is now rotated back in the opposite direction and the second arm emerges in a similar fashion.

Delay in birth of the head

- *Extended head.* If, when the body has been allowed to hang, the neck and hairline are not visible, it is probable that the head is extended. This may be dealt with by the use of forceps (if assisted by obstetrician in the hospital setting) or the Mauriceau–Smellie–Veit manoeuvre (can be used by either the midwife or obstetrician).

Complications

- Impacted breech
- Cord prolapse
- Birth injury:
  - superficial tissue damage
  - fractures of humerus, clavicle or femur or dislocation of shoulder or hip
  - Erb palsy
  - trauma to internal organs
  - damage to the adrenals
  - spinal cord damage or fracture of the spine
  - intracranial haemorrhage
  - fetal hypoxia
  - premature separation of the placenta
  - maternal trauma

The maternal complications of a vaginal breech birth are the same as those found in other operative vaginal births.

SHOULDER PRESENTATION

When the fetus lies with its long axis across the long axis of the uterus (*transverse lie*), the shoulder is most likely to present. Occasionally the lie is oblique but this does not persist, as the uterine contractions during labour make it longitudinal or transverse.

Causes

Maternal

- Lax abdominal and uterine muscles
- Uterine abnormality
- Contracted pelvis

Fetal

- Preterm pregnancy
- Multiple pregnancy
- Polyhydramnios
- Macerated fetus
- Placenta praevia

Antenatal diagnosis

Abdominal palpation

- The uterus appears broad and the fundal height is less than expected for the period of gestation.
- On pelvic and fundal palpation, neither head nor breech is felt. The mobile head is found on one side of the abdomen and the breech at a slightly higher level on the other.

Ultrasound

An ultrasound scan may be used to confirm the lie and presentation.

Diagnosis during labour

Abdominal palpation

- The findings are as previously mentioned but when the membranes have ruptured the irregular outline of the uterus is more marked.
- If the uterus is contracting strongly and becomes moulded around the fetus, palpation is very difficult.
- The pelvis is no longer empty, the shoulder being wedged into it.

Vaginal examination

- This should not be performed without first excluding placenta praevia.
- In early labour, the presenting part may not be felt.
- The membranes usually rupture early.
- If the labour has been in progress for some time, the shoulder may be felt as a soft irregular mass.
- It is sometimes possible to palpate the ribs, their characteristic grid-iron pattern being diagnostic.
- When the shoulder enters the pelvic brim, an arm may prolapse; this should be differentiated from a leg.

Possible outcomes of labour

If shoulder presentation persists in labour, birth must be by caesarean section to avoid obstructed labour and subsequent uterine rupture.

Management

Antenatal

- Identifying the cause is important before deciding on a course of management.
- Once placenta praevia or uterine abnormalities have been excluded, ECV may be attempted.
- If ECV fails, or if the lie is again transverse at the next antenatal visit, the woman is admitted to hospital while further investigations into the cause are made and frequently remains hospitalized until birth because of the risk of cord prolapse.

Intrapartum

- If a transverse lie is detected in early labour while the membranes are still intact, the obstetrician or competent health professional may attempt an ECV, followed, if this is successful, by a controlled rupture of the membranes.
- If the membranes have already ruptured spontaneously, a vaginal examination must be performed immediately to exclude cord prolapse.

Immediate caesarean section must be performed:
- if the cord prolapses
- when the membranes are already ruptured
- when ECV is unsuccessful
- when labour has already been in progress for some hours.

Complications

- Prolapsed cord
- Prolapsed arm
- Impacted shoulder presentation leading to obstructed labour, ruptured uterus and stillbirth

UNSTABLE LIE

The lie is defined as unstable when, after 36 weeks' gestation, instead of remaining longitudinal, it varies from one examination to another between longitudinal and oblique or transverse.

Causes

Conditions that increase the mobility of the fetus or prevent the head from entering the pelvic brim can cause an unstable lie.

Maternal causes include:
- lax uterine muscles in multigravidae
- contracted pelvis.

Fetal causes include:
- polyhydramnios
- placenta praevia.

Management

Antenatal

- Advise the woman to go to the labour ward as soon as labour commences or membranes rupture.
- Exclude placenta praevia.
- Attempts to correct the abnormal presentation by ECV may be made. If unsuccessful, caesarean section is considered.

Intrapartum

- Labour may be induced after 38 weeks' gestation, having first ensured that the lie is longitudinal.
- An empty bladder and rectum are important.
- A controlled rupture of the membranes is performed so that the head enters the pelvis.

The abdomen is palpated at frequent intervals to ensure that the lie remains longitudinal and to assess the descent of the head.

Complications

- If labour commences with the lie other than longitudinal, the complications are the same as for a transverse lie.

COMPOUND PRESENTATION

- A compound presentation is when a hand, or occasionally a foot, lies alongside the head.
- If diagnosed during the first stage of labour, medical aid must be sought.
- If, during the second stage, the midwife sees a hand presenting alongside the vertex, she could try to hold the hand back.

SUGGESTED READING

Guittier, M.G., Othenin-Girard, V., Irion, O., et al., 2014. Maternal positioning to correct occipito-posterior fetal position in labour: a randomised controlled trial. BMC Pregnancy Childbirth 14, 83. Available at: http://www.biomedcentral.com/1471-2393/14/83 (accessed 10 April 2016).

Walker, S., Scamell, M., Parker, P., 2016. Standards for maternity care professionals attending planned upright breech births: a Delphi study. Midwifery 34, 7–14. doi: 10.1016/j.midw.2016.01.007.

Szaboova, R., Sankaran, S., Harding, K., et al., 2014. PLD.23 Management of transverse and unstable lie at term. Arch. Dis. Child. Fetal Neonatal Ed. 99 (Suppl. 1), A112–A113. doi: 10.1136/archdischild-2014-306576.324. Available at: http://www.bmj.com (accessed 10 April 2016).

Useful website

National Institute for Health and Care Excellence. Available at: http://www.nice.org.uk Provides useful evidence guidelines for practice such as induction of labour.

Operative Births

OPERATIVE VAGINAL BIRTHS

Birth by forceps

Forceps might be employed to expedite birth in the following instances:

Fetal
- Malposition of the fetal head (occipitolateral and occipitoposterior).
- Presumed fetal compromise when the cervix is fully dilated.
- Assisted vaginal breech birth to facilitate the emergence of the after-coming head in order to control the birth of the vertex.
- Occasionally used to free the vertex from the pelvis at caesarean section birth.

Maternal
- Maternal distress/exhaustion or prolongation of the second stage of labour.
- Some medically significant conditions such as aortic valve disorder with major outflow obstruction.

Types of obstetric forceps

Wrigley forceps
- Designed for use in outlet lift-out when the head is on the perineum.
- Used for the after-coming head in an assisted vaginal breech birth.
- Can be employed at caesarean section to assist the birth of the fetal head.

Neville-Barnes or Simpson forceps
- Generally employed for a low or mid-cavity forceps birth when the sagittal suture is in the anteroposterior diameter of the cavity of the pelvis.

Kielland forceps
- More commonly used for the rotation and extraction of the fetal head that is in the deep transverse or the occipitoposterior position.

Box 22.1 **Some complications of forceps birth**

Maternal

- Trauma or soft tissue damage, which may occur to the perineum, vagina or cervix
- Haemorrhage from the above
- Dysuria or urinary retention, which may result from bruising or oedema to the urethra
- Painful perineum

Neonatal

- Marks on the baby's face caused by the pressure of the forceps; these resolve quite rapidly
- Excessive bruising
- Facial palsy

- Due to the risk of maternal genital tract trauma, only skilled obstetricians should use these forceps; they are increasingly being abandoned in many consultant-led units in resource rich countries.

Complications

These are listed in Box 22.1.

BIRTH BY VENTOUSE

The ventouse or vacuum extractor (made from metal or plastic) is essentially a suction cup that is connected via tubing to a vacuum source. It is applied to the fetal head to allow traction to be applied to assist the birth, can be used as an alternative to forceps, and is very much determined by the obstetrician's preference.

Relative contraindications to ventouse birth

- Suspected fetal macrosomia
- Excessive caput or moulding
- Prematurity – gestation < 34 completed weeks
- Poor maternal effort especially in the presence of maternal exhaustion where there is regional analgesia (epidural) with poor sensation
- Fetal bleeding disorders (e.g. alloimmune thrombocytopenia)

Absolute contraindications for both forceps and ventouse birth

- An operator inexperienced in instrumental vaginal births
- The vertex is ≥ 1/5th palpable abdominally
- The position of the fetal head (occipitoanterior/posterior or lateral) cannot be determined on vaginal examination
- Before full dilatation of the cervix (forceps only)

TYPES OF VENTOUSE

Soft or silicone cup design (Fig. 22.1A)
- is malleable, thus reducing incidence of maternal genital tract and fetal head trauma
- has a poorer success rate in achieving a vaginal birth than the metal cup.

Metal cup design (Bird or Malstrom)
- has a centrally placed traction chain with a laterally located vacuum conduit
- is available in a variety of diameters: 4, 5 and 6 cm.

Both the soft/silicone designs and the metal cups require the use of vacuum generated from an external source operated by a second practitioner. Consequently, they are less frequently used due to more recent advances in design that have removed the need for the external suction generators by incorporating the vacuum mechanism into 'hand held' pumps (e.g. Kiwi OmniCup), as illustrated in Fig. 22.1B.

Procedure

- Information and explanation is provided to obtain informed consent.
- The woman's legs are usually placed in the lithotomy position and the same precautions are observed as for a forceps birth.
- Adequate analgesia is assured prior to the bladder being emptied via catherization.
- Continuous electronic fetal heart rate monitoring is implemented throughout the procedure.
- Successful birth by ventouse is dependent on the location of the flexion point of the fetal head as the centre of the cup needs to be placed directly over this area.
- The operating vacuum pressure for almost all ventouse is usually between 0.6 and 0.8 kg/cm^2.
- When the vacuum is achieved, traction must be applied in the presence of a uterine contraction and subsequent maternal expulsive or bearing down efforts. Successful birth via ventouse is only realized with these two combined factors.

333

Fig. 22.1 (A) The soft cup ventouse; (B) the Kiwi OmniCup. (With permission from Marshall, J., Raynor, M. (Eds.), 2014. Myles Textbook for Midwives, 16th ed. Churchill Livingstone, London.)

- Traction is applied to follow the *curve of carus,* initially in a downward and backwards direction followed by a forward and upwards direction.
- The vacuum is released and the cup is removed at the crowning of the fetal head.
- Further maternal efforts result in the birth of the baby.

Complications

Prolonged traction will increase the likelihood of:

- scalp abrasions
- cephalhaematoma
- subaponeurotic bleeding.

CAESAREAN SECTION

Caesarean section (CS) is an operative procedure that is carried out under anaesthesia (regional or general), whereby the fetus, placenta and membranes are delivered through an incision in the abdominal wall and the uterus.

Preparation

Women expect to be actively involved in their care and the midwife must ensure that recent, valid and relevant information is provided.

The usual preoperative preparation is observed, including:

- The woman is fully informed and clear about the rationale for the procedure and consent has been obtained.
- An anaesthetic chart/preoperative assessment has been carried out.
- Measurement of weight has been taken.
- Baseline blood pressure, pulse, respiration and temperature has been observed.
- The woman is gowned, make-up and jewellery removed (wedding ring can be taped in line with local protocol).
- Every effort has been taken to ensure maternal safety such as the attachment of identification wristbands.
- Results are obtained of any blood tests that have been requested and a full blood count is carried out. Blood is grouped and saved.
- In the case of pre-eclampsia, urea and electrolyte levels has been examined and clotting factors assessed.
- With elective CS, the woman has fasted within the specified timeframe and taken the prescribed antacid therapy.
- To minimize discomfort the woman may choose to have her bladder catheterized in theatre once the regional or general anaesthetic is administered, or in her allocated hospital room where it may be more private.
- Infection control measures are implemented; the operative area of the skin is cleansed in accordance with local and national guidelines and intravenous antibiotics administered prior to skin

335

> Box 22.2 **Some indications for elective caesarean section**
>
> **Definite**
> - Cephalopelvic disproportion
> - Major degree of placenta praevia
> - High-order multiple pregnancy
>
> **Possible**
> - Breech presentation
> - Moderate to severe pre-eclampsia
> - A medical condition that warrants the exclusion of maternal effort
> - Diabetes mellitus
> - Intrauterine growth restriction
> - Antepartum haemorrhage
> - Certain fetal abnormalities (e.g. hydrocephalus)

incision. This approach is deemed more efficacious in preventing/minimizing infection than prophylactic antibiotics post-CS.

Positioning of the woman

As the woman will need to lie flat, it is essential that a wedge or cushion is used, or the table is tilted, to direct the weight of the gravid uterus away from the inferior vena cava and so avoid supine hypotensive syndrome.

Elective caesarean section

This implies that the decision to carry out the procedure has been taken during the pregnancy; therefore, before labour has commenced.

Indications for elective caesarean section are shown in Box 22.2.

Emergency caesarean section

This is carried out when adverse conditions develop during pregnancy or labour. Some examples of urgent/emergency reasons for caesarean birth are given in Box 22.3.

Vaginal birth after caesarean section (VBAC)

If the indication for caesarean section has been a non-recurring one (for example, placenta praevia), VBAC may be attempted after full discussion with, and agreement by the woman.

Box 22.3 **Some indications for emergency caesarean section**

- Antepartum haemorrhage
- Cord prolapse
- Uterine rupture (dramatic/scar dehiscence)
- Cephalopelvic disproportion diagnosed in labour
- Fulminating pre-eclampsia, eclampsia
- Failure to progress in the first or second stage of labour
- Fetal compromise if birth is not imminent

Criteria for successful VBAC are:
- Adequate supervision and care throughout labour to optimize and support the physiological processes involved.
- Continuous electronic fetal heart rate monitoring once the woman is in active labour.
- Ensuring that the progress of the labour is sufficient both in the descent of the presenting part and the dilatation of the cervix.
- All maternal vital signs (BP, temperature, pulse, respiration and temperature) are within normal parameters.
- There is clear liquor if the membranes rupture.
- The woman is fully informed of the benefits and risks.
- All the facilities for assisted birth are readily available.

Anaesthesia

Regional anaesthesia (epidural and intrathecal/spinal) normally remains the safer option for caesarean birth; however, general anaesthesia (GA) is sometimes required. Some reasons are:
- Regional anaesthesia is incompatible with any maternal coagulation disorder.
- GA can be more rapidly administered and is therefore invaluable when speed is of the essence, as when the fetus/woman is in serious jeopardy.
- Some women choose general rather than regional anaesthesia.

Mendelson syndrome

This is caused if acid gastric contents are inhaled and result in a chemical pneumonitis. This regurgitation may occur during the induction of a general anaesthetic. The acidic gastric contents damage the

337

alveoli, impairing gaseous exchange, and death may result if it becomes impossible to oxygenate the woman.

Prevention of Mendelson syndrome

Antacid therapy

- Prophylactic administration of antacids should be routine in all women having a planned or anticipated CS.
- A usual regimen is for women having an elective or anticipatory operation to be given two doses of oral ranitidine 150 mg approximately 8 hours apart.
- 30 ml sodium citrate should be administered orally immediately prior to the anaesthesia.

Cricoid pressure

- This is a technique applied during intubation to prevent acid reflux, achieved by applying pressure on the cartilaginous ring below the larynx, i.e. the cricoid, to occlude the oesophagus.

Complications associated with caesarean section

- Infection, e.g. wound, intrauterine, urinary tract and pelvic infections, thrombophlebitis
- Thromboembolic disorders
- Postpartum haemorrhage

Postoperative care

Immediate care

If GA used – maintain cardiopulmonary stability, airway management until airway control is achieved and woman is able to communicate effectively.

If the mother intends to breastfeed, skin-to-skin contact with the mother should be facilitated and assistance with breastfeeding provided as soon as possible and before the woman leaves the recovery room. Ideally, the baby should remain with the mother and they should be transferred to the postnatal ward together.

Observations

- Blood pressure and pulse should be recorded every 15 minutes in the immediate recovery period (for the first 30 minutes) then hourly thereafter if the observations remain stable.
- Temperature should be recorded every 2 hours.

- Lochia and the wound should be inspected every half hour.
- Following GA, level of consciousness and respirations should be monitored.
- Women who have had intrathecal (spinal) opioids will require hourly observation of respiration as a minimum, including sedation level and pain scores for at least 12 hours when Diamorphine (or other narcotic medication) has been administered.
- Women who have had epidural opioids or patient-controlled analgesia (PCA) with opioids will also require respiratory rate, sedation and pain score monitoring throughout the therapy and for at least 2 hours following discontinuation of the treatment.
- All observations must be recorded.

Analgesia and antiemetics

Analgesia is prescribed and given on a regular basis or as required, for example:
- ongoing epidural anaesthesia/analgesia.

PCA using opioid analgesics

- Analgesia, e.g. diclofenac (oral or rectal) or paracetamol (IV, oral or rectal) are the mainstays of postoperative analgesia in many Western high-income countries
- Nonsteroidal anti-inflammatory drugs (NSAIDs) can be used as an adjunct to other analgesics post-CS, as they help to reduce the need for opioids
- NSAIDs are contraindicated where there is a history of:
  - kidney disease
  - sensitivity to NSAIDs
  - peptic ulcer
  - asthma.

Antiemetics (e.g. cyclizine, prochlorperazine) are usually prescribed when opioids are in use.

Care following regional block

- Following epidural or spinal anaesthesia the woman may sit up as soon as she wishes, provided her blood pressure is not low.

Care in the postnatal ward

- Blood pressure, temperature and pulse are usually checked every 4 hours.

- The urinary catheter may remain in situ until the woman is able to get up to the toilet. Urinary output should be monitored after removal of the catheter. Any haematuria must be reported to the doctor.
- The wound and lochia must initially be observed at least hourly.
- Leg and breathing exercises are encouraged.
- Thrombo-embolic prophylaxis – prophylactic low-dose heparin and TED antiembolism stockings are often prescribed.
- Appropriate analgesia must be given as frequently as necessary.
- Help may be needed with care for the baby.
- The woman may value talking about her feelings.

KEY READING

Hook, C.D., Damos, J.R., 2008. Vacuum-assisted vaginal delivery. Am. Fam. Physician 78 (8), 953–960. Available at: http://www.aafp.org (accessed 13 April 2016).

Royal College of Obstetrician and Gynaecologists, 2015. Birth after caesarean section birth. Green-top guideline No. 45. Available at: http://www.rcog.org.uk (accessed 11 April 2016).

Useful websites

Advanced Life Support in Obstetrics (ALSO) produces a useful 'ABCDEFGHIJ' mnemonic via a poster that spells out the key principles to follow for birth by forceps/ventouse. Available at: https://nf.aafp.org/Shop/advanced-life-support-in-obstetrics/forceps-poster

National Institute for Health and Care Excellence provides helpful guidelines on caesarean section. Available at: http://www.nice.org.uk

Midwifery and Obstetric Emergencies

VASA PRAEVIA

The term *vasa praevia* is used when a fetal blood vessel lies over the os, in front of the presenting part. This occurs when fetal vessels from a velamentous insertion of the cord, or to a succenturiate lobe, cross the area of the internal os to the placenta.

Ruptured vasa praevia

When the membranes rupture in a case of vasa praevia, a fetal vessel may also rupture. This may result in exsanguination of the fetus unless birth occurs within minutes.

Diagnosis

- May be diagnosed antenatally via ultrasound scan.
  - Slight fresh vaginal bleeding, particularly if it commences at the same time as rupture of the membranes.
  - Vasa praevia may sometimes be palpated on vaginal examination when the membranes are still intact.
  - If it is suspected, a speculum examination should be made.
- Signs of fetal compromise disproportionate to blood loss.

Management

See Box 23.1.

PRESENTATION AND PROLAPSE OF THE UMBILICAL CORD

See Box 23.2 for definitions.

Predisposing factors

Any situation where the presenting part is neither well applied to the lower uterine segment nor well down in the pelvis may make it possible

---

Box 23.1 **Management of vasa praevia**

- Request urgent medical aid
- Continuous electronic monitoring of the fetal heart rate if in the hospital setting
- Arrange for immediate transfer if the mother is at home
- If the mother is in the first stage of labour and the fetus is still alive, an emergency caesarean section is carried out
- If in the second stage of labour, birth should be expedited; the mode of birth will be dependent on factors such as parity and fetal condition
- A paediatrician should be present at birth. If the baby is alive, haemoglobin (Hb) estimation will be necessary after resuscitation as a blood transfusion may be required
- Paired cord blood samples will be taken

Box 23.2 **Definitions**

Cord presentation

- The umbilical cord lies in front of the presenting part, with the fetal membranes still intact

Cord prolapse

- The cord lies in front of the presenting part and the fetal membranes are ruptured

Occult cord prolapse

- The cord lies alongside, but not in front of, the presenting part

---

for a loop of cord to slip down in front of the presenting part. Such situations include:

- high or ill-fitting presenting part
- high parity
- prematurity
- malpresentation
- multiple pregnancy
- polyhydramnios.

The contributory factors outlined previously are the same for both cord presentation and cord prolapse.

342

Box 23.3 **Management of cord presentation**

- Under no circumstances should the membranes be ruptured
- Summon medical aid
- Assess fetal wellbeing, using continuous electronic fetal monitoring if available
- Help the mother into a position that will reduce the likelihood of cord compression
- Caesarean section is the most likely outcome

Cord presentation

This is diagnosed on vaginal examination when the cord is felt behind intact membranes. It is, however, rarely detected but may be associated with aberrations in fetal heart monitoring such as decelerations, which occur if the cord becomes compressed.

Management

See Box 23.3.

Cord prolapse

Diagnosis

- Diagnosis is made when the cord is felt below or beside the presenting part on vaginal examination.
- A loop of cord may be visible at the vulva.
- Whenever there are factors present that predispose to cord prolapse, a vaginal examination should be performed immediately on spontaneous rupture of membranes.
- Bradycardia, variable decelerations and prolonged decelerations of the fetal heart are associated with cord compression, which may be caused by cord prolapse.

Immediate action and management

See Box 23.4.

SHOULDER DYSTOCIA

Definition

- The term 'shoulder dystocia' describes failure of the shoulders to traverse the pelvis spontaneously after birth of the head. A

343

Box 23.4 **Management of cord prolapse**

Immediate action

- Call for urgent assistance and record the time
- Effective communication/explanation to the woman of findings and emergency measures that will be implemented
- If an oxytocin infusion is in progress, this should be stopped
- A vaginal examination is performed to assess the degree of cervical dilatation and identify the presenting part and station. If the cord can be felt pulsating, it should be handled as little as possible
- Auscultate the fetal heart rate
- Relieve pressure on the cord
- The examiner's fingers remain in the woman's vagina and, especially during a contraction, to prevent the presenting part from compressing the umbilical cord
- Help the mother to change position so that her pelvis and buttocks are raised
  - The knee–chest position causes the fetus to gravitate towards the diaphragm, relieving the compression on the cord
  - Alternatively, help the mother to lie on her left side, with a wedge or pillow elevating her hips (exaggerated Sims position)
- The foot of the bed may be raised
- These measures need to be maintained until the birth of the baby, either vaginally or by caesarean section
- Consider inserting 500 ml of warm saline into the bladder to relieve the pressure/cord compression, especially useful if the woman is at home or midwife-led unit and transfer to an obstetric unit is required

Treatment

- Birth must be expedited with the greatest possible speed to reduce morbidity/mortality
- Caesarean section is the treatment of choice if the fetus is still alive and vaginal birth is not imminent
- In the second stage of labour, with a multiparous woman, the mother may be able to push and the birth expedited with the aid of an episiotomy if the presenting part is distending the perineum
- Where the presentation is cephalic, assisted birth may be achieved through ventouse or forceps
- A practitioner experienced in advanced resuscitation of the neonate should be present for the birth

universally accepted definition is not yet accounted for in the literature.
- The anterior shoulder becomes trapped behind or on the symphysis pubis, whilst the posterior shoulder may be in the hollow of the sacrum or high above the sacral promontory. This is, therefore, a bony dystocia, and traction at this point will further impact the anterior shoulder, impeding attempts at birth.
- It is a rare and unpredictable complication of vaginal births.

Risk factors

Antenatal

Antenatal risk factors provide an imprecise assessment of the likely occurrence of shoulder dystocia during labour. Therefore, its presentation in the majority of cases is unexpected and unpredictable. Several factors may be implicated such as:
- previous history of shoulder dystocia
- post-term pregnancy
- high parity
- maternal obesity (weight over 90 kg)
- fetal macrosomia (birth weight over 4000 g)
- maternal diabetes and gestational diabetes.

Intrapartum
- prolonged labour (first and second stages)
- oxytocin augmentation
- operative vaginal birth.

Warning signs during the second stage of labour

- The birth may have been uncomplicated initially.
- The head may have advanced slowly.
- The chin may have had difficulty in sweeping over the perineum.
- Slow advance of the baby's head/difficulty in freeing the face and chin from the vagina.
- Once the head is born, it may look as if it is trying to return into the vagina (the 'turtle sign').

Diagnosis

Shoulder dystocia is diagnosed when manoeuvres normally used by the midwife, such as gentle axial traction (i.e. traction that is in line with the fetal spine), fail to accomplish birth.

345

Management

See Box 23.5 and Figs 23.1–23.3.

Internationally, the mnemonic HELPERR is widely used in maternity emergencies drills and skills training (Box 23.6). An algorithm (Fig. 23.4) can also be a helpful aide memoire.

Box 23.5 **Management of shoulder dystocia**

- Summon help – an experienced obstetrician, an anaesthetist, a second midwife and a person proficient in neonatal resuscitation
- Attempt to disimpact the shoulders and accomplish birth. An accurate and detailed record of the type of manoeuvre(s) used, by whom, time implemented, the time taken, the amount of force used and the outcome of each attempted manoeuvre should be made
- The rule of thumb is to apply a manoeuvre for 30–60 seconds; if the baby is not born, move on to the next manoeuvre

External manoeuvres

- *Change in maternal position*, e.g. 'all fours'/Gaskin manoeuvre if woman in a different position
- *McRoberts manoeuvre*: will alter the tilt/angle of the pelvis and is a very effective manoeuvre in alleviating the problem in most cases. It involves helping the woman to lie flat and to bring her knees up to her chest as far as possible to rotate the angle of the symphysis pubis superiorly and use the weight of her legs to create gentle pressure on her abdomen, releasing the impaction of the anterior shoulder
- *Suprapubic pressure* (Fig. 23.1). Pressure is exerted on the side of the fetal back and towards the fetal chest to adduct the shoulders and push the anterior shoulder away from the symphysis pubis
  - Can be used with the McRoberts manoeuvre
  - It is important to position the hands over the supra-pubic area where the back is located

Internal (manipulative) manoeuvres

Where non-invasive/external manoeuvres have not been successful, direct manipulation of the fetus must now be attempted

- *Episiotomy*. May be necessary to create more space to gain access to the fetus
- *Rubin manoeuvre*. The posterior shoulder is pushed in the direction of the fetal chest, thus rotating the anterior shoulder away from the symphysis pubis into the oblique diameter

---

Box 23.5 **Management of shoulder dystocia – cont'd**

- *Woods manoeuvre* (Fig. 23.2). A hand is inserted into the vagina, pressure is exerted on the posterior fetal shoulder, and rotation is achieved
- *Reverse Woods manoeuvre*. Fingers on the back of the posterior shoulder apply pressure to rotate in opposite direction
- *Birth of the posterior arm* (Fig. 23.3). A hand is inserted into the vagina, and two fingers splint the humerus of the posterior arm, flex the elbow and sweep the forearm over the chest to birth the hand. If the rest of the birth is not then accomplished, the second arm can be birthed following rotation of the shoulder using either Woods or Rubin manoeuvre or by reversing the Løvset manoeuvre
- *Zavanelli manoeuvre*. If the manoeuvres described previously have been unsuccessful, the obstetrician as a last ditched effort may consider the Zavanelli manoeuvre
  - It requires the reversal of the mechanisms of birth so far achieved and reinsertion of the head into the vagina, which is no mean feat
  - The birth is then completed via caesarean section

Fig. 23.1 Correct application of suprapubic pressure for shoulder dystocia. (After Pauerstein C, 1987, with permission).

Continued

Box 23.5 **Management of shoulder dystocia – cont'd**

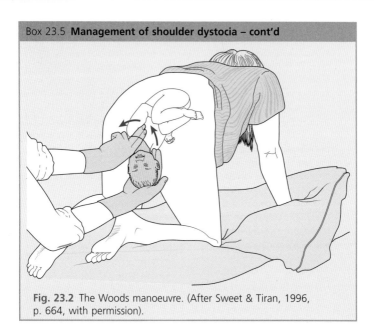

Fig. 23.2 The Woods manoeuvre. (After Sweet & Tiran, 1996, p. 664, with permission).

Complications associated with shoulder dystocia

A number of associated maternal and fetal/neonatal morbidities have been reported:

Maternal
- Postpartum haemorrhage
- Uterine rupture
- Possible psychological sequelae

Fetal
- Neonatal asphyxia
- Fracture of the clavicle or humerus
- Brachial plexus injury, e.g. Erb palsy
- Intrauterine death

Box 23.5 **Management of shoulder dystocia – cont'd**

Fig. 23.3 Birth of the posterior arm. (A) Location of the posterior arm. (B) Directing the arm into the hollow of the sacrum. (C) Grasping and splinting the wrist and forearm. (D) Sweeping the arm over the chest and delivering the hand.

Box 23.6 **The 'HELPERR' mnemonic**

- **H**elp
- **E**pisiotomy need assessed
- **L**egs in McRoberts position
- **P**ressure suprapubically
- **E**nter vagina (internal rotation)
- **R**emove posterior arm
- **R**oll over and try again

Fig. 23.4 Algorithm for the management of shoulder dystocia.

RUPTURE OF THE UTERUS

Rupture of the uterus is defined as:

- *Complete rupture* – involves a tear in the wall of the uterus with or without expulsion of the fetus.
- *Incomplete rupture* – involves tearing of the uterine wall but not the perimetrium.
- The life of both mother and fetus may be endangered in either situation.
- Dehiscence of an existing uterine scar may also occur.

Causes

- Antenatal rupture due to pre-existing uterine scar
- High parity and use of oxytocin with these women
- Obstructed labour
- Neglected labour, where there is previous history of caesarean section
- Extension of severe cervical laceration upwards into the lower uterine segment
- Trauma, as a result of a blast injury or an accident
- Use of prostaglandins to induce labour in the presence of an existing uterine scar

Signs of rupture of intrapartum the uterus

Complete rupture

- Severe and persistent abdominal pain accompanied by sudden maternal collapse especially in a previously non-scarred uterus
- Maternal tachycardia and tachypnoea
- Scar pain and tenderness (where there has been previous caesarean section)
- Abnormalities of the fetal heart rate and pattern
- Poor progress in labour
- Fresh vaginal bleeding
- Palpation of the fetus in the maternal abdomen as the presenting part regresses
- Possible cessation of uterine contractions

Incomplete rupture

- More commonly associated with previous caesarean section
- May have an insidious onset
- May only be detected at caesarean section or following the birth of the baby
- Blood loss tends to be scantier than a complete rupture

Management

- Immediate caesarean section
- Repair of the rupture or a hysterectomy, depending on the extent of the trauma and the mother's condition
- Management of any shock including fluid replacement therapy/ blood transfusion

AMNIOTIC FLUID EMBOLISM (AFE)/ ANAPHYLACTOID SYNDROME OF PREGNANCY

- A rare, unpredictable and unpreventable emergency with potentially catastrophic consequences if not speedily recognized as there are limited means to resuscitate the mother.
- It occurs when amniotic fluid enters the maternal circulation via the uterus or placental site.
- The presence of amniotic fluid in the maternal circulation triggers an anaphylactoid response.
- It should be suspected in cases of sudden collapse or uncontrollable bleeding.
- Early diagnosis and skilled management may lead to decreased maternal and fetal/neonatal mortality and morbidity rates.

Predisposing factors

AFE can occur at any gestation, labour and postpartum but is most common immediately following labour or:
- artificial rupture of the membranes
- placental abruption
- termination of pregnancy.

Signs and symptoms of AFE

Derangement in the following systems:
- Respiratory
  - Cyanosis
  - Dyspnea
  - Respiratory arrest
- Cardiovascular
  - Tachycardia
  - Hypotension
  - Change in colour of the skin – clammy to touch/shivering
  - Cardiac arrest
- Haematological
  - Haemorrhage from the placental site
  - Coagulopathy
- Neurological
  - Restlessness
  - Anxiety/panic/overwhelming feeling of gloom

- Altered level of consciousness
- Convulsions
- Fetal compromise

ACUTE INVERSION OF THE UTERUS

- A rare but potentially life-threatening complication of the third stage of labour that occurs within the first 24 hours of birth.

Classification of inversion

Inversion can be classified according to severity as follows:
- *First-degree.* The fundus reaches the internal os.
- *Second-degree.* The body or corpus of the uterus is inverted to the internal os.
- *Third-degree.* The fundus protrudes to or beyond the introitus and is visible.
- *Fourth-degree.* Total uterine and vaginal inversion are inverted beyond the introitus.

Causes

Causes of acute inversion are associated with uterine atony and cervical dilatation, and include:
- mismanagement in the third stage of labour, involving excessive cord traction to manage the birth of the placenta
- combining fundal pressure and cord traction to expel the placenta
- use of fundal pressure while the uterus is atonic, to birth the placenta
- pathologically adherent placenta
- spontaneous occurrence of unknown cause
- primiparity
- fetal macrosomia
- short umbilical cord
- sudden emptying of a distended uterus.

Warning signs and diagnosis

- Haemorrhage, the amount of which will depend on the degree of placental adherence to the uterine wall.
- Profound shock and sudden onset of pain.

> ## Box 23.7 **Management of acute inversion of the uterus**
>
> **Immediate action**
> - Summon immediate and appropriate medical support
> - Ensure adequate analgesia
> - Attempt to replace the uterus by:
>   - pushing the fundus with the palm of the hand, along the direction of the vagina, towards the posterior fornix. The uterus is then lifted towards the umbilicus and returned to position with a steady pressure (Johnson manoeuvre)
>   - giving hydrostatic pressure with warm saline
> - Insert an intravenous cannula and commence fluid therapy after obtaining blood for cross-matching
> - If the placenta is still attached, it should be left in situ as attempts to remove it at this stage may result in uncontrollable haemorrhage
> - Once the uterus is repositioned, the operator should keep the hand in situ until a firm contraction is palpated
> - Oxytocics should be given to maintain the contraction
>
> **Medical management**
> - If manual replacement fails, then medical or surgical intervention is required

- On abdominal palpation, an indentation of the fundus might be felt; however, if the degree of inversion is major the uterus will not be felt abdominally.
- A mass may be felt on vaginal examination.
- The fundus may be visible at the introitus.

Management

See Box 23.7.

BASIC LIFE-SUPPORT MEASURES

Before starting any resuscitation, assessment of any risk to the carer and the woman is needed. The basic principles of life support are:
- A – airway
- B – breathing
- C – circulation

- D – disability
- E – environment/examination.

The level of consciousness is established by shaking the woman's shoulders and enquiring whether she can hear.

- Summon urgent assistance.
- Lie the woman flat; if she is pregnant, position with a left lateral tilt to prevent aortocaval compression and check safety of surrounding area/environment/top-to-toe examination to identify the problem.
- Airway check and maintenance – remove any obstructions (e.g. mucus), tilt head back and lift chin upwards.
- Breathing – look for chest movements, listen and feel for breath.
- Circulation – check carotid pulse; if no pulse felt, commence cardiopulmonary resuscitation (CPR).

CPR

- Thirty chest compressions (rate of 100/min at a depth of 4–5 cm).
- Two mouth-to-mouth ventilations (insert airway if one available, rate of 10 breaths/min).
- Maintain ratio 30:2 (*note*: ratios may change in light of any new evidence; always follow national guidelines, e.g. Resuscitation Council guidelines).

SHOCK

Shock can be classified as follows:
- *hypovolaemic* – the result of a reduction in intravascular volume
- *cardiogenic* – impaired ability of the heart to pump blood
- *neurogenic* – occurs due to an insult to the nervous system
- *septic or toxic* – the result of a severe generalized infection.

Hypovolaemic shock

- Caused by any loss of circulating fluid volume that is not compensated for, as in haemorrhage, but may also occur when there is severe vomiting. The body reacts to the loss of circulating fluid in stages, as described in the following sections.

Initial stage

- The reduction in fluid or blood decreases the venous return to the heart.

- The ventricles of the heart are inadequately filled, causing a reduction in stroke volume and cardiac output.
- As cardiac output and venous return fall, the blood pressure is reduced. The drop in blood pressure decreases the supply of oxygen to the tissues and cell function is affected.

Compensatory stage

- The fall in cardiac output produces a response from the sympathetic nervous system through the activation of receptors in the aorta and carotid arteries.
- Blood is redistributed to the vital organs.
- Vessels in the gastrointestinal tract, kidneys, skin and lungs constrict. This response is seen as the skin becomes pale and cool.
- Peristalsis slows, urinary output is reduced and exchange of gas in the lungs is impaired as blood flow diminishes.
- The heart rate increases in an attempt to improve cardiac output and blood pressure.
- The pupils of the eyes dilate.
- The sweat glands are stimulated and the skin becomes moist and clammy.
- Adrenaline (epinephrine) is released from the adrenal medulla and aldosterone from the adrenal cortex.
- Antidiuretic hormone (ADH) is secreted from the posterior lobe of the pituitary. Their combined effect is to cause vasoconstriction, an increased cardiac output and a decrease in urinary output.
- Venous return to the heart will increase but, unless the fluid loss is replaced, will not be sustained.

Progressive stage

- This stage leads to multisystem failure.
- Compensatory mechanisms begin to fail, with vital organs lacking adequate perfusion.
- Volume depletion causes a further fall in blood pressure and cardiac output.
- The coronary arteries suffer lack of supply.
- Peripheral circulation is poor, with weak or absent pulses.

Final, irreversible stage of shock

- Multisystem failure and cell destruction are irreparable resulting in death.

Box 23.8 **Priorities in the management of hypovolaemic shock**

- Call for help
- Maintain the airway: If the woman is severely collapsed:
  - she should be turned on to her side and 40% oxygen administered at a rate of 4–6 L/min
  - insert airway if she is unconscious
- Replace fluids
  - Take blood for cross-matching and insert two wide-bore intravenous cannula to enable fluids and drugs to be administered swiftly
  - Crystalloid solutions (e.g. Hartmann's and Ringer's lactate) are given until the woman's condition has improved and to maintain intravascular volume, colloids such as gelatins and Hetastarch or blood are recommended after 2 L of crystalloid have been infused
- Ensure warmth
  - It is important to keep the woman warm, but not overwarmed or warmed too quickly, as this will cause peripheral vasodilatation and result in hypotension
- Arrest haemorrhage
  - The source of the bleeding needs to be identified and stopped
- Monitor vital signs

Management

The priorities are listed in Box 23.8.

Septic shock

- A distributive form of shock, where an overwhelming infection develops rendering the immune system ineffective, which sets off a series of reactions including:
  - inflammation
  - swelling
  - coagulopathy.
- One of the most common form of sepsis reported is that caused by beta-haemolytic *Streptococcus pyogenes* (Lancefield group A). This is a Gram-positive organism, responding to intravenous antibiotics, specifically those that are penicillin based.
- In the general population, infections from Gram-negative organisms such as *Escherichia coli*, *Proteus* or *Pseudomonas pyocyaneus* are

predominant; these are common pathogens in the female genital tract.

- The placental site is the main point of entry for an infection associated with pregnancy and childbirth. This may occur following:
  - prolonged rupture of fetal membranes
  - obstetric trauma or septic abortion, or in the presence of retained placental tissue
  - endotoxins present in the organisms release components that trigger the body's immune response, culminating in multiple organ failure.

Clinical presentation

- Often insidious onset.
- The mother may present with a sudden onset of tachycardia, pyrexia, rigours and tachypnoea.
- The mother may also exhibit a change in her mental state.
- Signs of shock, including hypotension, develop as the condition takes hold.
- Haemorrhage may develop as a result of disseminated intravascular coagulation.

Management

This is based on preventing further deterioration by restoring circulatory volume and eradication of the infection (Box 23.9) as outlined by

---

Box 23.9 **Management of septic shock**

- Implementation of the sepsis six 'bundle'
- Replacement of fluid volume will restore perfusion of the vital organs
- Satisfactory oxygenation is also needed
- Rigorous treatment with intravenous antibiotics, after blood cultures have been taken, is necessary to halt the illness
- Retained products of conception can be detected on ultrasound, and these can then be removed
- Monitor vital signs: temperature, pulse, respiration, blood pressure and urinary output
- Strict fluid balance chart

the internationally agreed sepsis six bundle. This is a 'bundle' of six elements of care that, when implemented as a group, lead to a more positive effect on outcomes than the implementation of the individual elements alone (see useful website section).

SUGGESTED READING

MBBRACE-UK. 2016. Saving lives, improving mothers' care. Surveillance of maternal deaths in the UK 2012–14 and lessons learned to inform maternity care from the UK and Ireland Confidential Enquiries into Maternal Deaths and Morbidity 2009–14. Available at: https://www.npeu.ox.ac.uk (accessed 18 Jan 2017).

Useful website

http://www.survivingsepsis.org. A very useful website for up-to-date information about sepsis and any changes to practice/definition from an international perspective.

Section | 4 |

Puerperium

Physiology and Care in the Puerperium

DEFINITIONS

Puerperium

- Physiologically it is seen as the fourth trimester, or the period following the birth of the placenta and membranes that continues for 6–8 weeks, when the reproductive organs return as close as possible to their pre-pregnant state and lactation is established for those women who are breastfeeding.
- Psychologically, newer evidence suggests that the process of recovery can take much longer as women adjust to their mothering role. In some instances, healing and recovery can take up to a year.

Postnatal period

- The period following labour during which the attendance of a midwife upon the woman and baby is required, being not less than 10 days and for a longer period if the midwife considers it necessary. This is not a universal definition but one that is standard within the United Kingdom.

MIDWIVES AND THE MANAGEMENT OF POSTPARTUM CARE

Aims of postnatal care

- To empower the mother (and her family) to care for herself and baby in a confident manner.
- To promote physical and psychological wellbeing and support the integration of the baby in the family unit.
- To provide public health information that supports breastfeeding, or guidance on safe formula feeding.

PHYSIOLOGICAL CHANGES

The uterus

- After the birth, oxytocin is secreted from the posterior lobe of the pituitary gland to act upon the uterine muscle and assist separation of the placenta.
- Following expulsion of the placenta and membranes, the walls of the now empty uterus are in apposition and act to compress the newly exposed placental site and effectively seal the exposed ends of the major blood vessels.
- The muscle layers of the myometrium are said to simulate the action of the 'living ligatures' that compress the large sinuses of the blood vessels exposed by placental separation. These occlude the exposed ends of the large blood vessels and contribute further to reduce blood loss.
- The uterus reduces in size through a number of key physiological processes:
  - *ischaemia*: vasoconstriction in the overall blood supply to the uterus results in the tissues being denied their previous blood supply, i.e. deoxygenation
  - *autolysis*: autodigestion of the ischaemic muscle fibres by proteolytic enzymes occurs, resulting in an overall reduction in their size
  - *phagocytosis:* there is phagocytic action of polymorphs and macrophages in the blood and lymphatic systems upon the waste products of autolysis, which are then excreted via the renal system in the urine
  - coagulation takes place through platelet aggregation and the release of thromboplastin and fibrin.
- Renewal of the uterine lining and renewal of the placental site involve different physiological processes. What remains of the inner surface of the uterine lining, apart from the placental site, regenerates rapidly to produce a covering of epithelium.
  - Partial coverage is said to have occurred within 7–10 days after birth;
  - Total coverage is complete by the 21st day.
- Once the placenta is expelled, the circulating levels of oestrogen, progesterone, human chorionic gonadotrophin and human placental lactogen are reduced. This leads to further physiological changes in muscle and connective tissues, as well as having a

major influence on the secretion of prolactin from the anterior pituitary gland.

- Once empty, the uterus can be likened to an empty sac, although it retains its muscular structure.
  - It is therefore important to remember that the uterus, although at this point markedly reduced in size, still retains the potential to be a much larger cavity.
  - This underpins the requirement to undertake immediate and then regular observations of fundal height, assessment of lochia and the degree of uterine contraction in the first few hours after the birth.
- Abdominal palpation of the uterus is usually performed soon after placental expulsion to ensure that the physiological processes described previously are beginning to take place.
- On abdominal palpation, the fundus of the uterus should be located centrally, at the same level or slightly below the umbilicus, and should be in a state of contraction, feeling firm under the palpating hand.
- The woman may experience some uterine or abdominal discomfort, especially where uterotonic drugs have been administered to augment the physiological process.

Involution

- This is the physiological process of the uterus returning to its non-pregnant state.
- A well-contracted uterus will gradually reduce in size until it is no longer palpable above the symphysis pubis.
- The rate at which this occurs and the duration of time taken have been demonstrated to be highly individual.
- The uterus should not be tender during this process, although the woman may be experiencing afterpains.
- The observations obtained by the midwife about the state of involution of the uterus should be placed into context alongside the colour, amount, odour and duration of lochia and the woman's general state of health at that time.

Lochia

- Lochia is the physiological vaginal discharge after the birth of the baby and expulsion of the placenta experienced by mothers in the initial 4–6 weeks postpartum, brought about by changes in the uterus and consisting mainly of blood and necrotic tissue.

- As involution progresses, the vaginal loss reflects this and changes from a predominantly fresh blood loss to one that contains stale blood products, lanugo, vernix and other debris from the unwanted products of the conception.
- The word lochia is plural and it is important to note that lochia varies from woman to woman, being lighter or darker in colour, but for any woman the shade and density tend to be consistent. Fig. 24.1 summarizes the different types of lochia.

Assessment of vaginal blood loss

The mother should be asked about the current vaginal loss:
- whether it is more or less than previously
- whether it is lighter or darker than previously
- whether she has any concerns about her vaginal loss.

It is of particular importance to record any clots passed and when these occurred and educate the mother about the importance of hand hygiene before and after changing her sanitary towels in order to reduce the risk of infection, especially sepsis.

Perineal pain

- Regardless of whether the birth resulted in actual perineal trauma, women who birth vaginally are likely to feel bruised and experience discomfort around the vaginal and perineal tissues for the first few days after the birth.
- Women who have undergone any degree of actual perineal injury will experience pain for several days until healing takes place.
- All women should be asked about discomfort in the perineal area, regardless of whether there is a record of actual perineal trauma.
- Where women appear to have no discomfort or anxieties about their perineum, it is not essential for the midwife to examine this area.
- For most women, the perineal wound gradually becomes less painful and healing should occur by 7–10 days after the birth.

Advice on what might help perineal pain

- Appropriate information and advice are important components in pain management and should take into account women's

Lochia rubra (approximately 3–4 days) (dark red lochia)	Lochia serosa (approximately 7–10 days) (pinkish-brown lochia)	Lochia alba (approximately 10–28 days) (whitish-yellow lochia)
Rubra means red Main constituents: • Red blood cells (RBCs) from healing placental site • Remnants of fetal cells • Meconium	Serosa denotes serous-like fluid Main constituents: • Less RBCs and more white blood corpuscles (WBCs) • Serous discharge fromplacental site • Cervical mucus	Alba means white Main constituents: • Decidual cells • WBCs • Epithelial cells • Cervical mucus

Fig. 24.1 The different types of lochia.

individual experiences of their pain and their preferences for its relief.

- Localized cooling and bathing: women may find soaking in a bath of great comfort to them regardless of any additive, and relief may be derived from the use of a bidet or cool water poured over the area that is tender.
- There is increasing interest in complementary therapeutic preparations and more and more research is being undertaken into their use. Essential oils such as lavender and tea tree have been found to be beneficial when used as bath additives or topical compresses. Homoeopathic remedies such as arnica can be applied topically or taken orally.
- Simple oral analgesia such as paracetamol that can be obtained at local pharmacy without a prescription can be very effective in managing mild to moderate pain.

Vital signs and general health

Observations of pulse, temperature, respiration and blood pressure are necessary. While monitoring the pulse rate, the midwife can also observe a number of related signs of wellbeing, as well as just listening to what the woman is saying. These include:

- respiratory rate
- overall body temperature
- any untoward body odour such as offensive lochia, infective perineal/ caesarean section wound
- skin condition
- overall colour and complexion.

Observation of temperature is unnecessary in women who are well and without symptoms that could be associated with an infection. Where the woman complains of feeling unwell with flu-like symptoms, or there are signs of possible infection, then the temperature and respirations must be taken.

Blood pressure

- Following the birth of the baby, a baseline recording of the woman's blood pressure will be made within 6 hours of birth.
- In the absence of any previous history of morbidity associated with hypertension, it is usual for the blood pressure to return to a normal range within 24 hours of the birth.
- Routine observation of blood pressure is not required without a clinical reason.

367

Circulation

- The body has to reabsorb excess fluid following the birth. For most women this results in passing large quantities of urine, particularly in the first day, as diuresis is increased.
- Women may also experience oedema of their ankles and feet and this swelling may be greater than that experienced in pregnancy. These are variations of normal physiological processes and should resolve within the puerperal time scale as the woman's activity levels also increase.
- Advice should be related to:
  - taking reasonable exercise
  - avoiding long periods of standing
  - elevating the feet and legs when sitting, where possible.
- Swollen ankles should be bilateral and not accompanied by pain; the midwife should note particularly if this is present in one calf only, as it could indicate pathology associated with a deep vein thrombosis.

Skin and nutrition

- Women who have suffered from urticaria of pregnancy or cholestasis of the liver should experience relief once the pregnancy is over.
- Women should be encouraged to maintain a balanced fluid intake and to eat a balanced diet that has a greater proportion of fresh food in it.

Urine and bowel function

- Minor disorders of urinary and bowel function are common. These may be associated with retention or incontinence of urine or constipation, or both.
- The midwife should explore the possible cause of this and decide whether it will resolve spontaneously or requires further investigation.

Exercise and healthy activity versus rest, relaxation and sleep

- Exploring each woman's level of activity will encourage advice in relation to appropriate exercise and, by association, nutritional intake and rest or relaxation and sleep.
- Undertaking regular pelvic floor exercises is of benefit to women's long-term health.

Afterpains

- Management of afterpains is by an appropriate analgesic; where possible, this should be taken prior to breastfeeding, as it is the production of oxytocin in relation to the let-down response that initiates the contraction in the uterus and causes pain.
- Pain in the uterus that is constant or present on abdominal palpation is unlikely to be associated with afterpains and further enquiry should be made into this. Women might also confuse afterpains with flatus pain, especially after an operative birth or where they are constipated. Relief of the cause is likely to relieve the symptoms.

FUTURE PUBLIC HEALTH ISSUES AND FUTURE FERTILITY

- A key public health role of the midwife is to promote physical and psychological health and wellbeing of mother and baby during the transitory postpartum period where there is much adjustment and change on the part of the mother, baby and family.
- Every effort must be made to reduce health inequalities. The midwife can do this by informing women and their family of agencies that can help to provide social and financial support.

Midwives need to be aware of a range of different needs with regard to women's health and newborn care and should be able to offer sensitive and appropriate advice on:

- sexual health/safe sexual practice
- family planning/spacing, including contraception where this is needed
- mental health
- safe infant feeding practice
- smoking cessation
- evidence-based information on safe sleeping and bed-sharing
- newborn screening programme
- hand hygiene/prevention of infection.

It is vital to educate women and their family on early warning signs of serious complications that will need reporting, e.g. pyrexia, sudden increase in lochia or offensive lochia, painful or hot breast(s), uterine tenderness or pain, fatigue/excessive tiredness, insomnia, severe headache, shortness of breath, chest pain and major changes to appetite.

There may also be safeguarding issues that the midwife needs to monitor and escalate such as:

- signs of domestic abuse
- child protection issues (e.g. risk of female genital mutilation).

SUGGESTED READING

Fletcher S., Grotegut C.A., James A.H., 2012. Lochia patterns among women: a systematic review. J. Womens Health 21 (12), 1290–1294. doi: 10.1089/jwh.2012.3668.

Salam, R.A., Mansoor, T., Mallick, D., et al., 2014. Essential childbirth and postnatal interventions for improved maternal and neonatal health. Reprod. Health 11 (Suppl. 1), S3. Available at: https://reproductive-health-journal.biomedcentral.com/articles/10.1186/1742-4755-11-S1-S3 (accessed 17 April 2016).

Useful website

World Health Organization. Available at: http://www.who.int. Useful information and recommendations on postnatal care can be accessed via this website, such as the publication of guides on pregnancy, childbirth, postpartum and newborn care.

Physical Problems and Complications in the Puerperium

In order to meet individual needs, a woman–centred approach to care in the postpartum period is essential. This period of recovery should be a seamless part of the continuation of the care the woman receives during pregnancy and labour. Knowledge of preceding factors such as socio-cultural background, pregnancy and labour complications, will help to inform individual care planning. This will assist physical and psychological recovery.

The role of the midwife in these cases is:

- to prevent and detect early any deviation from normal that may indicate a potentially pathological condition
- to provide timely referral of any woman with suspected underlying pathology for appropriate investigations and care.

IMMEDIATE UNTOWARD EVENTS FOR THE MOTHER FOLLOWING THE BIRTH OF THE BABY

Postpartum haemorrhage

Immediate (primary) postpartum haemorrhage (PPH)

- The most immediate and potentially life-threatening event occurring at the point of, or within 24 hours, of expulsion of the placenta and membranes.
- It presents as a sudden and excessive vaginal blood loss of 500 ml or more (see Ch. 19 for management).

Secondary or delayed PPH

- Defined as excessive or prolonged vaginal loss from 24 hours following birth of the placenta and membranes up to 12 weeks postpartum.
- Unlike primary PPH, which includes a specified volume of blood loss as part of its definition, no volume is defined for secondary PPH; management will depend on apparent clinical need.

> **Box 25.1 Secondary PPH**
>
> **Signs of secondary PPH**
> - Lochial loss is heavier than normal
> - Lochia returns to a bright red loss and may be offensive
> - Subinvolution of the uterus
> - Pyrexia and tachycardia
> - Haematoma formation
>
> **Treatment**
> - Call a doctor
> - Reassure the woman and her support person(s)
> - Rub up a contraction by massaging the uterus if it is still palpable
> - Express any clots
> - Encourage the mother to empty her bladder
> - Give an uterotonic drug, such as ergometrine maleate, by the intravenous or intramuscular route
> - Keep all pads and linen to assess the volume of blood lost
> - Antibiotics may be prescribed
> - If retained products of conception are seen on an ultrasound scan, it may be appropriate to transfer the woman to hospital and prepare her for theatre

- Regardless of the timing of any haemorrhage, it is most frequently the placental site that is the source.
- A cervical or deep vaginal wall tear or trauma to the perineum might be the cause in women who have recently given birth.
- Retained placental fragments or other products of conception are likely to inhibit the process of involution, or reopen the placental wound.
- Diagnosis is likely to be determined by the woman's condition and pattern of events and is also often complicated by the presence of infection (see Box 25.1).

Maternal collapse within 24 hours of the birth without overt bleeding

Consider:
- inversion of the uterus
- amniotic fluid embolism
- cerebrovascular accident.

Where no signs of haemorrhage are apparent, other causes must be considered (see Ch. 13).

POSTPARTUM COMPLICATIONS AND IDENTIFYING DEVIATIONS FROM THE NORMAL

- The woman may experience and report symptoms that might suggest early signs of pathology.
- The midwife needs to undertake a thorough assessment of the woman's physical and mental health/wellbeing to determine whether there are any signs of possible underlying morbidity and to determine the best course of action, including referral.

Fig. 25.1 suggests a model for linking together key observations that suggest potential risk of, or actual, morbidity.

- The central point, as with any personal contact, is the midwife's initial review of the woman's appearance, psychological state and vital signs.
  - A change in core body temperature ($< 36°C$ or rise in temperature above $38°C$) is usually considered to be of clinical significance (could signify sepsis). A mildly raised temperature may be related to normal physiological hormonal responses: e.g. the increasing production of breast milk.
  - A weak and rapid pulse rate in a woman who is in a state of collapse with signs of shock and a low blood pressure, but no evidence of vaginal haemorrhage, may indicate the formation of a haematoma. A rapid pulse rate in an otherwise well woman might suggest that she is anaemic but could also indicate increased thyroid or other dysfunctional hormonal activity.

The midwife needs to be alert to any possible relationship between the woman's vital signs and their potential cause.

Vulnerability to infection, potential causes and prevention

- The postpartum woman is vulnerable to infection; her vulnerability increases where conditions exist that enable harmful organisms to enter, thrive and reproduce, especially where there is access to and from entry points in the body, not least because of the healing placental site and the presence of lochia.
- Organisms are transferred between sources and potential hosts via:
  - *hands*
  - *air currents*

373

Uterus
On palpation feels poorly contracted
Wide, 'boggy', spongy
Fundus may be deviated to one side
Not progressively reducing in size
Tenderness felt on palpation
Vaginal loss heavier and fresher than previously
or scant but offensive
Passing clots

Breasts
Feel tight and tender
One segment is flushed
or reddened
One or both nipples have sore,
broken or discoloured/flaky skin
If breastfeeding, obtain a history
of feeding patterns and observe
a feed
Obtain swab for infection
(candidiasis)

General condition
Feeling unwell
Flu-like symptoms
A change in core body
temperature (< 36°C or rise in
temperature above 38°C)
Tachycardia >100 bpm
Pale, listless

Wounds
Inflammation and tenderness
around wound area
Poor healing or gaping at the
skin edge
Pain felt deeper in the wound site
Visible clear or purulent exudate
Remove sutures where these are
tight and pulling
Obtain a swab for culture
Review the wound environment
and method of cleansing the wound

Circulation
Respiratory collapse or severe breathlessness requires emergency assistance
Review for: Previous history of pulmonary embolism, DVT
Current history of epidural, prolonged labour, operative birth,
varicose veins, anaemia, obesity
Severe maternal illness requiring prolonged inactivity
Check use of preventative measures:
TED stockings, prophylactic heparin, degree of mobility attained
Look for signs of localised inflammation of varicose veins, pain in calf,
mild pyrexia

Fig. 25.1 Diagrammatic demonstration of the relationship between deviation from normal physiology and potential morbidity. *DVT,* Deep vein thrombosis.

- *formites (i.e. materials likely to carry infection, e.g. clothing and bed linen).*

Acquisition of infections

Infections can be acquired via the following means:

- Endogenous – the organism is already present in or on the body. For example:
  - *Streptococcus faecalis* (Lancefield group B – present in the vagina)
  - *Clostridium welchii* (present in the vagina)
  - *Escherichia coli* (present in the bowel)
  - Tuberculosis bacterium (might be reactivated after being dormant in the body)
- Exogenous – transfer of infective organisms from others, animals, body surfaces or the environment. For example:
  - Group A-haemolytic streptococcus (GAS) – spread by direct person-to-person contact, most likely through droplets of saliva or nasal secretions (e.g. coughing/sneezing); often implicated in puerperal sepsis.
  - Group B-haemolytic streptococcus – usually lives harmlessly in the digestive tract and vagina but can be transmitted via sexual activity.
  - *Chlamydia trachomatis* – a common sexually transmitted organism.
  - *Staphylococcus aureus* – a normal commensal that lives on the skin but can be transferred from one infected person or place to an uninfected one (more vulnerable when immuno-compromised) via nosocomial means or cross-infection (i.e. hospital–acquired).

Both the streptococcus and staphylococcus group of organisms are the most commonly cited bacteria responsible for the majority of puerperal infection, which is preventable.

Educating women and their family about the basic principles of good hand-washing/hygiene is the single most effective measure in staving off infection.

The uterus and vaginal loss following vaginal birth

Assessment of uterine involution is needed where the woman:

- is feeling generally unwell
- has abdominal pain

- has a vaginal loss that is markedly brighter red or heavier than previously
- is passing clots
- reports her vaginal loss to be offensive.

Where palpation of the uterus identifies deviation to one side, this might be the result of a full bladder. Where the woman had emptied her bladder prior to palpation, the presence of urinary retention must be considered, as catheterization of the bladder might be necessary.

Morbidity might be suspected where the uterus:

- fails to follow the expected progressive reduction in size
- feels wide or 'boggy' on palpation
- is less well contracted than expected.

The previously mentioned features might be described as *subinvolution* of the uterus, which can indicate postpartum infection, or the presence of retained products of the placenta/membranes, or both.

Treatment of uterine subinvolution:

- antibiotics
- use of uterotonic agent (e.g. syntometrine/ergometrine)
- hormonal preparations
- evacuation of the uterus (ERPC).

THE UTERUS AND VAGINAL LOSS FOLLOWING OPERATIVE BIRTH

In the early days following surgery, a woman who has had a caesarean section (CS) will have a different level of physical activity from a woman who has had a spontaneous vaginal birth.

- Initially the woman will be less mobile, which will affect the amount of lochia observed.
- Uterine palpation will be painful and is best undertaken 3–4 days post CS if clinically appropriate (e.g. she does not have heavier than expected lochia).

Wound problems

Perineal problems

Perineal pain

In order to respond appropriately and sensitively to the woman's report of perineal pain it is important that the midwife has a good comprehension of its aetiology, the effect of trauma and the physiological process and normal pattern of wound healing.

Severe perineal pain might be the result of:

- ineffective analgesia
- increased oedema in the surrounding tissues
- haematoma formation
- poor perineal repair technique resulting in sutures being too tight (the evidence-base recommends use of a loose, continuous and non-locking technique as highlighted in Ch. 15).

Haematoma

- This is the effusion of blood within the tissues leading to swelling; can be localized in the vagina and vulva.
- The blood contained within a haematoma can exceed 1000 ml and may significantly affect the overall state of the woman, who can present with signs of acute shock.
- Treatment is by evacuation of the haematoma and resuturing of the perineal wound, usually under general anaesthetic.

Inflammation and Oedema

- These can cause the stitches to feel excessively tight.
- Local application of cold packs, oral analgesia, as well as complementary medicines such as arnica and lavender, may bring relief but this practise is not currently evidence-based.
- Pain in the perineal area that occurs at a later stage, or pain that reoccurs might be associated with an infection.
  - The skin edges are likely to have a moist, puffy and dull appearance.
  - There may also be an offensive odour and evidence of pus in the wound.
  - A swab should be obtained for micro-organism culture and referral should be made to a medical practitioner.
  - Antibiotics might be commenced immediately when there is specific information about any infective agent.
- Advice should be given about cleaning the area, using cotton underwear, avoiding tights and trousers and changing sanitary pads frequently.
- Women should also be advised to avoid using perfumed bath additives or talcum powder.
- If the perineal area fails to heal or continues to cause pain by the time the initial healing process should have begun, resuturing or refashioning might be advised. There is currently ongoing research and a Cochrane review on this subject that hopefully will provide recommendations to guide practice in the future.

- Providing the women have had an uncomplicated vaginal birth, most should be pain free and able to resume sexual intercourse within a few weeks after the birth; some discomfort might still be present, depending on the degree of trauma experienced and the healing process.

Evidence suggest that a substantial proportion of women continue to experience problems up to 12 months post-birth and do not report these to health care professionals. It is therefore important that midwives inform women of the need to seek help and advice from their family doctor should any problems arise.

Caesarean section wounds

It is now common practice for women undergoing an operative birth to be given prophylactic antibiotics at the time of the surgery. This has been demonstrated to reduce the incidence of subsequent wound infection and endometritis significantly.

- It is usual for the wound dressing to be removed after the first 24 hours, as this also aids healing and reduces infection.
- Providing the woman with information about wound care is vital especially after bathing/showering and if the woman is obese.
- Hydration and nutrition play a crucial part in the wound healing process.
- A wound that is hot, tender and inflamed and is accompanied by pyrexia is highly suggestive of an infection. Where this is observed, the midwife needs to:
  - obtain a swab for micro-organism culture
  - complete a full assessment of all vital signs
  - seek medical advice
  - complete all relevant documentation.
- Haematoma and abscesses can also form underneath the wound, and women may identify increased pain around the wound where these are present. Rarely, a wound may need to be probed to reduce the pressure and to allow infected material to drain, reducing the likelihood of the formation of an abscess.

Circulation problems

Globally, pulmonary embolism remains a major cause of maternal death. Women at higher risk include those with the factors listed in Box 25.2.

Women who undergo surgery and have these pre-existing factors should be:

- provided with TED stockings during, or as soon as possible after, the birth
- prescribed prophylactic thromboprophylaxis in the form of low molecular weight heparin (e.g. enoxaparin sodium [Clexane]) until normal mobility returns.

Clinical signs that women might report include the following conditions (the most common to the most serious):

- Signs of circulatory problems related to varicose veins usually include localized inflammation or tenderness around the varicose vein, sometimes accompanied by mild pyrexia. This is superficial thrombophlebitis, which is usually resolved by applying support to the affected area and administering anti-inflammatory drugs, where these are not contraindicated and do not conflict with other medication being taken or with breastfeeding.
- Unilateral oedema of an ankle or calf, accompanied by stiffness or pain and a positive Homan's sign, might indicate a deep vein thrombosis that has the potential to cause a pulmonary embolism. Urgent medical referral must be made to confirm the diagnosis and commence anticoagulant or other appropriate therapy.
- The most serious outcome is the development of a pulmonary embolism. The first sign might be the sudden onset of breathlessness, which may not be associated with any obvious clinical sign of a blood clot. Women with this condition are likely to become seriously ill and could suffer respiratory collapse with very little prior warning.
- Some degree of oedema of the lower legs, ankles and feet can be viewed as being within normal limits where it is not accompanied by calf pain (especially unilaterally), pyrexia or raised blood pressure.

Box 25.2 **Risk factors for postpartum pulmonary embolism**

- Previous history of pulmonary embolism
- Deep vein thrombosis
- Varicose veins
- Epidural anaesthetic
- Anaemia
- Prolonged labour
- Operative birth

379

Hypertension

- Women who have had previous episodes of hypertension in pregnancy may continue to demonstrate this postpartum.
- There is still a clinical risk that mothers with clinical signs of pregnancy-induced hypertension can develop eclampsia in the hours and days following the birth, although this is a relatively rare outcome in the normal population. For these women, the medical advice should cover:
  - optimal systolic and diastolic levels, i.e. < 140 mmHg (systolic) and < 90 mmHg (diastolic)
  - instructions for treatment with antihypertensive drugs if the blood pressure (BP) exceeds these levels.
- Occasionally, some women can develop postpartum pre-eclampsia without a previous history of proteinuria and raised blood pressure.
- Some degree of BP monitoring should continue if there has been a history of hypertension in pregnancy.
- BP monitoring must be undertaken whenever there are signs of a clinical need to do so.
- Postpartum women who present with signs associated with pre-eclampsia, will need their BP checked, coupled with urinalysis and medical advice.
- For women with essential hypertension, management of their overall medical condition will be reviewed postpartum by their usual caregivers.

Headache

Concern about postpartum morbidity should centre around careful history taking to determine:

- the severity, duration and frequency of the headaches
- the medication (if any) being taken to alleviate the headache and its efficacy
- maternal mental wellbeing (e.g. sleep pattern, fatigue, hydration/nutritional status any stress/distress being experienced – headaches might also be precursor of psychological distress)
- if a regional analgesia/anaesthetic was administered, medical advice should be sought via the anaesthetist. Headaches from a dural tap typically arise once the woman has become mobile after the birth; these headaches are at their most severe when the woman

is standing, lessening when she lies down. They are often accompanied by:

- neck stiffness
- vomiting
- visual disturbances.

- These headaches are very debilitating and are best managed by stopping the leakage of cerebrospinal fluid (CSF) by the insertion of 10–20 ml of blood into the epidural space; this should resolve the clinical symptoms. If women have returned home after the birth, they would need to return to the hospital to have this procedure carried out.

Backache

- Many women experience pain or discomfort from backache in pregnancy as a result of separation or diastasis of the abdominal muscles (rectus abdominis diastasis, RAD).
- It might be sufficient to:
  - give advice on skeletal support to attain a good posture when feeding and lifting
  - suggest a feasible personal exercise plan and how to achieve this
  - discuss a range of relaxation techniques.
- Where backache is causing pain that affects the woman's activities of daily living, referral can be made to local physiotherapy services.
- Pelvic girdle pain experienced during pregnancy should resolve spontaneously during the puerperium.

Urinary problems

- Urinary problems can take a toll on women's physical and psychosocial health/wellbeing with short and long-term consequences.
- Approximately 19% of women experience urinary problems post-birth.
- Stress incontinence is most commonly reported, even though some women experience frequency, urgency and urge incontinence.
- Epidural or spinal anaesthetic can have an effect on the neurological sensors that control urine release and flow; acute retention may develop.
- Women who sustain damage to the pelvic floor or urethral lacerations may experience urinary difficulty.

- Urinary retention carries the risk of:
  - infection
  - increased vaginal blood loss as the uterus might be impeded in its ability to contract and retract effectively.

Assessment

- A full bladder might be detected by the midwife as a result of abdominal palpation of the uterus.
- Abdominal tenderness in association with other urinary symptoms – for example, poor output, dysuria or offensive urine, pyrexia or general flu-like symptoms – might indicate a urinary tract infection.
  - A mid-stream specimen of urine for laboratory investigation is necessary in cases of suspected infection.
- Very rarely, urinary incontinence might be a result of a urethral fistula following complications from the labour or birth.
- Urinary problems may cause embarrassment and reluctance for the woman to divulge such information. Encouraging her to keep a bladder diary for the initial days of the puerperium can help to capture important information.
- Pelvic floor exercises and referral to a physiotherapist might be appropriate.
- Specific enquiry about these issues should be made when women attend their 6–8-week postnatal examination.

It is important to note the literature has identified that ongoing urinary problems can undermine a woman's health and might be the precursor to depression.

Bowels and constipation

- Normal bowel pattern should return within days of the birth.
- Bowel problems have serious implications for a woman's physical, social and mental health.
- Approximately 3–10% of women experience faecal incontinence.
- Flatus incontinence, passive leakage, urge and faecal incontinence are usually related to neurological or muscular dysfunction or both.
- Constipation and haemorrhoids pose challenges:
  - approximately 44% of postpartum women experience constipation;
  - approximately 20–25% of women will suffer from haemorrhoids.

- Women who have haemorrhoids or difficulty with constipation should be given:
  - advice on diet and hydration
  - instructions on the use of appropriate aperients to soften the stools
  - topical applications to reduce the oedema and pain especially in the presence of perineal trauma.
- It is also a matter of concern if women experience a loss of bowel control or faecal incontinence. It is important to determine the nature of the incontinence and distinguish it from an episode of diarrhoea (in the absence of any laxatives being used).
- Women who identify any change to their prepregnant bowel pattern by the end of the puerperal period should have this reviewed.
- The woman should consult her family doctor in the presence of deviation from normal.

Anaemia

- Due to the competing demands of the developing fetus during pregnancy, iron-deficiency anaemia is very common, even among women who are well-nourished, putting women at risk of anaemia postpartum.
- Where it is evident that a larger than normal blood loss has occurred, red blood cell volume, serum ferritin and haemoglobin (Hb) can be assessed and appropriate treatment provided to reduce the effects of anaemia.
- Where the Hb level is < 90 g/L and the woman is symptomatic, a blood transfusion might be appropriate; oral iron and appropriate dietary advice are advocated when women decline a blood transfusion or when the Hb level is less than 110 g/L.
- If Hb values have not been assessed, clinical symptoms such as lethargy, tachycardia, breathlessness or pale mucous membranes may suggest anaemia; a blood profile should then be considered.

Breast problems

Regardless of whether women are breastfeeding, they may experience tightening and enlargement of their breasts towards the 3rd or 4th day, as hormonal influences encourage the breasts to produce milk.

- For women who are breastfeeding, the general advice is to feed the baby and avoid excessive handling of the breasts.
- Simple analgesics may be required to reduce discomfort.

383

- For women who are not breastfeeding, the advice is to ensure that the breasts are well supported but that the support is not too restrictive; again, taking regular analgesia for 24–48 hours should reduce any discomfort.
- Heat and cold applied to the breasts via a shower or soaking in the bath may temporarily relieve acute discomfort.
- The use of chilled dark-green cabbage leaves might be useful though the evidence in this area is spurious.
- Problems such as engorgement and mastitis are preventable through good positioning and attachment when the baby is breastfeeding and to ensure effective emptying of the breasts.

SUGGESTED READING

Bain, E., Wilson, A., Tooher, R., et al., 2014. Prophylaxis for venous thromboembolic disease in pregnancy and the early postnatal period. Cochrane Database Syst. Rev. (2), CD001689. doi: 10.1002/14651858. CD001689.pub3.

Useful website

National Perinatal Epidemiology Unit. Available at: https:// www.npeu.ox.ac.uk. Reports on the triennial Confidential Enquiries into Maternal Deaths in the UK can be accessed from this site.

Perinatal Mental Health

Perinatal mental health (PNMH) is a key public health issue because:

- The full range of PNMH disorders can complicate pregnancy and the postpartum year.
- The incidence of affective (mood) disorder, particularly the most severe, increases in the postpartum period.
- PNMH disorders disrupt mother-baby relationship and affect the whole family.
- Women who have had a serious mental illness such as puerperal psychosis (a bipolar state) and severe depression have a $1:2$ to $1:3$ risk of a recurrence postpartum.
- Suicide is still a leading cause of indirect maternal deaths in some resource rich countries such as the UK.
- Early identification is important; every pregnant woman should be screened for a history of mental illness at the first antenatal contact with the midwife via sensitive enquiry.

STRESS/ANXIETY AND DOMESTIC ABUSE

- Women are affected emotionally and socially on many levels.
- Women in abusive relationships are particularly vulnerable.
- Approximately 30% of domestic violence and abuse begins or escalates during pregnancy or following childbirth.

Tokophobia

This is an emerging field in the context of maternity care. It is best described as a morbid fear of pregnancy/childbirth that has a complex array of psychosocial factors linked to its root cause such as:

- domestic abuse
- communication difficulties
- previous traumatic sexual/birth experience
- nulliparity
- lack of social support
- pre-existing mental illness.

The literature describes three types of tokophobia:

1. *Primary tokophobia* – relates to nulliparous women who avoid pregnancy.

2. *Secondary tokophobia* – develops as a consequence of a previous traumatic birth experience, which can include miscarriage, abortion and intrauterine fetal death/stillbirth.
3. *Tokophobia* – develops as a feature of depression.

THE TRANSITION TO MOTHERHOOD

- Postnatally, parents may find coping with the demands of a new baby, infant feeding, financial constraints and adjusting to changes in roles and relationships particularly testing emotionally.
- Disturbed sleep is inevitable. Soreness and pain from perineal trauma will affect libido; so too will the feelings of exhaustion, despair and unhappiness that may be associated with the round-the-clock demands of caring for a new baby.

NORMAL EMOTIONAL CHANGES DURING PREGNANCY, LABOUR AND THE PUERPERIUM

It is perfectly normal for women to have periods of self-doubt and crises of confidence. They may experience fluctuations between positive and negative emotions, as described in the following sections.

First trimester

- Pleasure, excitement, elation
- Dismay, disappointment
- Ambivalence
- Emotional lability
- Increased femininity

Second trimester

- A feeling of wellbeing
- A sense of increased attachment to the fetus
- Stress and anxiety about antenatal screening and diagnostic tests
- Increased demand for knowledge and information
- Feelings relating to the need for increasing detachment from work commitments

Third trimester

- Loss of or increased libido
- Altered body image

- Psychological effects from physiological discomforts such as backache and heartburn
- Anxiety about labour (e.g. pain)
- Anxiety about fetal abnormality
- Increased vulnerability to major life events

Labour

For many women, labour will be greeted with varied emotional responses such as:
- great excitement and anticipation to utter dread
- fear of the unknown
- fear of technology, intervention (hospital birth)
- fear of hospitals, illness and death
- tension, fear and anxiety about pain and lack of control
- concerns about the baby and ability of their partner to support/cope
- a fear of lack of privacy or embarrassment.

Women's perceptions of control during labour are influenced by:
- continuity of care by the midwife
- one-to-one care in labour
- not being left for long periods
- being involved in decision making.

The puerperium

Normal emotional changes are complex and may encompass the following:
- Relief labour is over – others may convey a cool detachment from events.
- Contradictory and conflicting feelings from joy and elation to exhaustion and helplessness.
- Closeness to partner and/or baby or disinterest.
- Desire for prolonged skin-to-skin contact and early breastfeeding.
- Fear of the unknown and realization of overwhelming responsibility.
- Exhaustion and increased emotionality.
- Pain (e.g. perineal, nipples).
- Increased vulnerability and indecisiveness.
- Loss of libido, disturbed sleep, anxiety.

Postnatal 'blues'

- A common and transient emotional phase experienced by 50–80% of women depending on parity.
- Technically, it is not a form of mental illness per se as many women are affected but may act as a precursor to such illness.
- Typical onset occurs between 3 and 4 days postpartum, but may last up to a week or more, though rarely persisting for longer than a few days.
- The features of this state are mild and transitory and may include a state in which women usually experience labile emotions.
- The actual aetiology is unclear but hormonal influences seem to be implicated, as the period of increased emotionality appears to coincide with the production of breastmilk.
- A self-limiting state that requires the midwife to be extra vigilant as persistent features could be indicative of depressive illness.

Emotional distress associated with traumatic birth events

Over recent years the label 'post-traumatic stress disorder' (PTSD) has emerged in midwifery practice. Many women will eventually overcome the stress, pain and trauma that might have been their birth experience. However, others may find their birth experience blights their life and affects relationships with their partner and baby.

PNMH DISORDERS

Definition

Perinatal mental illness is now an accepted term used internationally. It encompasses those conditions that complicate pregnancy, childbirth and the postnatal period. This includes not only those illnesses that develop at this time, but also pre-existing disorders such as schizophrenia, bipolar illness and depression.

- Midwives are recommended to routinely ask at early pregnancy assessment about previous mental health problems, their severity and care by using a validated risk assessment tool such as the Whooley questions:
  - During the past months, have you often been bothered by feeling down, depressed or hopeless? (yes/no)

- During the past months, have you often been bothered by having little interest or pleasure in doing things? (yes/no)

A third question should be considered if the woman answers 'yes' to initial question:

- Is this something you feel you need or want help with? (yes/no)

Types of PNMH disorders

PNMH disorders encompass a broad spectrum of mental illness and are conventionally grouped into the following categories:

- Serious mental illness, for example:
  - schizophrenia
  - bipolar illness
  - major unipolar depressive illness.
- Mild to moderate psychiatric disorders, for example:
  - mild to moderate depressive illness
  - anxiety disorders
  - panic disorders
  - obsessive compulsive disorder
  - post-traumatic stress disorder.
- Adjustment reactions (e.g. distressing reactions to death, adversity).
- Substance misuse (e.g. dependence on alcohol or drugs).
- Personality disorders – should only be used for those with persistent severe problems(e.g. maintaining satisfactory relationships); controlling their behaviour.
- Learning disability when people have lifetime evidence of intellectual and cognitive impairment.

PNMH in pregnancy

- New onset PNMH disorders in pregnancy are mostly accounted for by mild depressive illnesses, mixed anxiety and depression or anxiety states.
- Most conditions are likely to improve as pregnancy progresses.
- Caution needs to be exercised before the implementation of pharmacological intervention.
- New onset psychosis in pregnancy is relatively rare but if the condition appears it requires urgent and expert treatment.

Women with pre-existing serious PNMH disorders (e.g. bipolar and major unipolar depression) require individualized care plans as follows:

- Well, stable, not on medication – risk of becoming psychotic postnatally – will therefore need referral to/ psychiatric review.
- Relatively well and stable but taking medication – need expert advice on risks and benefits of treatment.
- Chronically mentally ill and on medication – need careful monitoring by maternity, mental health teams and social services.

PNMH disorders after birth

Conventionally, three postpartum disorders are described:
- the postnatal 'blues'
- puerperal psychosis
- postnatal depression.

As previously highlighted, the blues is a common dysphoric, self-limiting state, occurring in the first week postpartum.

Puerperal psychosis

- Psychosis is often accompanied by mania and/or depressive symptoms in the immediate postnatal period.
- It can become very severe extremely quickly.
- It is the most severe form of postpartum affective disorder, albeit rare (affects 2 : 1000 women).
- It is a psychiatric emergency.
- It has a sudden onset, the majority presenting in the first 14 days postpartum, most commonly between day 3 and day 7.

Features may include:
- restlessness and agitation
- confusion and perplexity
- suspicion and fear, even terror
- insomnia
- episodes of mania making the woman hyperactive (e.g. talking rapidly and incessantly, and being very overactive and elated)
- neglect of basic needs (e.g. nutrition and hydration)
- psychotic features: hallucinations and morbid delusional thoughts (may involve thoughts of self-harm)
- major behavioural disturbance
- profound depressive mood.

Care and management should be based on:
- preventive measures preconception and antenatal
- interprofessional collaboration
- care in a specialist PNMH mother and baby unit.

Postnatal depressive illness (PND)

Mild to moderate forms

- The ubiquitously used term 'PND' only applies to a nonpsychotic depressive illness of mild to moderate severity with a gradual onset; usually arises within 3 months of childbirth.
- Affects approximately 10–15% of mothers.
- The Whooley questions can easily be used during every contact the midwife has with the woman during the antenatal and postnatal period.
- Where a screening tool such as the Edinburgh Postnatal Depression Scale (EPDS) is used, a score of 14 is said to correlate with a clinical diagnosis of major depression (Box 26.1). However, the National Screening Committee (NSC) in the UK, cautions that the EPDS is not a diagnostic tool. Instead the NSC recommends that there should be evidence from quality randomized controlled trials to demonstrate that a screening programme could reduce mortality or morbidity to justify its use.

Box 26.1 **Value and limitations of the Edinburgh Postnatal Depression Scale as a screening tool**

Value

- Useful screening tool
- Acceptable to women
- Takes minutes to complete and score
- Results can be discussed immediately, leading to early identification of problems
- A score of 12 + may indicate that the woman may have depression
- Provides women with tangible 'permission' to talk, be listened to and have feelings validated

Limitations

- Not a diagnostic tool
- May lead to misdiagnosis, i.e. false positives and medicalization of low moods and situational distress
- Depression about depression
- Only predictive, not diagnostic
- Is not a magic wand
- Does not and should not replace clinical judgement
- Does not give women the opportunity to describe symptoms fully

---

Severe depressive illness

- An early-onset condition that develops over 2–4 weeks, unlike the abrupt onset of puerperal psychosis.
- The more severe illnesses tend to present by 4–6 weeks postpartum but the majority tend to present later, between 8 and 12 weeks postpartum.
- Affects approximately 3% of women.

Main clinical features of severe depression

- Insomnia
- 'Biological syndrome' of sleep disturbance – waking early in the morning; the woman will feel most depressed and her symptoms will be worst at the start of the day (diurnal variation of mood).
- Impaired concentration, disturbed thought processes, indecisiveness and an inability to cope with everyday life.
- Emotional detachment and profound lowering of mood.
- Loss of ability to feel pleasure (anhedonia), especially from activities enjoyed in the past.
- Feelings of guilt, unworthiness linked to feelings of incompetence – being a 'bad' mother.
- In approximately one-third of women, distressing intrusive obsessional thoughts and ruminations.
- Commonly, extreme anxiety and even panic attacks.
- Impaired appetite and weight loss.
- In a small number, a depressive psychosis and morbid, delusional thoughts and hallucinations.

TREATMENT OF PNMH DISORDERS

There are three components to management:

1. psychological treatment and social intervention
2. pharmacological treatment
3. services and resources.

Some or all three treatment interventions will be required.

Pharmacological treatment

Given that there is a paucity of systematic research into the efficacy and risks of pharmacological intervention in the management of depression in the postpartum period, balancing risk to the fetus against the risk of not treating the mother is a challenge. Women should be actively supported to breastfeed their baby, if this is their wish.

General principles

- Whenever possible, conception and birth should be medication free.
- Most new episodes of mental illness in pregnancy are early and improve as pregnancy progresses with appropriate psychosocial interventions.
- Liaison between the midwife, general practitioner, obstetrician, psychiatrist, community mental health nurse, health visitor and, where necessary, social worker is of great importance.
- No medication is of proven safety.

Medications that carry a significant risk of teratogenesis have been shown to affect 1–2% of exposed pregnancies, so may be considered of low risk. Nevertheless, they may contribute to fetal demise, intrauterine growth restriction, organ dysgenesis and adverse effects on the neonate, such as withdrawal.

- Serious mental illness requires robust treatment; the more serious the illness is, the more likely it is that the risks of not treating outweigh the risks of treating.
- Babies more than 12 weeks old are at low risk of exposure to antidepressants in breast milk.
- Breast milk levels will reflect the serum levels of the medication. Therefore, women should be advised to avoid feeding at times of peak plasma level, and preferably should time their medication after a feed and before the baby's longest sleep.
- The baby should be monitored for any deleterious effects, particularly weight gain and drowsiness.

A summary of key recommendations for best practice is given in Box 26.2.

Antidepressants

- *Tricyclic antidepressants* (e.g. imipramine, lofepramine, amitriptyline, dosulepin) have shown no harmful effects in pregnancy but babies are at risk of withdrawal effects.
- *Selective serotonin reuptake inhibitors* (SSRIs) (e.g. fluoxetine, paroxetine, citalopram) have given concerns as to their use in early pregnancy. This risk has to be balanced with potential reoccurrence of the woman's condition.

393

Box 26.2 **Summary of key recommendations for best practice**

Prevention of PNMH disorders

- Prepare couples realistically to aim for achievable birth expectations and to deal ably with the demands and challenges of parenthood
- Recognize the value of interagency networking to afford more responsive helplines and points of contact for parents in crisis
- Develop an evidence base of effective mental health promotion strategies
- Be aware that the risk of recurrence of a severe mental illness is at its greatest in the first 30 days postpartum
- Antenatally, screen for risk factors that may culminate in antenatal or postnatal depression: personal or family history of mental illness, history of substance (drug or alcohol) abuse, domestic violence, and self-harm and suicidal traits
- Be vigilant with record keeping to ensure good communication and continuity of care. Promote good liaison between members of the interprofessional team
- Avoid misdiagnosis and prevent errors and missed opportunities in care by employing the correct terminology. Use of the umbrella term 'PND' to describe all types of postpartum mental health problems must cease; use it only when referring to nonpsychotic depressive illness of mild to moderate severity that has an onset following childbirth

Standards and targets

- Set national targets for perinatal mental health services
- Develop clear care pathways for women with a history of mental health problems, substance abuse and abusive relationships
- Set targets to establish the incidence of antenatal depression and reduce the prevalence of postnatal depression; one way of achieving this is to standardize the criteria used for screening

Services

- Improve access to perinatal mental health services
- Increase consultants specializing in perinatal mental health problems
- Increase specialist activities to avoid risk of mother and baby being admitted to a general psychiatric ward
- Form a strategy group reflective of all key members of the multiprofessional team to review services for the childbearing woman with perinatal mental health problems
- Ensure interprofessional and interagency collaboration, especially within the primary and secondary care sectors

> Box 26.2 **Summary of key recommendations for best practice – cont'd**
>
> **Research, education and training**
> - Evaluate perinatal mental health services
> - Develop interprofessional or interagency education programmes to aid learning and to improve and understand lines of communication or delineate professional boundaries
> - Distinguish between psychology and pathology in order to avoid or reduce inappropriate referrals

Tricyclic antidepressants or sertraline should be the antidepressants of choice during breastfeeding.

Antipsychotics

- As antipsychotic medication passes through the placenta and into breast milk, the dose should be reduced as far as possible.
- Examples of anti-psychotics are:
  - trifluoperazine, chlorpromazine and haloperidol (older and 'typical' group)
  - clozapine, olanzapine and risperidone (newer and 'atypical' group).

Mood stabilizers

- Used to treat bipolar illness (including puerperal psychosis).
- Lithium carbonate is not recommended in pregnancy or while breastfeeding.
- Close monitoring is essential if it has to be taken.
- Abrupt cessation is associated with substantial risk of recurrence of the condition.

Anticonvulsants

- Used as mood stabilizers for > 30 years.
- Newer groups include lamotrigine and topiramate.
- All anticonvulsants are associated with a risk of fetal teratogenesis.
- Folic acid reduces the risk of neural tube defects.

SUGGESTED READING

Bosanquet, K., Bailey, D., Gilbody, S., et al. (2015) Diagnostic accuracy of the Whooley questions for the identification of depression: a diagnostic meta-analysis. Available at: http://bmjopen.bmj.com/content/5/12/e008913.full.pdf+html (accessed 24 April 2016).

Howard, L.M., Megnin-Viggars, O., Symington, I., Pilling, S., 2014. Antenatal and postnatal mental health: summary of updated NICE guidance. BMJ 349, g7394. http://dx.doi.org/10.1136/bmj.g7394 (accessed 24 April 2016).

National Institute for Health and Care Excellence, 2014. Antenatal and postnatal mental health: clinical management and service guidance. CG192. Available at: https://www.nice.org.uk/guidance/cg192/resources/antenatal-and-postnatal-mental-health-clinical-management-and-service-guidance-35109869806789 (accessed 24 April 2016).

Useful websites

National Institute for Health and Care Excellence. Available at: https://www.nice.org.uk

The International Association for Perinatal Mental Health. Available at: http://marcesociety.com

Section | 5 |

The Newborn Baby

The Baby at Birth and Neonatal Resuscitation

A newborn baby's survival is dependent on adaptations in cardiopulmonary circulation and other physiological adjustments to replace placental function and maintain homeostasis. Birth is also the commencement of the reciprocal dynamic parent(s)/baby relationship.

ADAPTATION TO EXTRAUTERINE LIFE

Commences with:
- intermittent diminution of the oxygen supply during uterine contractions (vaginal births or emergency operative births for women who labour)
- compression followed by decompression of the head and chest, and extension of the limbs, hips and spine during a vaginal birth
- the baby emerging into the world to a lighter, noisier, cooler and dry environment.

Simultaneously, the baby has to make major adjustments in the respiratory and circulatory systems, as well as controlling body temperature.

Respiratory and cardiovascular changes are interdependent and concurrent.

Pulmonary adaptation

- Prior to birth, the fetus makes 'breathing' movements and the lungs will be mature enough, both biochemically and anatomically, to produce surfactant and will have adequate numbers of alveoli for gas exchange.
- The fetal lung is full of fluid, which is excreted by the lung itself. During a vaginal birth, this fluid leaves the alveoli, either by being squeezed via the air passages and out of the mouth and nose, or by moving across the alveolar walls into the pulmonary lymphatic vessels and into the thoracic duct, or to the lung capillaries.
- Stimuli to respiration include the mild hypercapnia, hypoxia and acidosis that result from normal labour, due partially to the

intermittent cessation of maternal–placental perfusion with contractions.

- The rhythm of respiration changes from episodic shallow fetal respiration to regular deeper breathing, as a result of a combination of chemical and neural stimuli: notably, a fall in pH and partial pressure of arterial oxygen (PaO_2) and a rise in partial pressure of arterial carbon dioxide ($PaCO_2$).
- Other stimuli include cold, light, noise, touch and pain.
- Considerable negative intrathoracic pressure of up to 9.8 kPa (100 cm water) is exerted as the first breath is taken.
- Pressure exerted to effect inhalation diminishes with each breath taken until only 5 cm water pressure is required to inflate the lungs. This is an effect of surfactant, which lines the alveoli, lowering surface tension and thus permitting residual air to remain in the alveoli between breaths.
- Surfactant is a complex of lipoproteins and proteins produced by the alveolar type 2 cells (*pneumocytes*) in the lungs; it is primarily concerned with the reduction in surface tension at the alveolar surface, thus reducing the work of breathing.

Cardiovascular adaptation

- The baby's circulatory system must make major adjustments in divert deoxygenated blood to the lungs for reoxygenation.
- With the expansion of the lungs and lowered pulmonary vascular resistance, virtually all the cardiac output is sent to the lungs.
- Oxygenated blood returning to the heart from the lungs increases the pressure within the left atrium.
- Pressure in the right atrium is lowered because blood ceases to flow through the cord.
- A functional closure of the foramen ovale takes place. During the first days of life this closure is reversible and reopening may occur if pulmonary vascular resistance is high (e.g. when crying) resulting in transient cyanotic episodes in the baby.
- The septa usually fuse within the first year of life to form the interatrial septum, though in some individuals, perfect anatomical closure may never be achieved.
- Contraction of the muscular walls of the ductus arteriosus takes place; this is thought to occur because of sensitivity of the muscle of the ductus arteriosus to increased oxygen tension and reduction in circulating prostaglandin.

- Because of altered pressure gradients between the aorta and pulmonary artery, a temporary reverse left-to-right shunt through the ductus arteriosus may persist for a few hours, though there is usually functional closure of this temporary structure within 8–10 hours of birth.
- The remaining temporary structures of the fetal circulation – the *umbilical vein, ductus venosus and hypogastric arteries* – close functionally within a few minutes after birth and constriction of the cord. Anatomical closure by fibrous tissue occurs within 2–3 months, resulting in the formation of the ligamentum teres, ligamentum venosum and the obliterated hypogastric arteries. The proximal portions of the hypogastric arteries persist as the superior vesical arteries.

Thermal adaptation

- The baby enters a much cooler atmosphere, the birthing room temperature of 21°C contrasting sharply with an intrauterine temperature of 37.7°C. Heat loss can be rapid, and takes place through the mechanisms listed in Box 27.1.
- The heat-regulating centre in the baby's brain has the capacity to promote heat production in response to stimuli received from thermoreceptors. However, this is dependent on increased metabolic activity, compromising the baby's ability to control body temperature, especially in adverse environmental conditions.
- The baby has a limited ability to shiver and is unable to increase muscle activity voluntarily to generate heat. Therefore, the baby must depend on his or her ability to produce heat by metabolism.

Brown fat and thermogenesis

- The neonate has brown adipose tissue, which assists in the rapid mobilization of heat resources (namely, free fatty acids and glycerol) in times of cold stress. This mechanism is called non-shivering thermogenesis.
- Babies derive most of their heat production from the metabolism of brown fat.
- The term baby has sufficient brown fat to meet minimum heat needs for 2–4 days after birth, but cold stress results in increased oxygen consumption as the baby strives to maintain sufficient heat for survival.
- Brown fat uses up to three times as much oxygen as other tissue, with the undesired effect of diverting oxygen and glucose from vital centres such as the brain and cardiac muscle.

Box 27.1 **Mechanisms of heat loss in the newborn baby**

Evaporation

- Amniotic fluid evaporates from the skin. Each millilitre that evaporates removes 560 calories of heat. The baby's large surface area:body mass ratio potentiates heat loss, especially from the head, which comprises 25% of body mass

Poor insulation

- The subcutaneous fat layer is thin, allowing rapid transfer of core heat to the skin and the environment

Conduction

- Conduction takes place when the baby is in contact with cold surfaces

Radiation

- Heat radiates to cold objects in the environment that are not in contact with the baby

Convection

- This is caused by currents of cool air passing over the surface of the body

- In addition, cold stress causes vasoconstriction, thus reducing pulmonary perfusion, and respiratory acidosis develops as the pH and PaO_2 of the blood decrease and the $PaCO_2$ increases, leading to respiratory distress, exhibited by tachypnoea, and grunting respirations. This, together with the reduction in pulmonary perfusion, may result in the reopening or maintenance of the right-to-left shunt across the ductus arteriosus.
- Anaerobic glycolysis (i.e. the metabolism of glucose in the absence of oxygen) results in the production of acid, compounding the situation by adding a metabolic acidosis.
- Protraction of cold stress should be avoided.
- The peripheral vasoconstrictor mechanisms of the baby are unable to prevent the fall in core body temperature that occurs within the first few hours after birth. It is important, therefore, to minimize heat loss at birth.

IMMEDIATE CARE OF THE BABY AT BIRTH

Prevention of heat loss

It is important to provide an ambient temperature in the range 21–25°C. The baby's temperature can drop by as much as 3–4.5°C within the first minute. Measures to conserve heat include:

- drying the baby at birth
- avoiding draughts to maintain the room temperature as already detailed
- removing wet towels
- encouraging skin-to-skin contact with the mother
- wrapping the baby in dry, pre-warmed towels.

The midwife must have knowledge of the sources of heat loss highlighted in Box 27.1.

Clearing the airway

- As the baby's head is born, any excess mucus may be wiped gently from the mouth. Care must be taken to avoid touching the nares, as such action may stimulate reflex inhalation of debris in the trachea.
- Although fetal pulmonary fluid is present in the mouth, most babies will achieve a clear airway unaided. Only rarely will it be necessary to clear the airway with the aid of a soft suction catheter attached to low-pressure (10 cm water) mechanical suction.
  - If suction is necessary, it is important to aspirate the oropharynx prior to the nasopharynx so that, if the baby gasps as the nasal passages are aspirated, mucus or other material is not drawn down into the respiratory tract.
  - Suction at the back of the pharynx can result in vagal stimulation, with laryngospasm and bradycardia.

Cutting the umbilical cord

- A Cochrane systematic review highlighted the beneficial neonatal outcomes of delayed cord clamping (e.g. increased early haemoglobin concentration and iron level).
- Delayed clamping and cutting of the cord is also advocated in preterm babies.

Table 27.1 The Apgar score

	Score		
Sign	**0**	**1**	**2**
Heart rate	Absent	< 100 bpm	> 100 bpm
Respiratory effort	Absent	Slow, irregular	Good or crying
Muscle tone	Limp	Some flexion of limbs	Active
Reflex response to stimulus	None	Minimal grimace	Cough or sneeze
Colour	Blue, pale	Body pink, extremities blue	Completely pink

The score is assessed at 1 minute and 5 minutes after birth. Medical aid should be sought if the score is less than 7. 'Apgar minus colour' score omits the fifth sign. Medical aid should be sought if the score is less than 6.

Identification

- The time of birth and sex of the baby are noted and recorded.
- Babies born in a hospital setting must be readily identifiable from one another via identification labels in accordance with local and national protocols.

Immediate neonatal assessment at birth

At 1 minute and 5 minutes after the birth, an assessment is made of the baby's general condition using the crude measure of the Apgar score (Table 27.1).

- The assessment at 1 minute is important for the further management of resuscitation.
- An assessment at 5 minutes provides a record of response to resuscitation and immediate care needs.
- The higher the score, the better the outcome for the baby. A mnemonic – APGAR – for the Apgar score is given in Box 27.2.

Continued early care

Prior to leaving the mother's home or transferring the baby to the ward, the midwife undertakes an initial detailed examination of the baby in the presence of the parent(s), to detect early any malformations and to provide the parents with health education information about

> Box 27.2 **A mnemonic for the Apgar score**
>
> - **A**ppearance, i.e. colour
> - **P**ulse, i.e. heart rate
> - **G**rimace, i.e. response to stimuli
> - **A**ctive, i.e. tone
> - **R**espirations

the neonatal screening programme, including the more detailed Neonatal and Infant Physical Examination (NIPE). In the UK, this assessment is performed within 24–72 hours of birth by a NIPE practitioner (i.e. a midwife who has undertaken the NIPE programme or a doctor). Information about general neonatal care is also provided. Fig. 27.1 summarizes the key issues involved in the initial examination of the neonate at birth by the midwife.

- Ensure the umbilical cord is securely clamped via application of a disposable plastic clamp (or rubber band or three cord ligatures) placed not too close to the skin but approximately 2–3 cm from the umbilicus.
- Check and record the baby's temperature.
- It is not necessary to bath the baby immediately after birth. This and other non-urgent procedures should be deferred to minimize thermal stress.

Vitamin K

- To prevent vitamin K deficiency-related bleeding (VKDB) prophylaxis by the administration of vitamin K preparation via oral or intramuscular route is recommended but is not a universal practice.
- Administration of vitamin K to neonates can be the oral or parenteral (intramuscular) route, depending on parental choice and consent.
- Vitamin K is fat soluble and can only be absorbed from the intestine in the presence of bile salts.
- The body's capacity to store vitamin K is very low and the half-life of the vitamin K-dependent coagulation factors is short.
- A single dose (1.0 mg) of intramuscular vitamin K after birth has been found to be effective in the prevention of classic VKDB.

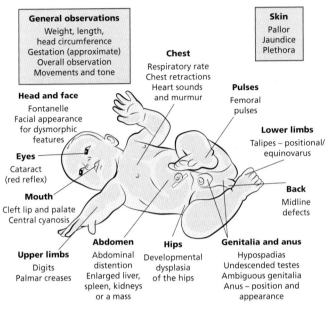

General observations
Weight, length,
head circumference
Gestation (approximate)
Overall observation
Movements and tone

Skin
Pallor
Jaundice
Plethora

Chest
Respiratory rate
Chest retractions
Heart sounds
and murmur

Pulses
Femoral
pulses

Head and face
Fontanelle
Facial appearance
for dysmorphic
features

Lower limbs
Talipes – positional/
equinovarus

Eyes
Cataract
(red reflex)

Back
Midline
defects

Mouth
Cleft lip and palate
Central cyanosis

Upper limbs
Digits
Palmar creases

Abdomen
Abdominal
distention
Enlarged liver,
spleen, kidneys
or a mass

Hips
Developmental
dysplasia
of the hips

Genitalia and anus
Hypospadias
Undescended testes
Ambiguous genitalia
Anus – position and
appearance

Fig. 27.1 Initial neonatal examination.

FAILURE TO ESTABLISH RESPIRATION AT BIRTH

Although the majority of babies gasp and establish respirations within 60 seconds of birth, some do not, mainly as a consequence of intrauterine hypoxia.

Intrauterine hypoxia

Possible causes include:
- maternal cardiac or respiratory disease
- eclamptic fit
- delayed intubation for induction of general anaesthesia
- hypertension
- hypotension due to haemorrhage or shock
- hypertonic uterine action
- prolapsed or compressed umbilical cord

405

- abnormal fetal cardiac function
- reduced fetal haemoglobin, e.g. Rhesus incompatibility, ruptured vasa praevia.

The fetus responds to hypoxia by accelerating the heart rate in an effort to maintain supplies of oxygen to the brain.

The consequences of hypoxia are:

- Glucose depletion stimulating anaerobic glycolysis and resulting in a metabolic acidosis.
- Cerebral vessels dilate and some brain swelling may occur.
- Reduced peripheral circulation.
- Fetal acidosis may lead to:
  - depletion of cardiac glycogen reserves
  - fetal bradycardia
  - relaxation of the anal sphincter with passage of meconium into the liquor
  - gasping breathing movements triggered by hypoxia may result in the aspiration of meconium-stained liquor into the lungs, which presents an additional problem after birth.
- The length of time during which the fetus or neonate is subjected to hypoxia determines the outcome.
- The initial response of gasping respirations is followed by a period of apnoea lasting 1.5 minutes – *primary apnoea*. If this is not resolved by means of intervention techniques, it is followed by a further episode of gasping respirations. These accelerate while diminishing in depth until, approximately 8 minutes after birth, respirations cease completely – *secondary apnoea*.
- The essential difference between primary and secondary apnoea is the baby's circulatory status.
- During primary apnoea, the circulation and heart rate are maintained and such babies respond quickly to simple resuscitation measures.
- In secondary apnoea, the circulation is impaired, the heart rate is slow and the baby looks shocked (Table 27.2).

Respiratory depression

- Obstruction of the baby's airway by mucus, blood, liquor or meconium is one of the most common reasons for a baby failing to establish respirations.
- Depression of the respiratory centre may be due to:
  - the effects of drugs administered to the mother, e.g. opiates or diazepam

Table 27.2 Degrees of respiratory depression

Mildly depressed	Severely depressed
Heart rate not severely depressed (60–80 bpm)	Slow feeble heart rate (< 40 bpm)
Short delay in onset of respiration	No attempt to breathe
Good muscle tone	Poor muscle tone
Responsive to stimuli	Limp, unresponsive to stimuli
Deeply cyanosed	Pale, grey
Apgar score 5–7	Apgar score < 5
No significant deprivation of oxygen during labour (primary apnoea)	Oxygen lack has been prolonged before or after delivery, circulatory failure is present, baby is shocked (secondary apnoea)

- cerebral hypoxia during labour or traumatic birth
- immaturity of the baby, which causes mechanical dysfunction because of underdeveloped lungs, lack of surfactant and a soft pliable thoracic cage
- intranatal pneumonia, which can inhibit successful establishment of respirations and should be considered, especially if the membranes have been ruptured for some time
- severe anaemia, caused by fetomaternal haemorrhage or Rhesus incompatibility, which diminishes the oxygen-carrying capacity of the blood
- respiratory function, which may be compromised by major congenital malformations, particularly those of the central nervous system or within the respiratory tract
- a congenital malformation such as choanal or tracheal atresia which may be present (choanal atresia should be suspected when a baby is pink when crying but becomes cyanosed at rest).

RESUSCITATION OF THE NEWBORN

The aims of resuscitation are to:
- establish and maintain a clear airway, by ventilation and oxygenation

---

Box 27.3 Resuscitation equipment

- Resuscitaire with overhead radiant heater (switched on) and light, piped oxygen, manometer, suction and clock timer
- Two straight-bladed infant laryngoscopes, spare batteries and bulbs (size 0 and 1)
- Neonatal endotracheal tubes (2.0, 2.5, 3.0 and 3.5 mm) and connectors
- Neonatal airways (sizes 0, 00 and 000)
- Suction catheters (sizes 6, 8 and 10FG)
- Neonatal bag and mask and facemasks of assorted sizes (clear, soft masks)
- Magill forceps
- Endotracheal tube introducer
- Syringes (1 ml, 2 ml, 5 ml and 20 ml) and assorted needles
- Drugs: Naloxone hydrochloride 1 ml ampoules 400 µg/ml (adult Narcan)
- Adrenaline (epinephrine) 1:10 000 and 1:1000
- THAM (tris-hydroxymethyl-amino-methane) 7%
- Sodium bicarbonate 4.2%
- Dextrose 10%
- Vitamin K_1 1 mg ampoules
- Normal saline 0.9%
- Stethoscope
- Cord clamps
- Warmed dry towels
- Adhesive tape for tube fixation

- ensure effective circulation
- correct acidosis
- prevent hypothermia, hypoglycaemia and haemorrhage.

All equipment necessary for advanced resuscitation of the neonate must be ready and easily accessible for use (Box 27.3).

- As soon as the baby is born, the clock timer of the resuscitaire should be started. The Apgar score is assessed in the normal manner at 1 minute. In the absence of any respiratory effort, resuscitation measures are commenced.

408

Table 27.3 Resuscitation action plan

A	Anticipation	Assessment (Apgar)	Airway – clear debris
B	Breathing	Bag + mask	
C	Circulation	Cardiac massage	Caring – warmth, comfort
D	Doctor	Drugs	Documentation
E	Explanation	Environment	Endotracheal tube
F	Follow-up care	Family	

- As discussed earlier, if necessary, the baby's upper airways may be cleared by gentle suction of the oropharynx and nasopharynx and the presence of a heart beat verified.
- The baby is dried quickly, transferred to a well-lit resuscitaire and placed on a flat, firm surface at a comfortable working height and under a radiant heat source to prevent hypothermia.
- The baby's shoulders may be elevated on a small towel, which causes slight extension of the head and straightens the trachea. Hyperextension may cause airway obstruction owing to the short neck of the neonate and large, ill-supported tongue.

Table 27.3 details the action plan that should be implemented for resuscitation of the neonate. Readers are directed to the Resuscitation Council (UK) for an example of the most up to date guideline and algorithm for the resuscitation of babies at birth by accessing the following link: https://www.resus.org.uk/resuscitation-guidelines/resuscitation-and-support-of-transition-of-babies-at-birth.

External cardiac massage

- Chest compressions should be performed if the heart rate is less than 60 bpm, or between 60 and 100 bpm and falling despite adequate ventilation.
- The most effective way of performing chest compressions is to:
  - encircle the baby's chest with your fingers on the baby's spine and your thumbs on the lower mid-sternum (Fig. 27.2)
  - depress the chest at a rate of 100–120 times per minute, at a ratio of three compressions to one ventilation, and at a depth of one-third (2–3 cm) of the baby's chest.

(Excessive pressure over the lower end of the sternum may cause rib, lung or liver damage.)

Sternum

Fig. 27.2 External cardiac massage.

Use of drugs by the medical team

- If the baby's response is slow or he/she remains hypotonic after ventilation is achieved, consideration will be given to the use of drugs.
- In specialist obstetric units, pulse oximetry may be employed to monitor hypoxia and blood obtained through the umbilical artery or vein to ascertain biochemical status. Results will enable appropriate administration of resuscitation drugs, as discussed in the following section.

Naloxone hydrochloride

- Caution must be exercised with its use; employed only in specific circumstances by the doctor.
- It is a powerful opioid antagonist for the reversal of the effects of maternal narcotic drugs given in the preceding 3 hours.
- Ventilation should be established prior to its use.
- *It must not be given to apnoeic babies.*
- A dose of up to 100 µg/kg body weight may be administered intramuscularly for prolonged action.
- As opioid action may persist for some hours, the midwife must be alert for signs of relapse when a repeat dose may be required.
- *It should not be administered to babies of narcotic-addicted mothers, as this may precipitate acute withdrawal.*

Sodium bicarbonate

- Not recommended for brief periods of cardiopulmonary resuscitation.
- Once tissues are oxygenated by lung inflation with 100% oxygen and cardiac compression, the acidosis will self-correct unless asphyxia is very severe.
- Given by slow intravenous injection if the heart rate is < 60 bpm despite effective ventilation, chest compression and two intravenous doses of adrenaline (epinephrine).
- It should be given slowly and cautiously to avoid the attendant risk of intracranial haemorrhage.
- *It should not be given prior to ventilation being established.*
- In some resource rich countries, THAM 7% (tris-hydroxymethyl-amino-methane) 0.5 mmol/kg may be used in preference to sodium bicarbonate.

Adrenaline (epinephrine)

- Often used if the heart rate is < 60 bpm despite 1 minute of effective ventilation and chest compression.
- Can be administered intravenously or via an endotracheal tube that is already in situ.

Dextrose solution

- Hypoglycaemia is not usually a problem unless resuscitation has been prolonged.

> Box 27.4 **Key points for practice**
>
> - Anticipation of problems
> - Checking of resuscitation equipment
> - Starting clock
> - Suctioning
> - Keeping baby warm
> - Apgar score
> - Bag and mask ventilation
> - Endotracheal ventilation
> - Cardiac massage
> - Drugs
> - Other problems

- A solution of dextrose 10% 3 ml/kg may be given intravenously to correct a blood sugar of less than 2.5 mmol/L.

Observations and after-care

- Constant vigilance and observations are required.
- Throughout the resuscitation procedure the baby's response is monitored and recorded. An accurate written record detailing the resuscitation events is essential.
- The endotracheal tube may be left in place for a few minutes after the baby starts to breathe spontaneously. Suction may be applied through the endotracheal tube as it is removed.
- Explanation must be given to the parent(s) about the resuscitation and the need for transfer to hospital (if the baby was born at home) or to the neonatal unit. The principles of resuscitation of the newborn are applicable wherever and whenever apnoea occurs.
- The midwife must be able to implement emergency care while awaiting medical assistance (Box 27.4 and Table 27.3).

SUGGESTED READING

Fulton, C., Stoll, K., Thordarson, D., 2016. Bedside resuscitation of newborns with an intact umbilical cord: experiences of midwives from British Columbia. Midwifery 34, 42–46. doi: 10.1016/j.midw.2016.01.006.

McDonald, S.T., Middleton, P., Dowswell, T., et al., 2013. Effect of timing of umbilical cord clamping of term infants on maternal and neonatal outcomes. Cochrane Database Syst. Rev. (7), CD004074, doi: 10.1002/1465/858.pub3.

Useful website

http://www.nrls.npsa.nhs.uk. The National Reporting and Learning System (NRLS) combines the work of the National Patient Safety Authority (NPSA) in England and Wales to provide a comprehensive database of patient safety information to identify and address patient safety issues under the auspices of the NHS Commissioning Board Special Health Authority.

The Normal Baby

GENERAL CHARACTERISTICS

Appearance

Salient points relating to the newborn baby's general appearance are listed in Box 28.1.

Physiology

Respiratory system

- The normal baby has a respiratory rate of 40–60 breaths per minute.
- Breathing is diaphragmatic, the chest and abdomen rising and falling synchronously.
- The breathing pattern is erratic. Respirations are shallow and irregular, being interspersed with brief 10- to 15-second periods of apnoea. This is known as periodic breathing.
- Babies are obligatory nose breathers and do not convert automatically to mouth breathing when nasal obstruction occurs.
- Babies have a lusty cry, which is normally loud and of medium pitch.

Cardiovascular system and blood

- The heart rate is rapid: 110–160 beats per minute.
- Blood pressure fluctuates from 50–55/25–30 mmHg to 80/50 mmHg in the first 10 days of life.
- The total circulating blood volume at birth is 80 ml/kg body weight.
- The haemoglobin (Hb) level is high (13–20 g/dl), of which 50–85% is fetal Hb.
- Breakdown of excess red blood cells in the liver and spleen predisposes to jaundice in the first week.
- Vitamin K-dependent clotting factors II (prothrombin), VII, IX and X are low.
- Platelet levels equal those of the adult but there is a reduced capacity for adhesion and aggregation.

> Box 28.1 **The appearance of the newborn baby**
>
> - Weight is highly variable but is normally approximately 3.5 kg
> - Length is in the region of 50 cm from the crown of the head to the heels
> - Occipitofrontal head circumference is 34–35 cm
> - In an attitude of flexion, with arms extended, babies' fingers reach upper thigh level
> - Vernix caseosa, a white sticky substance, is present on the baby's skin at birth
> - Lanugo, downy hair, covers areas of the skin
> - Colour is according to ethnic origin
> - Cartilage of the ears is well formed
> - Milia, distended glands in the skin, are often found over nose and cheeks

Temperature regulation

- The baby's normal core temperature is 36.5–37.3 °C.
- A healthy, clothed, term baby will maintain this body temperature satisfactorily, provided the environmental temperature is sustained between 18 and 21 °C, nutrition is adequate and movements are not restricted by tight swaddling.

Renal system

- The glomerular filtration rate is low and tubular reabsorption capabilities are limited.
- The baby is not able to concentrate or dilute urine very well in response to variations in fluid intake nor compensate for high or low levels of solutes in the blood.
- The first urine is passed at birth or within the first 24 hours, and thereafter with increasing frequency as fluid intake rises.
- The urine is dilute, straw coloured and odourless.
- Cloudiness of the urine caused by mucus and urates may be present initially until fluid intake increases.
- Urates may cause pink staining, which is insignificant.

Gastrointestinal system

- The mucous membrane of the mouth is pink and moist.
- The teeth are buried in the gums and ptyalin secretion is low.

- Small epithelial pearls are sometimes present at the junction of the hard and soft palates.
- Sucking pads in the cheeks give them a full appearance.
- Sucking and swallowing reflexes are coordinated.
- The stomach has a small capacity (15–30 ml), which increases rapidly in the first weeks of life.
- The cardiac sphincter is weak, predisposing to regurgitation or posseting.
- Gastric acidity, equal to that of the adult within a few hours after birth, diminishes rapidly within the first few days and by the 10th day the baby is virtually achlorhydric, which increases the risk of infection.
- Gastric emptying time is normally 2–3 hours.
- The gut is sterile at birth but is colonized within a few hours.
- Bowel sounds are present within 1 hour of birth.
- Meconium, present in the large intestine from 16 weeks' gestation, is passed within the first 24 hours of life and is totally excreted within 48–72 hours.
- Features of meconium, the first stool of the newborn, is blackish–green in colour, is tenacious and contains bile, fatty acids, mucus and epithelial cells.
- From the 3rd–5th neonatal day the stools undergo a transitional stage and are brownish–yellow in colour.
- Once feeding is established, yellow faeces are passed.
- The consistency and frequency of stools reflect the type of feeding.
- Breast milk results in loose, bright yellow and inoffensive acid stools. The stools of the bottle-fed baby are paler in colour, semi-formed and less acidic, and have a slightly sharp smell.
- Physiological immaturity of the liver results in low production of glucuronyl transferase for the conjugation of bilirubin. This, together with a high level of red cell breakdown and stimulation of hepatic blood flow, may result in a transient jaundice which is manifest on the 3rd to 5th days.
- Glycogen stores are rapidly depleted, so early feeding is required to maintain normal blood glucose levels (2.6–4.4 mmol/L).
- Feeding stimulates liver function and colonization of the gut, which assists in the formation of vitamin K.

Immunological adaptations

- Neonates demonstrate a marked susceptibility to infections.
- The baby has some immunoglobulins at birth.

- There are three main immunoglobulins – IgG, IgA and IgM.
- Only IgG is small enough to cross the placental barrier. It affords immunity to specific viral infections. At birth the baby's levels of IgG are equal to or slightly higher than those of the mother. This provides passive immunity during the first few months of life.
- IgM and IgA do not cross the placental barrier but can be manufactured by the fetus. Levels of IgM at term are 20% those of the adult, taking 2 years to attain adult levels (elevation of IgM levels at birth is suggestive of intrauterine infection).
- Breast milk, especially colostrum, provides the baby with IgA passive immunity.
- The thymus gland, where lymphocytes are produced, is relatively large at birth and continues to grow until 8 years of age.

Reproductive system: genitalia and breasts

- In boys, the testes are descended into the scrotum by 37 weeks. The urethral meatus opens at the tip of the penis and the prepuce is adherent to the glans.
- In girls born at term, the labia majora normally cover the labia minora. The hymen and clitoris may appear disproportionately large.
- In both sexes, withdrawal of maternal oestrogens results in breast engorgement sometimes accompanied by secretion of 'milk' by the 4th or 5th day. Baby girls may develop pseudomenstruation for the same reason. Both boys and girls have a nodule of breast tissue around the nipple.

Skeletomuscular system

- The muscles are complete, subsequent growth occurring by hypertrophy rather than by hyperplasia.
- The long bones are incompletely ossified to facilitate growth at the epiphyses. The bones of the vault of the skull also reveal lack of ossification. This is essential for growth of the brain and facilitating moulding during labour. Moulding is resolved within a few days of birth.
- The posterior fontanelle closes at 6–8 weeks.
- The anterior fontanelle remains open until 18 months of age, making assessment of hydration and intracranial pressure possible by palpation of fontanelle tension.

PSYCHOLOGY AND PERCEPTION

- The newborn baby is alert and aware of his or her surroundings when awake.

Special senses

Vision

- Babies are sensitive to bright lights, which cause them to frown or blink.
- Newborns demonstrate a preference for bold black and white patterns and the shape of the human face, focusing at a distance of approximately 15–20 cm.
- No tears are present in the eyes of the newborn; therefore, they become infected easily.

Hearing

- Newborn babies' eyes turn towards sound. On hearing a high-pitched sound, they first blink or startle and then become agitated, and are comforted by low-pitched sounds. They prefer the sound of the human voice to other sounds.

Smell and taste

- Babies prefer the smell of milk to that of other substances and show a preference for human milk.
- They turn away from unpleasant smells and show preference for sweet taste, as demonstrated by vigorous and sustained sucking and a speedy grimacing response to bitter, salty or sour substances.

Touch

- Babies are acutely sensitive to touch, enjoying: skin-to-skin contact, baby massage, immersion in water, stroking, cuddling and rocking movements.

Sleeping and waking

- Sleeping and waking rhythms show marked variations. Initially, waking periods are related to hunger, but within a few weeks the waking periods last longer and meet the need for social interaction.

Crying

- The crying repertoire of babies distinguishes different needs and is the way in which they communicate discomfort and summon assistance. With experience, it is possible to differentiate the cry and identify the need, which may be hunger, thirst, pain, general discomfort (for example, wanting a change of position or feeling too cold or too hot), boredom, loneliness or a desire for physical and social contact.

EXAMINATION AT BIRTH

The reader is advised to refer again to Fig. 27.1 in Chapter 27, which provides a visual summary of the newborn examination conducted by the midwife at birth.

Colour and respirations

- Babies are obligatory nose breathers; bilateral nasal obstruction is of major significance if due to bilateral choanal atresia, which is a major medical emergency.
- Observe the colour of the baby's skin and mucous membranes. In the normal baby, the lips and mucous membranes are pink and well perfused.

Face, head and neck

- Each eye should be visualized to confirm that it is present and that the lens is clear. The eyes open spontaneously if the baby is held in an upright position. Any slight oedema or bruising is noted but may be insignificant. The normal space between the eyes is up to 3 cm.
- The skull should be palpated to determine the degree of moulding by the amount of over-riding of the bones at the sutures and fontanelles. The bones should feel hard in a term baby.
- A wide anterior fontanelle and splayed sutures may indicate hydrocephalus or immaturity.
- An oedematous swelling, caput succedaneum, may be noted overlying the part of the vertex that was presenting during labour.
- The short thick neck of the baby must be examined to exclude the presence of swellings and to ensure that rotation and flexion of the head are possible.

419

The mouth

- The mouth can be opened easily by pressing against the angle of the jaw. This allows visual inspection of the tongue, gums and palate.
- The palate should be high arched and intact, and the uvula should be central.
- As stated earlier, epithelial pearls (Epstein pearls) may be observed. They are of no significance, though occasionally mistaken for infection, and they disappear spontaneously.
- The palate should be palpated for any submucous cleft. A normal baby will respond by sucking the finger.
- A tight frenulum will give the appearance of tongue-tie; no treatment is necessary for this.

The ears

- The ears are inspected, noting their position.
- The upper notch of the pinna should be level with the canthus of the eye.
- Patency of the external auditory meatus is verified.
- Accessory auricles, small tags of tissue, are sometimes noted lying in front of the ear.
- Ear malformations can be associated with chromosomal anomalies and syndromes, and should be reported to a paediatrician.

Chest and abdomen

- Chest and abdominal movements are synchronous. The respirations may still be irregular at this stage.
- The space between the nipples should be noted, widely spaced nipples being associated with chromosomal abnormality.
- The shape of the abdomen should be rounded.
- Haemostasis of the umbilical cord is vital. A blood loss of 30 ml from a baby is equivalent to almost 0.5 L of blood from an adult.
- Normally, three cord vessels are present. Absence of one of the arteries is occasionally associated with renal anomalies and must be reported to the paediatrician.

Genitalia and anus

- If the neonate's sex is uncertain, the paediatrician will initiate investigations.

Limbs and digits

- The hands should be opened fully, as any accessory digits may be concealed in the clenched fist.
- The feet are examined for any malformations such as talipes equinovarus, as well as for any extra digit(s).
- The axillae, elbows, groins and popliteal spaces should also be examined for any malformation.
- Normal flexion and rotation of the wrist and ankle joints should be confirmed.

Spine

- With the baby lying prone, the midwife should inspect and palpate the baby's back. Any swellings, dimples or hairy patches may signify an occult spinal defect.

Temperature

- The baby's temperature may be taken, normally in the axilla (underarm), tympanum (ear) or groin. The normal baby's skin temperature should range from 36.5 to 37.3 °C.

Documentation

- The midwife records her findings in the case notes. Any abnormalities are brought to the attention of the paediatrician, or GP if birth occurs at home or a birth centre/midwife-led unit.

OBSERVATION AND GENERAL CARE

- In the hospital setting the identification bands, previously mentioned in Chapter 27, must remain on the baby until mother and baby are transferred home.
- During the first few hours after birth, the midwife should observe the baby frequently for any colour changes, patency of airway and haemorrhage from the umbilical cord.
- Temperature should also be monitored to ensure that it is maintained within the normal range.

Neonatal care

- In caring for the normal baby, it is important to ensure protection from:
  - airway obstruction
  - hypothermia

- infection
- injury and accident.

Prevention of airway obstruction

- It is important for a baby to sleep in the supine position (on the back) with the feet at the foot of the cot. This is one of the key public health messages to parents to help prevent/reduce the risk of sudden infant death (see Ch. 30).

Prevention of hypothermia

- Where possible, the room temperature should be maintained at 18–21°C.
- Bath water should be warm (36°C), and wet clothing should be changed as soon as possible.
- It is essential also to avoid overheating.
- Parents should be advised to take account of environmental temperature when dressing their baby. Swaddling should be avoided but if used, it should be loose enough to permit easy movement of baby's arms and legs.

Prevention of infection

- Members of staff who are liable to be a source of infection should not handle babies and friends and relatives who have colds or sore throats (especially children) should not visit.
- Hand washing before and after handling babies is essential.

Skin care

- Promotion of skin integrity is enhanced by avoiding friction against hard fabrics or soiled or wet clothing.
- The timing of the first bath is not critical, although it has been suggested that removal of blood and liquor reduces the risk of transmission of HIV and other organisms to staff.
- Daily bathing is not essential.
- The baby's eyes do not need to be cleansed unless a discharge is present.
- Attention should be paid to the washing and drying of skin flexures to prevent excoriation.
- The buttocks must be washed and dried carefully at every nappy change. Sore buttocks may occur if the stools are loose, if there is protracted delay in changing a soiled nappy or if the skin is traumatized by overenthusiastic rubbing. Regular use of a barrier

cream is recommended by some but may interfere with the 'one-way' membrane in disposable nappies.

- Cleanliness of the umbilical cord is essential.
- Hand washing is required before and after handling the cord.
- No specific cord treatment is required, although a wide variety of preparations have been used to promote early separation. Cleansing with tap water and keeping the cord dry have been shown to promote separation.
- The cord clamp or ligature may be removed on the third day, provided the cord is dry and necrosed. From a cultural perspective, a minority of women choose lotus birth (non-severance of the umbilical cord), believing it to be a spiritual and non-violent practice. Currently there is no evidence to support the potential benefits/risks of this practice.

Vaccination and immunization
- BCG vaccination may be given during the early neonatal period in some areas where early protection is desirable.
- Vaccination against hepatitis B and poliomyelitis may also be given in some parts of the world.

Prevention of injury and accident
- Advice should also be given to parents about baby care and safety in the home. This should address such issues as:
  - bed sharing
  - the use of cat nets
  - fireguards
  - cooker guards
  - stair gates
  - pram brakes
  - car seats.
- 'Smoking', 'back-to-sleep' and 'feet-to-foot' advice should be included.

Assessing the baby's wellbeing
- At every contact the mother is asked about the baby's health and feeding.
- Examination of the baby is at the discretion of the midwife and when the mother has any concerns.
- Weight loss is normal in the first few days but more than 10% body weight loss is deemed abnormal and requires investigation.

- Most babies regain their birth weight in 7–10 days, thereafter gaining weight at a rate of 150–200 g per week.

FULL EXAMINATION WITHIN 72 HOURS OF BIRTH

- This is usually performed by a competent professional (usually paediatrician or midwife) (Box 28.2).

Blood tests

- Certain inborn errors of metabolism and endocrine disorders are detected by means of a blood test, obtained from a heel prick made with a stilette on the lateral aspect of the heel to avoid nerves and blood vessels. Commonly, blood is dripped onto circles on an absorbent card, onto which full details of the baby's identity are entered.
- For detection of phenylketonuria, hypothyroidism and cystic fibrosis the baby must have had at least 4–6 days of milk feeding, and if for any reason the baby or mother is receiving antibiotics, this information should be recorded on the card.
- Some centres also test routinely for galactosaemia and haemaglobinopathies

PROMOTING FAMILY RELATIONSHIPS

Parent–infant attachment

- Parents develop their relationship with their babies in individual ways and at their own pace. It is suggested that the parents' relationship with one another is enhanced when the woman's partner is encouraged to be involved in discussions, choices and decisions about baby care and to share the responsibility for care.

Promoting confidence and competence

- Total care should be delegated to the parents as soon as possible. In hospital, especially, procedures can be rendered unnecessarily complicated for new mothers.

Promoting communication

- The increasing interest in baby massage in recent years capitalizes on the knowledge that the baby is sensitive and responsive to

Box 28.2 **Examination of the baby within 72 hours of birth**

Appearance

- Activity
- Behaviour
- Breathing
- Colour
- Cry
- Posture

Skin

- Colour
- Texture
- Rashes
- Birthmarks

Head

- Symmetry and facial features
- Face
- Fontanelles
- Mouth
- Eyes
- Ears
- Neck

Neck, limbs and joints

- Proportions
- Symmetry
- Digits
- Movements

Heart

- Position
- Rate
- Rhythm
- Sounds
- Murmurs
- Femoral pulses

Lungs

- Rate
- Effort
- Sounds

Abdomen

- Shape
- Palpation for organ enlargement
- Umbilical cord

Genitalia and anus

- Sex clear
- Complete and patent
- Testes descended or not
- Meconium within 24 hours
- Urinary output

Spine

- Length felt for integrity and skin cover

Central nervous system

- Behaviour
- Tone
- Movements
- Posture
- Reflexes as appropriate

Hips

- Barlow and Ortolani manoeuvres
- Symmetry of limbs

Feeding

- Ask mother, carers

Measurements

- Weight
- Length
- Head circumference

touch. Grapeseed or equivalent oil is used rather than baby oils, which stick to the skin.

- Aromatherapy oils should not be used, as the extent of their absorption is not known.

SUGGESTED READING

Ball, H.L., Howel, D., Bryant, A., et al., 2016. Bed-sharing by breastfeeding mothers: who shares and what is the relationship with breastfeeding duration? Acta Paediatr. 105 (6), 628–634. doi: 10.1111/apa.13354.

Graves, B.W., Haley, M.M., 2013. Newborn transition. J. Midwifery Womens Health 58 (6), 662–670.

Useful websites

http://www.unicef.org.uk. Provides useful resources for parents and health care professionals such as a checklist for breastfeeding mothers on how many wet and dirty nappies to expect each day in the initial neonatal period.

http://cpd.screening.nhs.uk/newbornbloodspot. Professional education and training programme on newborn blood spot screening can be located on this website.

Chapter | 29 |

Infant Feeding

ANATOMY AND PHYSIOLOGY OF THE BREAST

- The breasts are compound secreting glands, composed mainly of glandular tissue, which is arranged in lobes. Each lobe is divided into lobules that consist of alveoli and ducts.
- The alveoli contain acini cells, which secrete the components of milk and are surrounded by myoepithelial cells, which contract and propel the milk out.
- Small lactiferous ducts, carrying milk from the alveoli, unite to form larger ducts.
- Myoepithelial cells are oriented longitudinally along the ducts; under the influence of oxytocin, these smooth muscle cells contract and the tubule becomes shorter and wider.
- The nipple is composed of erectile tissue and plain muscle fibres, which have a sphincter-like action in controlling the flow of milk.
- Surrounding the nipple is an area of pigmented skin called the areola, which contains Montgomery glands. These produce a sebum-like substance, which acts as a lubricant during pregnancy and throughout breastfeeding.
- The breast is supplied with blood from the internal and external mammary arteries with corresponding venous drainage.
- Lymph drains freely between the two breasts and into lymph nodes in the axillae and the mediastinum.
- During pregnancy, oestrogens and progesterone induce alveolar and ductal growth, as well as stimulating the secretion of colostrum. When the levels of placental hormones fall, this allows the already high levels of prolactin to initiate milk secretion. Continued production of prolactin is caused by the baby feeding at the breast, with concentrations highest following night feeds.
- Prolactin is particularly important in the initiation of lactation. As lactation progresses, the milk removal becomes the driving force behind milk production, due to a protein feedback inhibitor of lactation. This protein accumulates in the breast as the milk accumulates and it exerts negative feedback control on the continued

production of milk. Removal of this autocrine inhibitory factor, by removing the milk, allows milk production to be stepped up again.

- Milk release is under neuroendocrine control. Tactile stimulation of the breast also stimulates the oxytocin, causing contraction of the myoepithelial cells. This process is known as the 'let-down' or 'milk ejection' reflex and makes the milk available to the baby. This occurs in discrete pulses throughout the feed and may well trigger the bursts of active feeding.

- In the early days of lactation this reflex is unconditioned. Later, it becomes a conditioned reflex, which can be enhanced or suppressed by environmental factors.

PROPERTIES AND COMPONENTS OF BREAST MILK

- Human milk varies in its composition. The most dramatic change in the composition of milk occurs during the course of a feed. At the beginning of the feed the baby receives a high volume of relatively low-fat milk.

- As the feed progresses, the volume of milk decreases but the proportion of fat in the milk increases, sometimes to as much as five times the initial value.

- The baby's ability to obtain this fat-rich milk is *not* determined by the length of time spent at the breast, but by the quality of attachment to the breast. The baby needs to be well attached so that he or she can use the tongue to maximum effect, stripping the milk from the breast, rather than relying solely on the mother's milk ejection reflex.

Fats and fatty acids

- For the human infant, with a unique and rapidly growing brain, it is the fat and not the protein in human milk that has particular significance. Ninety-eight per cent of the lipid in human milk is in the form of triglycerides: three fatty acids linked to a single molecule of glycerol.

- Over 100 fatty acids have so far been identified, approximately 46% being saturated fat and 54% unsaturated fat.

- Fat provides the baby with more than 50% of calorific requirements. It is utilized very rapidly because *the milk itself* contains the enzyme

(bile salt-stimulated lipase) needed for fat digestion, but in a form that only becomes active when it reaches the infant's intestine.
- Pancreatic lipase is not plentiful in the newborn, so a baby who is not fed human milk is less able to digest fat.

Carbohydrate

- The carbohydrate component of human milk is provided chiefly by lactose, which supplies the baby with approximately 40% of calorific requirements.
- Lactose is converted into galactose and glucose by the action of the enzyme lactase and these sugars provide energy to the rapidly growing brain.
- Lactose enhances the absorption of calcium and also promotes the growth of lactobacilli which increase intestinal acidity, thus reducing the growth of pathogenic organisms.

Protein

- Human milk contains less protein than any other mammalian milk. Human milk is whey dominant (the whey being mainly alpha-lactalbumin) and forms soft, flocculent curds when acidified in the stomach.

Vitamins

- All the vitamins required for good nutrition and health are supplied in breast milk, although the actual amounts vary from mother to mother.

Fat-soluble vitamins

Vitamin A
- This is present in human milk as retinol, retinyl esters and beta-carotene. It gives colostrum its yellow colour as colostrum contains twice the amount present in mature human milk.

Vitamin D
- This is the name given to two fat-soluble compounds: calciferol (vitamin D2) and cholecalciferol (vitamin D3).
- Vitamin D3 plays an essential role in the metabolism of calcium and phosphorus in the body and prevents rickets in children. Adults can obtain these substances from dietary sources and the conversion of 7-dehydrocholesterol in the skin to vitamin D3 from exposure to sunlight.

429

- For light-skinned babies, exposure to sunlight for 30 minutes per week wearing only a nappy, or 2 hours per week fully clothed but without a hat, will keep vitamin D requirements within the lower limits of the normal range.
- The babies of dark-skinned mothers living in temperate zones and preterm babies may be at risk of vitamin D deficiency. This is because vitamin D is produced mainly from exposure to sunlight. Darker skin contains more melanin than lighter skin, which offers some natural protection from the damaging UV rays of the sun. However, this means more time has to be spent in the sun before endogenous synthesis of Vitamin D in the skin occurs. Populations that reside in northern latitudes, such as the UK, have reduced sunlight/exposure to the sun and have difficulty producing enough vitamin D.
- Coupled to the this, the blanket use of sunscreen and a tendency of some families to live more 'indoors' leave many vulnerable to vitamin D deficiency. A paper in the Lancet journal has highlighted that rickets in the UK is at an all-time high for 50 years in children who have been hospitalized.

Vitamin E

- Although vitamin E is present in human milk, its role is uncertain. It appears to prevent the oxidization of polyunsaturated fatty acids and may prevent certain types of anaemia to which preterm infants are susceptible.

Vitamin K

- This vitamin (83% of which is present as alpha-tocopherol) is essential for the synthesis of blood-clotting factors. It is present in human milk and absorbed efficiently.
- Because it is fat soluble, it is present in greater concentrations in colostrum and in the high-fat hind-milk, although the increased volume of milk as lactation progresses means that the infant obtains twice as much vitamin K from mature milk as from colostrum.

Water-soluble vitamins

- Unless the mother's diet is seriously deficient, breast milk will contain adequate levels of all the vitamins.

- An improved diet is always more beneficial than artificial supplements. With some vitamins, particularly vitamin C, a plateau may be reached where increased maternal intake has no further impact on breast milk composition.

Minerals and trace elements

Iron

- Normal term babies are usually born with a high haemoglobin (Hb) level (16–22 g/dl), which decreases rapidly after birth. The iron recovered from Hb breakdown is utilized again.
- Babies also have ample iron stores, sufficient for at least 4–6 months.
- Although the amounts of iron are lower than those found in formula, the bioavailability of iron in breast milk is very much higher: 70% of the iron in breast milk is absorbed.
- Only 10% of iron is absorbed from formula.

Zinc

- A deficiency of this essential trace mineral may result in failure to thrive and typical skin lesions. Although there is more zinc present in formula than in human milk, the bio-availability is greater in human milk.
- Breastfed babies maintain high plasma zinc values when compared with formula-fed infants, even when the concentration of zinc is three times that of human milk.

Calcium

- Calcium is more efficiently absorbed from human milk than from formula milks because of human milk's higher calcium:phosphorus ratio.
- Infant formulae, which are based on cow's milk, inevitably have a higher phosphorous content than human milk.

Other minerals

- Human milk has significantly lower levels of calcium, phosphorus, sodium and potassium than formula.
- Copper, cobalt and selenium are present at higher levels. The higher bioavailability of these minerals and trace elements ensures that the infant's needs are met while also imposing a lower solute load on the neonatal kidney than do breast milk substitutes.

431

Anti-infective factors

Leucocytes

- During the first 10 days of life there are more white cells per ml in breast milk than there are in blood.
- Macrophages and neutrophils are among the most common leucocytes in human milk and they surround and destroy harmful bacteria by their phagocytic activity.

Immunoglobulins

- Five types of immunoglobulin have been identified in human milk: IgA, IgG, IgE, IgM and IgD.
- IgA is the most important, it is both synthesized and stored in the breast. Although some IgA is absorbed by the infant, much of it is not. Instead it coats the intestinal epithelium and protects the mucosal surfaces against entry of pathogenic bacteria and enteroviruses.
- IgA affords protection against:
  - *Escherichia coli*
  - salmonellae
  - shigellae
  - streptococci
  - staphylococci
  - pneumococci
  - poliovirus
  - the rotaviruses.

Lysozyme

- This kills bacteria by disrupting their cell walls. The concentration of lysozyme increases with prolonged lactation.

Lactoferrin

- This binds to enteric iron, thus preventing potentially pathogenic *E. coli* from obtaining the iron needed for survival.
- It also has antiviral activity (HIV, cytomegalovirus, herpes simplex virus), acting by interfering with virus absorption and/or penetration.

Bifidus factor

- The bifidus factor in human milk promotes the growth of Gram-positive bacilli in the gut flora, particularly *Lactobacillus bifidus*, which discourages the multiplication of pathogens.

432

Hormones and growth factors

- Epidermal growth factor (and insulin-like growth factor) found in breast milk and colostrum stimulate the baby's digestive tract to mature more quickly and strengthen the barrier properties of the gastrointestinal epithelium.
- Once the initially leaky membrane lining the gut matures, it is less likely to allow the passage of large molecules and becomes less vulnerable to micro-organisms.
- The timing of the first feed also has a significant effect on gut permeability, which drops markedly if the first feed takes place soon after birth.

MANAGEMENT OF BREASTFEEDING

The first feed

- In accordance with UNICEF baby friendly standards, skin-to-skin contact promotes early feeding and a good start to mothering, which contributes to the success of breastfeeding.
- The first feed should be supervised by the midwife, who will be able to guide the mother on attachment and positioning.
- The feed should proceed without pain and the baby be allowed to terminate the feed spontaneously.
- One of the UNICEF baby friendly standards is that the midwife should be able to apply knowledge of physiology and the principle of reciprocity to empower and support mothers to keep their babies in close proximity so that they can be responsive to their feeding and comfort cues.

Attachment and positioning

The baby's body should be *turned towards* the mother's body so that he/she is coming up to her breast at the same angle as her breast is coming down to him/her. Useful information and videos on attachment and positioning can be accessed via UNICEF website at: http://www.unicef.org.uk/BabyFriendly/Resources/AudioVideo/Positioning-and-attachment/

- If the baby's nose is opposite the mother's nipple before the baby is brought to the breast and his/her neck is slightly extended, the baby's mouth will be in the correct relationship to the nipple.
- In determining good attachment, UNICEF identifies four cardinal signs:

- ensure baby's mouth is wide open
- more of the areola can be viewed above the baby's mouth than below
- the baby's lower lip is turned outwards
- the baby's chin is touching the mother's breast.

Once attached correctly the baby will feed in a rhythmical way taking deep sucks while attached to the breast with some pausing between sucking.

Feeding behaviour

- When babies first go to the breast, they feed vigorously, with few pauses. As the feed progresses, pausing occurs more frequently and lasts longer.
- Pausing is an integral part of the baby's feeding rhythm and should not be interrupted. The change in the pattern probably relates to milk flow.
- If the baby is not satiated after feeding from the first breast, the baby *should be offered* the second breast after being given the opportunity to bring up wind.
- Provided that the baby starts each feed on alternate sides, both breasts will be used equally.
- If the baby does not release the breast or will not settle after a feed, the most likely reason is that he or she was not correctly attached to the breast and was therefore unable to strip the milk efficiently.
- Other reasons for coming off the breast are:
  - The baby may need to let go and pause if the milk flow is very fast.
  - The baby may have swallowed air with the generous flow of milk that occurs at the beginning of a feed and needs an opportunity to burp.
- There is no justification for imposing either one breast per feed or both breasts per feed as a feeding regime.

Timing and frequency of feeds

- It is not unusual in the first day or two for the baby to feed infrequently, and to have 6- to 8-hour gaps between good feeds, each of which may be quite long. This is normal and provides the mother with the opportunity to sleep if she needs to.
- As the milk volume increases, the feeds tend to become more frequent and a little shorter. It is unusual for a baby to feed less

often than six times in 24 hours from the 3rd day, and most babies ask for between six and eight feeds per 24 hours by the time they are a week old.

- Babies who feed infrequently may be consuming less milk than they need, and/or they may be unwell.
- To achieve successful breast-feeding, the new UNICEF baby friendly standards place emphasis on the education of mothers in terms of positioning, attachment, and hand expression, and on mothers understanding the importance of the reciprocal relationship with their baby, including responsive feeding. The terms 'baby-led' feeding and 'feeding on demand' are no longer employed.
- Responsive feeding simply means the mother responds early to the feeding cues of the baby (e.g. baby starting to awake from sleep, licking his/her lips, rooting or making sucking noises or even finger sucking). The mother might also feel that her breasts are full and need emptying.
- Breastfeeding involves offering the breasts for feeds as well as comfort.
- The feeding technique and the weight should be monitored.

Expressing breast milk

All breastfeeding mothers should know how to hand-express milk. The situations where expressing is appropriate are listed in Box 29.1.

Box 29.1 **Appropriate situations for expressing breast milk**

- There is concern about the interval between feeds in the early newborn period (expressed colostrum should always be given in preference to formula to healthy term babies)
- There are problems in attaching the baby to the breast
- The baby is separated from the mother, owing to prematurity or illness
- There is concern about the baby's rate of growth or the mother's milk supply (expressing to top up with the mother's own milk may be necessary in the short term while the cause of the problem is resolved)
- Later in lactation, the mother may need to be separated from her baby for periods (occasionally or regularly)

Care of the breasts

- Daily washing is all that is necessary for breast hygiene. The normal skin flora is beneficial to the baby.
- Brassieres may be worn to provide comfortable support and are useful if the breasts leak and breast pads (or breast shells) are used.

Breast problems

Sore and damaged nipples

- The cause is almost always trauma from the hard palate of the baby's mouth and tongue, which results from incorrect attachment of the baby to the breast. Correcting this will provide immediate relief from pain and will also allow rapid healing to take place. Epithelial growth factor, contained in fresh human milk and saliva, may aid this process.
- 'Resting' the nipple is not advised as, although this enables healing to take place, it makes the continuation of lactation much more complicated.
- Nipple shields should only be used with extreme caution, and never before the mother has begun to lactate.

Other causes of soreness

- Infection with *Candida albicans* (thrush) can occur, although it is not common during the first week.
- The sudden development of pain, when the mother has had a period of trouble-free feeding, is suggestive of thrush. The nipple and areola are often inflamed and shiny, and pain typically persists throughout the feed. The baby may show signs of oral or anal thrush. Both mother and baby should receive concurrent fungicidal treatment.

One breast only

- It is perfectly possible to feed a baby well using just one breast, as each breast works independently.

Anatomical variations

These are described in Box 29.2.

> ## Box 29.2 **Anatomical nipple variations**
>
> ### Long nipples
>
> - These can lead to poor feeding because the baby is able to latch on to the nipple without drawing breast tissue into his or her mouth
> - The mother may need to be shown how to help the baby to draw in a sufficient portion of the breast
>
> ### Short nipples
>
> - As the baby has to form a teat from both the breast and nipple, short nipples should not cause problems
> - The mother should be reassured
>
> ### Abnormally large nipples
>
> - If the baby is small, his/her mouth may not be able to get beyond the nipple and on to the breast
> - Lactation could be initiated by expressing, either by hand or by pump, provided that the nipple fits into the breast cup
> - As the baby grows and the breast and nipple become more protractile, breastfeeding may become possible
>
> ### Inverted and flat nipples
>
> - If the nipple is deeply inverted it may be necessary to initiate lactation by expressing
> - Attempts to attach the baby to the breast are delayed until lactation is established and the breasts have become soft and the breast tissue more protractile

Problems with breastfeeding

Engorgement

- This condition occurs on approximately the 3rd or 4th day postpartum.
- The breasts are hard (often oedematous), painful and sometimes flushed.
- The mother may be pyrexial.
- Engorgement is usually an indication that the baby is not in step with the stage of lactation.
- Engorgement may occur if feeds are delayed or restricted or if the baby is unable to feed efficiently due to poor positioning/attachment technique.

- Management should be aimed at enabling the baby to feed well. In severe cases the only solution will be hand expression. This will reduce the tension in the breast and *will not* cause excessive milk production.
- The mother's fluid intake should not be restricted, as this has no direct effect on milk production.
- The use of hot and cold compresses might bring relief, as well as the use of simple analgesia such as paracetamol for the relief of pain and pyrexia.

Deep breast pain

- In most cases this responds to improvement in breastfeeding technique and is thus likely to be due to raised intraductal pressure caused by inefficient milk removal.
- Although it may occur during the feed, it typically occurs afterwards and thus can be distinguished from the sensation of the let-down reflex, which some mothers experience as a fleeting pain.
- Very rarely, deep breast pain may be the result of ductal thrush infection.

Mastitis

- Mastitis means inflammation of the breast.
- In the majority of cases it is the result of milk stasis, not infection, although infection may supervene.
- Typically, one or more adjacent segments of the breast tissue are inflamed and appear as a wedge-shaped area of redness and swelling.
- In some cases, flu-like symptoms, including shivering attacks or rigours, may occur.

Non-infective (acute intramammary) mastitis

- This condition results from milk stasis.
- It may occur during the early days as the result of unresolved engorgement or at any time when poor feeding technique results in the milk from one or more segments of the breast not being efficiently removed by the baby.
- It occurs much more frequently in the breast that is opposite the mother's preferred side for holding her baby.
- It is extremely important that breastfeeding from the affected breast continues; otherwise milk stasis will increase further and provide ideal conditions for pathogenic bacteria to replicate.

Infective mastitis

- The main cause of superficial breast infection is damage to the epithelium, which allows bacteria to enter the underlying tissues.
- The damage results from incorrect attachment of the baby to the breast, which has caused trauma to the nipple.
- The mother therefore urgently needs help to improve her technique, as well as the appropriate antibiotic.
- Multiplication of bacteria may be enhanced by the use of breast pads or shells.
- In spite of antibiotic therapy, abscess formation may occur.
- Infection may also enter the breast via the milk ducts if milk stasis remains unresolved.

Breast abscess

- A fluctuant swelling develops in a previously inflamed area.
- Pus may be discharged from the nipple. Simple needle aspiration may be effective or incision and drainage may be necessary.
- It may not be possible to feed from the affected breast for a few days but milk removal should continue and breastfeeding should recommence as soon as practicable to reduce the chances of further abscess formation.
- A sinus that drains milk may form but it is likely to heal in time.

Blocked ducts

- Lumpy areas in the breast are not uncommon – the mother is usually feeling distended glandular tissue. If they become very firm and tender (and sometimes flushed), they are often described as 'blocked ducts'.
- The solution is to improve milk removal (improved attachment, and possibly milk expression as well) and to treat the accompanying pain and inflammation.
- Massage, which is often advocated to clear the imagined 'blockage', may make matters worse by forcing more milk into the surrounding tissue.

White spots

- Very occasionally, a ductal opening in the tip of the nipple may become obstructed by a white granule or by epithelial overgrowth.
- White granules appear to be caused by the aggregation and fusion of casein micelles, to which further materials become added. This

hardened lump may obstruct a milk duct as it slowly makes its way down to the nipple, where it may be removed by the baby during a feed or expressed manually.

- Epithelial overgrowth seems to be the more common cause of a physical obstruction. A white blister is evident on the surface of the nipple, and it effectively closes off one of the exit points in the nipple, which leads from one or more milk-producing sections of the breast.
- This problem may also be resolved if the baby feeds. Alternatively, after the baby has fed (and the skin is softened), the spot may be removed with a clean fingernail, a rough flannel or a sterile needle.
- True blockages of this sort tend to recur, but once the woman understands how to deal with them, progression to mastitis can be avoided.

Feeding difficulties due to the baby

Cleft lip

- Provided that the palate is intact, the presence of a cleft in the lip should not interfere with breastfeeding because the vacuum that is necessary to enable the baby to attach to the breast is created between the tongue and the hard palate, not the breast and the lips.

Cleft palate

- Babies are only able to obtain milk as the result of the mother's milk ejection reflex.
- Because of the cleft, the baby is unable to create a vacuum and thus form a teat out of the breast and nipple.
- The use of an orthodontic plate has limited success. The mother should be encouraged to put the baby to the breast – for comfort, pleasure or food – provided that she is aware that expressed breast milk will also be required.

Tongue-tie (ankyloglossia)

- If the baby cannot extend the tongue over the lower gum he or she is unlikely to be able to draw the breast deeply into the mouth, which is necessary for effective feeding. Sometimes this is because the tongue is short, and sometimes this is because the frenulum, the whitish strip of tissue which attaches the tongue to the floor of the mouth, is preventing it. As the baby lifts the tongue, the tip becomes heart shaped as the frenulum pulls on it.

- Frenotomy is only recommended in some cases after assessment; 50% of babies with tongue-tie who are breast-fed will not encounter any difficulties.

Blocked nose

- As highlighted in Chapter 28, babies normally breathe through their noses.
- If there is an obstruction, babies have great difficulty with feeding because they have to interrupt the process in order to breathe.

Down syndrome

- Babies with this condition can be successfully breastfed, although extra help and encouragement may be necessary initially.

Prematurity

- Preterm babies who are sufficiently mature to have developed sucking and swallowing reflexes may successfully breastfeed.
- Those too immature to breastfeed may be able to cup feed, as an alternative to being tube fed.

Contraindications to breastfeeding

Medication

- Breastfeeding may have to be suspended temporarily following the administration of certain drugs or following diagnostic techniques.
- Breast milk expression must continue to maintain lactation.

Cancer

- If the mother has cancer, the treatment she receives will make it impossible to breastfeed without harming the baby.
- If the mother has had a mastectomy, she may feed successfully from the other breast.
- Following a lumpectomy for cancer, she may also be able to breastfeed. She should seek advice from her surgeon.

Breast surgery

- Neither breast reduction nor augmentation are an inevitable contraindication to breastfeeding and much depends on the technique used.

HIV infection

- HIV may be transmitted in breast milk.
- In developed countries, where artificial feeding is relatively safe, the mother may be advised not to breastfeed if she is HIV positive.
- In countries where artificial feeding is a significant cause of infant morbidity and mortality, exclusive breastfeeding may be the safer option.

Weaning from the breast

- When the mother or the baby decides to stop breastfeeding, feeds should be tailed off gradually.
- Breastfeeds may be omitted, one at a time, and spaced further apart.
- UNICEF and World Health Organization highlight the importance of exclusive breastfeeding for at least 6 months. Therefore, adding supplementary foods within this timeframe is not recommended.
- If the mother is using solid food to give the baby 'tastes' and the experience of different textures before weaning, these should be given after the breastfeed. Solid foods given before the breastfeed (weaning) will result in the baby taking less milk from the breast and thus less will be produced.

Complementary and supplementary feeds

- *Complementary feeds* (or 'top-ups') are feeds given *after* a breastfeed.
- Complementary feeds of breast milk substitutes are not recommended, except for medical indications.
- Approximately 10% of newborns are at risk for hypoglycaemia, and may thus need a higher calorific intake straight from birth than their mothers are able to provide. Where possible, this should be human milk, from an approved human milk bank.
- Babies who are well but sleepy, jaundiced, unsettled or difficult to attach should, if necessary, be given their mother's own expressed milk in addition to being offered the breast.
- If complementary feeds are clinically indicated and the mother is unable to express sufficient milk, donor milk from a human milk bank could be used.
- *Supplementary feeds* are feeds given *in place of* a breastfeed. There can be no justification for their use, except in extreme circumstances (such as severe illness or unconsciousness).

Artificial feeding

Most breast milk substitutes (infant formula) are modified cow's milk. The two main components used are:

- skimmed milk (a by-product of butter manufacture)
- whey (a by-product of cheese manufacture).

Breast milk substitutes may contain fats from any source, animal or vegetable (except from sesame and cotton seeds), provided that they do not contain more than 8% trans isomers of fatty acids. They may also contain, among other things, soya protein, maltodextrin, dried glucose syrup and gelatinized and precooked starch.

There are two main types of formula:

- whey dominant
- casein dominant.

Whey-dominant formulae

- A small amount of skimmed milk is combined with demineralized whey.
- The ratio of proteins in the formulae approximates to the ratio of whey to casein found in human milk (60:40).
- Whey-dominant formula feeds should only be used up to 6 months. These feeds are more easily digested than the casein-dominant formulae.

Casein-dominant formulae

- Although these are sold as being suitable for use from birth, more of the protein present is in the form of casein (20:80), which forms large relatively indigestible curds in the stomach.

Babies intolerant of standard formulae

Hydrolysate formulae.

- If breastfeeding is not possible, there are (prescription-only) alternatives that carry less risk of allergy than standard formulae – hydrolysates – some of which are designed to treat an existing allergy.
- Others are designed for preventative use in bottle-fed babies who are at high risk of developing cow's milk protein allergy.

Whey hydrolysates.

- These are made from the whey of cow's milk (rather than whole milk) and these are potentially more useful for highly allergenic babies.

443

Amino acid-based formulae or elemental formulae.
- This has a completely synthetic protein base providing the essential and non-essential amino acids, together with fat, maltodextrin, vitamins, minerals and trace elements.

Soya-based formulae.
- These are no longer recommended because of concerns about the possible effects of phyto-oestrogen compounds and the possibility of unavoidably high levels of manganese and aluminium.

Preparation of an artificial feed

- All powdered formula available in the UK is now reconstituted using 1 scoop (provided with the powder) to 30 ml water.
- Many of the major UK manufacturers of formula now produce ready-to-feed cartons.
- Reconstituted formula should be prepared as required due to the growth of pathogenic bacteria in stored reconstituted formula.

The water supply

- It is essential that the water used is free from bacterial, radioactive contamination and any harmful chemicals.
- It is generally assumed in high resource countries that boiled tap water will meet these criteria, but from time to time this is shown not to be the case.
- If bottled water is used, a still, non-mineralized variety suitable for babies must be chosen and it should be boiled as usual.
- Softened water is usually unsuitable.

Sterilization of feeding equipment

- The effective cleaning of all utensils should be demonstrated and the method of sterilization discussed.
- If boiling is to be used, full immersion is essential and the contents of the pan must be boiled for 10 minutes.
- If cold sterilization using a hypochlorite solution is the method of choice, the utensils must be fully immersed in the solution for the recommended time.
- The manufacturer's advice should be followed with regard to rinsing items that have been removed from the solution. If the item is to

be rinsed, previously boiled water should be used, not water direct from the tap.
- Both steam and microwave sterilization is now possible, but the mother should check that her equipment can withstand it.

Bottle teats
- Parents will find it helpful to have several teats with holes of different sizes so that they can be changed throughout the feed as necessary.
- A useful test for the correct hole size is to turn the bottle upside down; the feed should drip at a rate of approximately one drop per second.

Feeding the baby with the bottle
- Mothers should be warned about the dangers of 'bottle propping', and told that the baby must never be left unattended while feeding from a bottle.
- The principles of responsive feeding also apply to babies who are being artificially fed, with emphasis on the mother–baby dynamic relationship and communication.
- Modern formulae do not, when correctly prepared, cause hypernatraemia. There is therefore no need to give babies extra water.
- The stools and vomit of a formula-fed baby have an unpleasant sour smell.
- The stools tend to be more formed than those of a breastfed baby and, unlike a breastfed baby, there is a real risk that an artificially fed baby may become constipated.

THE BABY-FRIENDLY HOSPITAL INITIATIVE

This is an initiative that was launched in 1991 by the World Health Organization (WHO) and UNICEF to encourage hospitals to promote practices that are supportive of breastfeeding. It was focused around the 'Ten Steps' (Box 29.3), with which all hospitals that wish to achieve 'baby-friendly' status must comply. The evidence for the Ten Steps is contained in the WHO document of the same name, published in 1998. The new UNICEF Baby Friendly Standards can be viewed at: https://www.unicef.org.uk/babyfriendly/

Box 29.3 **The ten steps (WHO and UNICEF baby-friendly initiative)**

- Have a written breastfeeding policy that is routinely communicated to all healthcare staff
- Train all healthcare staff in the skills necessary to implement this policy
- Inform all pregnant women about the benefits and management of breastfeeding
- Help mothers initiate breastfeeding soon after birth
- Show mothers how to breastfeed and how to maintain lactation, even if they should be separated from their infants
- Give newborn infants no food or drink other than breast milk, unless medically indicated
- Practise rooming-in, allowing mothers and infants to remain together 24 hours a day
- Encourage breastfeeding on demand
- Give no artificial teats or dummies to breastfeeding infants
- Foster the establishment of breastfeeding support groups and refer mothers to them on discharge from hospital or clinic

SUGGESTED READING

Goldacre, M., Hall, N., Yeates, D.G.R., 2014. Hospitalisation for children with rickets in England: a historical perspective. Lancet 383 (9917), 597–598. Available from: http://www.thelancet.com/journals/lancet/article/PIIS0140-6736%2814%2960211-7/fulltext (accessed 26 July 2016).

Power, R.F., Murphy, J.F., 2014. Tongue-tie and frenotomy in infants with breastfeeding difficulties: achieving a balance. Arch. Dis. Child. doi: 10.1136/archdischild-2014-306211.

Useful websites

http://www.unicef.org

http://www.who.int

The Healthy Low-Birth-Weight Baby

CLASSIFICATION OF BABIES BY WEIGHT AND GESTATION

- Definitions of low birth weight are based upon weight alone and do not consider the gestational age of the baby.
- Likewise, definitions of gestational age disregard any considerations of birth weight.
- It is the *relationship* between these two separate considerations of weight (for assessment of growth) and gestational age (for assessment of maturity) that is of great importance and can be plotted on centile charts (Fig. 30.1).
- Growth charts should be derived from studies of local populations.

Weight

- The following nomenclature based on birth weight is based on *the international statistical classification of diseases and related health problems* issued by the World Health Organization:
  - Very low-birth-weight (VLBW) babies are those weighing less than 1500 g (up to and including 1499 g) at birth.
  - Extremely low-birth-weight (ELBW) babies are those who weigh less than 1000 g (up to and including 999 g) at birth.

Gestational age

- A preterm baby is born before completion of the 37th week of gestation, calculated from the first day of the last menstrual period.

Small for gestational age (SGA)

- SGA babies are defined as having a birth weight below the 10th centile for gestational age or < 2 standard deviations below mean (the 50th centile) for gestational age.

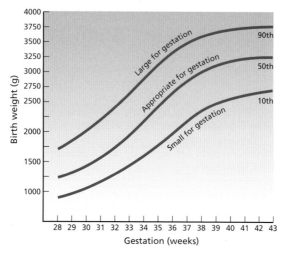

Fig. 30.1 A centile chart, showing weight and gestation. (From Simpson 1997, with permission of Baillière Tindall.)

Intrauterine growth restriction (IUGR)

- This is failure of normal fetal growth caused by multiple adverse effects on the fetus.

CAUSES OF INTRAUTERINE GROWTH RESTRICTION

- Fetal growth is regulated by maternal, placental and fetal factors and represents a mix of genetic mechanisms and environmental influences through which growth potential is expressed.
- The mechanisms that appear to limit fetal growth are multifactorial and can be maternal, fetal or placental, although several factors might be interrelated.

Asymmetric growth (sometimes called acute)

- Fetal weight is reduced out of proportion to length and head circumference. This is thought to be caused by extrinsic factors, such as pregnancy-induced hypertension, that adversely affect fetal nutrition.

Box 30.1 **Appearance of the baby with asymmetric intrauterine growth restriction**

- Head looks disproportionately large compared to the body
- Head circumference is usually within normal parameters
- Bones are within gestational norms for length and density
- Anterior fontanelle may be larger than expected, due to diminished membranous bone formation
- Abdomen looks 'scaphoid', or sunken due to shrinkage of the liver and spleen
- There is decreased subcutaneous fat deposition
- Skin is loose, which can give the baby a wizened, old appearance
- Vernix caseosa is frequently reduced or absent as a result of diminished skin perfusion
- Unless severely affected, these babies appear hyperactive and hungry with a lusty cry

Appearance

See Box 30.1.

Symmetric growth (chronic)

- This is due either to decreased growth potential of the fetus as a result of congenital infection or chromosomal/genetic defects (intrinsic), or to extrinsic factors that are active early in gestational life (e.g. the effects of maternal smoking or poor dietary intake) or a combination of both intrinsic and extrinsic factors.

Appearance

See Box 30.2.

- Symmetric growth (genetically small) babies are small normal babies and should be treated in accordance with their gestational age.

THE PRETERM BABY

- Birth occurs before the end of the 37th gestational week, regardless of birth weight.

> **Box 30.2 Appearance of the baby with symmetric intrauterine growth restriction**
>
> - Head circumference, length and weight are all proportionately reduced for gestational age
> - Babies are diminutive in size
> - They do not appear wasted, and have subcutaneous fat appropriate for their size
> - Skin is taut
> - Babies are generally vigorous and less likely to be hypoglycaemic or polycythaemic
> - They may suffer major congenital abnormalities and can be a source of infection to carers, as a result of transplacental infection

- Most of these babies are appropriately grown; some are SGA, whilst a small number are macrosomic or large for gestational age (LGA) (these tend to be babies of mothers with diabetes).

See Box 30.3 for causes of preterm labour.

Characteristics of the preterm baby

The appearance at birth of the preterm baby will depend upon gestational age (Box 30.4).

MANAGEMENT AT BIRTH OF THE HEALTHY LOW-BIRTH-WEIGHT BABY

- Current cot availability in the neonatal intensive care unit (NICU), transitional care unit (as applicable) and postnatal ward should be known.

See Chapter 27 for information on preparation of the birth environment/ neonatal resuscitation equipment.

On cutting the cord, leave an extra length, in case access to the umbilical vessels is necessary later.

- The Apgar score is traditionally scored at 1 and 5 minutes.
- Clear identification labels placed on the LBW baby is particularly important because separation of mother and baby could happen at any time if the baby's condition becomes unstable.
- A detailed but expedient examination of the baby should be carried out.

Box 30.3 **Causes of preterm labour**

Spontaneous causes

- 40% unknown
- Multiple gestation
- Hyperpyrexia as a result of viral or bacterial infection
- Premature rupture of the membranes caused by maternal infection
- Maternal short stature
- Maternal age and parity
- Poor obstetric history; history of preterm labour
- Cervical incompetence
- Poor social circumstances

Elective causes

- Pregnancy-induced hypertension, pre-eclampsia, chronic hypertension
- Maternal disease: renal, cardiac
- Placenta praevia, abruptio placenta
- Rhesus incompatibility
- Congenital malformation
- IUGR

Box 30.4 **Appearance of the preterm baby**

- Posture appears flattened with hips abducted, knees and ankles flexed
- Babies are generally hypotonic with a weak and feeble cry
- Head is in proportion to the body
- The skull bones are soft with large fontanelles and wide sutures
- Chest is small and narrow and appears underdeveloped due to minimal lung expansion during fetal life
- Abdomen is prominent because the liver and spleen are large and abdominal muscle tone is poor
- Umbilicus appears low in the abdomen because linear growth is cephalocaudal (more apparent nearer to the head than the feet)
- Subcutaneous fat is laid down from 28 weeks' gestation; therefore, its presence and abundance will affect the redness and transparency of the skin
- Vernix caseosa is abundant in the last trimester and tends to accumulate at sites of dense lanugo growth, i.e. face, ears, shoulders, sacral region

Continued

> **Box 30.4 Appearance of the preterm baby – cont'd**
>
> - Ear pinna is flat with little curve, the eyes bulge, the orbital ridges are prominent
> - Nipple areola is poorly developed and barely visible
> - Cord is white, fleshy and glistening
> - Plantar creases are absent before 36 weeks
> - In girls, the labia majora fail to cover the labia minora; in boys, the testes descend into the scrotal sac in approximately the 37th gestational week

- Once it is established that the baby is healthy, the midwife may attempt to normalize care by emphasizing to the parents the importance of preventing cold stress and promoting skin-to-skin contact in line with international guidelines.
- Ensure that the baby is thoroughly dried before skin-to-skin contact is attempted.
- The baby's body temperature should be maintained between 36.5°C and 37.3°C.

CARE OF THE HEALTHY LOW-BIRTH-WEIGHT BABY

- Many of the care issues relevant to the LBW baby apply to both the preterm and SGA infant.

Principles of thermoregulation

- Thermoregulation is the balance between heat production and heat loss.
- The prevention of cold stress, which may lead to hypothermia (body temperature < 36°C), is critical for the intact survival of the LBW baby.
- Newborn babies are unable to shiver, move very much or ask for an extra blanket, and therefore rely upon physical adaptations that generate heat by raising their basal metabolic rate and utilizing brown fat deposits.
- As body temperature falls, tissue oxygen consumption rises as the baby attempts to raise its metabolic rate by burning glucose to generate energy and heat.

- Care measures should aim to provide an environment that supports thermoneutrality.

Thermoregulation and the healthy mature SGA baby

- Rapid heat loss due to the large head to body ratio and large surface area is exaggerated, particularly in the asymmetrically grown SGA baby.
- Wide sutures and large fontanelles add to the heat-losing tendency.
- These babies often have depleted stores of subcutaneous fat, which is used for insulation. Their raised basal metabolic rate helps them to produce heat, but their high energy demands in the presence of poor glycogen stores and minimal fat deposition can soon lead to hypoglycaemia and then hypothermia.
- Once the baby is thoroughly dried, a prewarmed hat will minimize heat loss from the head.

Thermoregulation and the healthy preterm baby

- All preterm babies are prone to heat loss because their ability to produce heat is compromised by their immaturity, so factors like their large surface area to weight ratio, their varying amounts of subcutaneous fat and their ability to mobilize brown fat stores will be affected by their gestational age.
- During cooling, the immature heat-regulating centres in the hypothalamus and medulla oblongata fail, to different degrees, to recognize and marshal adequately coordinated homeostatic controls.
- Preterm babies are often unable to increase their oxygen consumption effectively through normal respiratory function, and their calorific intake is often inadequate to meet increasing metabolic requirements.
- Furthermore, their open resting postures increase their surface area and insensible water losses.
- Babies under 2.0 kg may need incubator care when the baby is not in skin-to-skin contact with either parent.
- The warm conditions in an incubator can be achieved either by heating the air to 30–32 °C (air mode) or by servo-controlling the baby's body temperature at a desired set point (36 °C). In servo mode, a thermocouple is taped to the upper abdomen and the incubator heater maintains the skin at that site to a preset

constant. Babies are clothed with bedding, in a room temperature of 26 °C.

- Most preterm babies between 2.0 and 2.5 kg will be cared for in a cot, in a room temperature of 24 °C.

Hypoglycaemia and the healthy LBW baby

- Hypoglycaemia refers to a low blood glucose concentration; it is more likely to occur in conditions where babies become cold or where the initiation of early feeding (within the first hour) is delayed.
- The aim is to maintain the true blood sugar above 2.6 mmol/dl. However, this does not mean that every LBW baby should be *routinely* screened. Well LBW babies who show no clinical signs of hypoglycaemia, are responsively fed, taking nutritive feeds on a regular basis, and are maintaining their body temperature do not need screening for hypoglycaemia.
- If a baby, despite being fed, presents with clinical signs of hypoglycaemia, a venous sample should be taken by the paediatrician to assess true blood sugar.
- A blood glucose that remains < 2.6 mmol/dl, despite the baby's further attempts to feed by breast or to take colostrum by cup, may warrant transfer to the NICU, because glucose by intravenous bolus may be necessary to correct the metabolic disturbance.
- In addition, consideration should be given as to whether there may be some underlying medical condition.

Hypoglycemia and the healthy mature SGA baby

- Asymmetrically grown babies have reduced glycogen stores in liver and skeletal muscles.
- Their greater brain to body mass and a tendency towards polycythaemia increase their energy demands, which in turn increase glucose requirements.
- Mature SGA babies with an asymmetric growth pattern will usually feed within the first half an hour of birth and demand feeds 2–3 hourly thereafter.
- Their susceptibility to hypoglycaemia is relatively short-lived and is limited to the first 48 hours following birth.
- If the baby is taking formula milk, feeds are usually calculated at 90 ml/kg on the first day, with 30 ml increments per day thereafter.

Hypoglycaemia and the preterm baby

- The preterm baby may be sleepier, and attempts to take the first feed may reflect gestational age.
- Total feed requirements (60 ml/kg on the first day, with 30 ml/kg increments per day thereafter) may not be taken directly from the breast and supplementary feeds can be given by cup.

Feeding the low-birth-weight baby

- Both preterm and SGA babies benefit from human milk because it contains long-chain polyunsaturated omega 3 fatty acids, which are thought to be essential for the myelination of neural membranes and retinal development.
- Preterm breast milk has:
  - a higher concentration of lipids, protein, sodium, calcium and immunoglobulins
  - a low osmolarity
  - lipases and enzymes that improve digestion and absorption.

The baby is normally able to co-ordinate breathing with sucking and swallowing reflexes between 32 and 36 weeks.

- Preterm babies are limited in their ability to suck by their weak musculature and flexor control, which is important for firm lip and jaw closure.
- Before 32 weeks, most healthy preterm babies will need to be tube-fed on a regular basis, usually on a 3-hourly regime with breast milk, hind-milk or formula milk.
- Tube feeding has the advantage that the tube can be left in situ during a cup feed or breastfeed and has been shown to eliminate the need to introduce bottles into a breastfeeding regime.
- Several problems have been identified with tube feeding:
  - Nasal and oral gastric tubes encourage milk lipid adherence to their inside surfaces and reduce the amount of fat calories available to the baby.
  - Babies are preferential nose breathers and the presence of a nasogastric tube will take up part of their available airway.
  - Prolonged use has been associated with delay in the development of sucking and swallowing reflexes simply because the mouth is bypassed.

Cup feeding has been used, therefore, in favour of tube feeding in order to:

- provide the baby with a positive oral experience
- stimulate saliva and lingual lipases to aid digestion
- accelerate the transition from naso/oral gastric feeding to breastfeeding without the introduction of bottles and teats.

Certain behaviours, such as licking and lapping, are well established *before* sucking and swallowing:

- Between 32 and 34 weeks' gestation, cup feeding can act as the main method of feeding, with the baby taking occasional complete breastfeeds.
- From 35 weeks' onwards, cup feeding can be gradually replaced by complete breastfeeding.

An unrushed feed can take up to an hour to complete. Feeding frequency can vary between 6 and 10 feeds per day.

THE CARE ENVIRONMENT: PROMOTING HEALTH AND DEVELOPMENT

- The ideal environment should provide a cycle of day and night, regular nourishment, rest, stimulation and loving attention.
- The mother's desire to be involved is seen as an *essential* element in the success of caring for LBW babies on postnatal wards. Parents can be reassured that by paying attention to their baby's behavioural cues, they can work with his or her capabilities; this is responsive parenting.

Handling and touch

- Kangaroo mother care (KMC) is used to promote closeness between a baby and mother and involves placing the nappy-clad baby upright between the maternal breasts for skin-to-skin contact. The LBW baby remains beneath the mother's clothing for varying periods of time that suit the mother.
- KMC, according to a Cochrane systematic review, is an efficacious and innocuous means of caring for the LBW baby especially in resource-poor countries.

Noise and light hazards

- Noise should be kept to a minimum.
- In dimmed lighting conditions, preterm babies are more able to improve their quality of sleep and alert status.

- Reduced light levels at night will help to promote the development of circadian rhythms and diurnal cycles.
- Screens to shield adjacent babies from phototherapy lights are essential.

Sleeping position

- Preterm babies have reduced muscle power and bulk, with flaccid muscle tone; therefore, their movements are erratic, weak or flailing. Without support they may, to differing degrees, develop head, shoulder and hip flattening, which in turn can lead to poor mobility.
- Nesting the more immature preterm babies into soft bedding, in addition to the use of close flexible boundaries, helps to keep their limbs in midline flexion.
- However, it is vital that they are nursed in a supine position to prevent asphyxia.

Sudden infant death syndrome (SIDS)

- There is a need to remind parents constantly of the risk factors and safety procedures (feet-to-foot sleeping position, smoke-free room) associated with SIDS, alongside teaching them to keep their babies warm.
- The midwife needs to explain that families should take into consideration time of year, gestational age and postnatal age.
- Parental training on 'what to do if my baby stops breathing' should be offered to parents but the decision to receive training should be their choice.

The prevention of infection

- LBW babies, particularly preterm ones, are especially vulnerable to infections caused by immaturity of their host defence systems.

The provision of neonatal care: the question of venue and facilities

- The decision to transfer a healthy LBW baby to a postnatal ward, a transitional unit or a NICU will depend upon the baby's gestational age and weight. In addition, the availability of facilities and level of staffing are also taken into account.

SUGGESTED READING

Carberry, A.E., Gordon, A., Bond, D.M., et al., 2014. Customised versus population-based growth charts as a screening tool for detecting small for gestational age infants in low-risk pregnant women. Cochrane Database Syst. Rev. (5), CD008549. doi: 10.1002/14651858.CD008549 .pub3.

Conde-Agudelo, A., Díaz-Rossello, J.L., 2014. Kangaroo mother care to reduce morbidity and mortality in low birthweight infants. Cochrane Database Syst. Rev. (4), CD002771. doi: 10.1002/14651858.CD002771. pub3.

Flenady, V., Wojcieszek, A.M., Middleton, P., et al., 2016. Stillbirths: recall to action in high-income countries. Lancet 387 (10019), 691–702.

Useful websites

http://www.who.int

http://www.lullabytrust.org.uk/sids

http://www.sidsandkids.org/

Recognizing the Ill Baby

ASSESSMENT OF THE INFANT

Immediately after birth, all infants should be examined for any gross congenital malformations or evidence of birth trauma. They should also have their weight and gestational age plotted on a standard growth chart.

History

Maternal health

Maternal morbidity can have a negative effect on pregnancy. Influencing factors may include a variety of medical conditions such as:
- anaemia
- pregnancy-induced hypertension
- infection such as pyelonepheritis
- history of epilepsy
- maternal diabetes
- history of substance abuse
- history of sexually transmitted diseases.

Fetal wellbeing and health

The following are examples of factors that may have a critical influence on the wellbeing of the neonate:
- small for gestational age (SGA)
- poor intrauterine growth
- evidence of congenital malformations detected on ultrasound.

Perinatal and birth complications

Labour and birth may also have an effect on the general welfare of the neonate in the following ways:
- prolonged prelabour rupture of membranes
- abnormal fetal heart rate pattern/pathological cardiotocograph (CTG)
- meconium-stained liquor

- difficult or rapid birth
- caesarean section and the reason for this mode of birth.

PHYSICAL ASSESSMENT

The skin

The presence of meconium on the skin, usually seen in the nail beds and around the umbilicus, is frequently associated with neonates who have cardiorespiratory problems. The skin of all babies should be examined for:

- pallor
- plethora
- cyanosis
- jaundice
- rashes.

Pallor

A pale, mottled baby is an indication of poor peripheral perfusion. At birth this can be associated with low circulating blood volume or with circulatory adaptation and compensation for perinatal hypoxaemia. The anaemic neonate appearance is usually pale pink, white or, in severe cases where there is vascular collapse, grey. Other presenting signs are:

- tachycardia
- tachypnoea
- poor capillary refill.

The most likely causes of anaemia in the newborn period are listed in Box 31.1.

Pallor can also be observed in infants who are hypothermic or hypoglycaemic. Problems associated with pallor include:

- anaemia and shock
- respiratory disorders

Box 31.1 **Common causes of anaemia in the newborn period**

- A history in the baby of haemolytic disease of the newborn
- Twin-to-twin transfusions in utero (which can cause one baby to be anaemic and the other polycythaemic)
- Maternal antepartum or intrapartum haemorrhage

- cardiac anomalies
- sepsis (where poor peripheral perfusion might also be observed).

Plethora

The baby's colour may indicate an excess of circulating red blood cells (polycythaemia). This is defined as a venous haematocrit greater than 70%. Newborn infants can become polycythaemic if they are recipients of:
- twin-to-twin transfusion in utero
- a large placental transfusion.

Other infants at risk are:
- SGA babies
- infants of diabetic mothers
- chromosomal disorders (e.g. Down syndrome)
- neonatal hypothyroidism.

Hypoglycaemia is commonly seen in plethoric neonates because red blood cells consume glucose. The baby can exhibit a neurological disorder; irritability, jitteriness and convulsions can occur. Other problems that may manifest are:
- apnoea
- respiratory distress
- cardiac failure
- necrotizing enterocolitis.

Cyanosis

- The mucous membranes are the most reliable indicators of central colour in all babies, and if the tongue and mucous membranes appear blue, this indicates low oxygen saturation levels in the blood, usually of respiratory or cardiac origin.
- Episodic central cyanotic attacks may be an indication that the infant is having a convulsion.
- Peripheral cyanosis of the hands and feet is common during the first 24 hours of life; after this time, it may be a non-specific sign of illness.

Jaundice (see Ch. 35)

- Early-onset jaundice (occurring in the skin and sclera within the first 12 hours of life) is abnormal and needs investigating.
- If a jaundiced baby is unduly lethargic, is a poor feeder, vomits or has an unstable body temperature, this may indicate infection and action should be taken to exclude this.

Surface lesions and rashes

Rashes (Box 31.2) are quite common in newborn babies but most are benign and self-limiting.

Other factors that affect the appearance of the skin

- If the neonate is dehydrated, the skin looks dry and pale and is often cool to touch. If gently pinched, it will be slow in retracting.

Box 31.2 Surface lesions and rashes in the newborn baby

Milia

- White or yellow papules seen over the cheeks, nose and forehead
- Invariably disappear spontaneously over the first few weeks of life

Miliaria

- Clear vesicles on the face, scalp and perineum, caused by retention of sweat in unopened sweat glands
- Appear on the chest and around areas where clothes can cause friction
- Treatment is to care for the infant in a cooler environment or remove excess clothing

Petechiae or purpura rash

- Can occur in neonatal thrombocytopenia, a condition of platelet deficiency that usually presents with a petechial rash over the whole of the body
- There may also be prolonged bleeding from puncture sites and/or the umbilicus and bleeding into the gut
- Thrombocytopenia may be found in infants with:
  - Congenital infections, both viral and bacterial
  - Maternal idiopathic thrombocytopenia
  - Drugs (administered to mother or neonate)
  - Severe Rhesus haemolytic disease

Bruising

- Can occur extensively following breech extractions, forceps and ventouse birth
- Bleeding can cause a decrease in circulating blood volume, predisposing the baby to anaemia or, if the bruising is severe, hypotension

---

Box 31.2 **Surface lesions and rashes in the newborn baby – cont'd**

Erythema toxicum

- A rash that consists of white papules on an erythematous base
- Occurs in approximately 30–70% of neonates
- Is benign and should not be confused with a staphylococcal infection, which will require antibiotics
- Diagnosis can be confirmed by examination of a smear of aspirate from a pustule, which will show numerous eosinophils (white cells indicative of an allergic response, rather than infection)

Thrush

- A fungal infection of the mouth and throat
- Very common in neonates, especially if they have been treated with antibiotics
- Presents as white patches seen over the tongue and mucous membranes and as a red rash on the perineum

Herpes simplex virus

- If acquired in the neonatal period, this is a most serious viral infection
- Transmission in utero is rare; the infection usually occurs during birth
- 70% of affected babies will produce a rash, which appears as vesicles or pustules

Umbilical sepsis

- Can be caused by a bacterial infection
- Until its separation, the umbilical cord can be a focus for infection by bacteria that colonize the skin of the newborn
- If periumbilical redness occurs or a discharge is noted, it may be necessary to commence antibiotic therapy to prevent an ascending infection

Bullous impetigo

- A condition which makes the skin look as though it has been scalded
- Caused by streptococci or staphylococci
- Presents as widespread tender erythema, followed by blisters that break, leaving raw areas of skin
- Particularly noticeable around the nappy area but may also cause umbilical sepsis, breast abscesses, conjunctivitis and, in deep infections, involvement of the bones and joints

- Other signs of dehydration are pallor or mottled skin, sunken fontanelle or eyeball sockets, and tachycardia.

Respiratory system

It is important to observe the baby's breathing when he or she is at rest and when active. The midwife should always start by observing skin colour and then carry out a respiratory inspection, taking into account whether the baby is making either an extra effort or insufficient effort to breathe.

Respiratory inspection

- The respiration rate should be between 40 and 60 breaths per minute (bpm) but will vary between levels of activity.
- As stated in previous chapters, neonates are primarily nose breathers and obstructions of the nares may lead to respiratory distress and cyanosis.
- The chest should expand symmetrically. If there is unilateral expansion and breath sounds are diminished on one side, this may indicate that a pneumothorax has occurred.
- Babies at risk of pneumothorax or other air leaks are:
  - preterm neonates with respiratory distress
  - term neonates with meconium-stained amniotic fluid
  - infants who require resuscitation at birth.

Increased work of breathing

- Tachypnoea is an abnormal respiratory rate at rest above 60 bpm.
- Note any inspiratory pulling in of the chest wall above and below the sternum or between the ribs (retraction).
- If nasal flaring is also present, this may indicate that there has been a delay in the lung fluid clearance or that a more serious respiratory problem is developing.
- Grunting, heard either with a stethoscope or audibly, is an abnormal expiratory sound. The grunting baby forcibly exhales against a closed glottis to prevent the alveoli from collapsing.

These neonates may require help with their breathing, either by intubation or continuous positive airway pressure (CPAP) ventilation.

Apnoea

- Apnoea is cessation of breathing for 20 seconds or more. It is associated with pallor, bradycardia, cyanosis, oxygen desaturation or a change in the level of consciousness.

> **Box 31.3 Causes of apnoea in the newborn baby**
>
> - Hypoxia
> - Pneumonia
> - Aspiration
> - Pneumothorax
> - Metabolic disorders, e.g. hypoglycaemia, hypocalcaemia, acidosis
> - Anaemia
> - Maternal drugs
> - Neurological problems, e.g. intracranial haemorrhage, convulsions, developmental disorders of the brain
> - Congenital anomalies of the upper airway

- Disorders that can cause apnoea, other than the type found in preterm babies, are listed in Box 31.3.

Body temperature

The normal body temperature range for term neonates is 36.5 to 37.3°C (see Ch. 28).

Hypothermia

Hypothermia is defined as a core temperature below 36°C. This can cause complications such as:
- increased oxygen consumption
- lactic acid production
- apnoea
- decrease in blood coagulability
- hypoglycaemia (most common).

In preterm babies, cold stress may also cause a decrease in surfactant secretion and synthesis.

- When neonates are exposed to cold, they will at first become very restless; then, as their body temperature falls, they adopt a tightly flexed position to try to conserve heat.
- The sick or preterm baby will tend to lie supine in a frog-like position with all surfaces exposed, which maximizes heat loss.
- Hypoglycaemia is a common feature of neonates with increased energy expenditure associated with thermoregulation and this can cause them to have jittery movements of the limbs, even though they are often quiet and often limp.

465

Hyperthermia

- Hyperthermia is defined as a core temperature above 38°C.
- The usual cause of hyperthermia is overheating of the environment but it can also be a clinical sign of sepsis, brain injury or drug therapy.
- If babies are too warm, they become restless and may have bright red cheeks. They will attempt to regulate their temperature by increasing their respiratory rate, and this can lead to an increased fluid loss by evaporation through the airways.
- Other problems caused by hyperthermia are:
  - hypernatraemia
  - jaundice
  - recurrent apnoea.

Cardiovascular system

- The normal heart rate of a newborn baby is 110–160 bpm with an average of 130 bpm.
- Cardiovascular dysfunction should be suspected in neonates who commonly present with lethargy and breathlessness during feeding.
- It can be very difficult to identify babies with congenital heart disease because the clinical picture of tachycardia, tachypnoea, pallor or cyanosis may be suggestive of a respiratory problem or sepsis.
- Persistent pulmonary hypertension of the newborn is usually seen in term or post-term babies who have a history of hypoxia or asphyxia at birth.
  - They are slow to take their first breath or are difficult to ventilate. Respiratory distress and cyanosis are seen before 12 hours of age.
  - Hypoxaemia is usually profound and may suggest cyanotic heart disease.
- Risk factors include:
  - meconium-stained amniotic fluid
  - nuchal cord
  - placental abruption
  - acute blood loss
  - maternal sedation.
- Cyanosis can be a prominent feature in some cardiac defects but not all. Box 31.4 lists signs that may be indicative of congenital heart disease.

Box 31.4 Warning signs suggestive of congenital heart disease

- Cyanosis (often out of proportion to the degree of respiratory distress)
- Persistent tachypnoea
- Persistent tachycardia at rest
- Poor feeding: neonates may be breathless and sweaty during the feed or after feeding; they may not complete their feeds and subsequently fail to thrive
- A sudden gain in weight leading to clinical signs of oedema; usually noted as the baby having puffy feet or eyelids and, in males, the scrotum being swollen
- A very loud systolic murmur: invariably significant
- Evidence of cardiac enlargement on X-ray, persisting beyond 48 hours of life
- Enlargement of the liver

- Cardiac shock may resemble early septicaemia, pneumonia or meningitis.
- The first indication of an underlying cardiac lesion may be the presence of a murmur heard on routine examination. However, a soft localized systolic murmur with no evidence of any symptoms of cardiac disease is usually of no significance.

Central nervous system

Abnormal postures, which include neck retraction, frog-like postures, hyperextension or hyperflexion of the limbs or jittery or abnormal involuntary movements, along with a high-pitched or weak cry, could be indicative of neurological impairment and need investigation.

Neurological disorders

Neurological disorders found at or soon after birth may be either prenatal or perinatal in origin. They include:

- congenital abnormalities: hydrocephaly, microcephaly, encephalocele, chromosomal anomalies
- hypoxic–ischaemic cerebral injuries
- birth traumas: skull fractures, spinal cord and brachial plexus injuries, subdural and subarachnoid haemorrhage

> Box 31.5 **Neurological disorders recognized in the neonatal period**
>
> - *Infection*: meningitis, herpes simplex, viral encephalitis
> - *Hypoxia*: birth asphyxia, respiratory distress, apnoeic episodes
> - *Metabolic disorders*: acidosis, hypoglycaemia, hyponatraemia, hypernatraemia, hypothermia, hypocalcaemia, hypomagnesaemia
> - *Drug withdrawal*: narcotics, barbiturates, general anaesthesia
> - *Intracranial haemorrhages/intraventricular haemorrhage (IVH)*
> - *Secondary bleeding*: intracranial haemorrhage from thrombocytopenia or disseminated intravascular coagulation

- infections passed on to the fetus: toxoplasmosis, rubella, cytomegalovirus (CMV), syphilis.

Neurological disorders that appear in the neonatal period need to be recognized promptly to minimize brain damage. The most common are listed in Box 31.5.

Seizures

Seizures in the newborn period can be extremely difficult to diagnose, as they are often very subtle and easily missed (Table 31.1).

The most common causes of seizure activity are:

- asphyxia
- metabolic disturbance
- intracranial/intraventricular haemorrhage
- infection
- malformation/genetic defect.

Hypotonia (floppy infant)

The term hypotonia describes the loss of body tension and tone. As a result, the neonate adopts an abnormal posture which is noticeable on handling.

The causes of hypotonia include:

- maternal sedation
- birth asphyxia
- prematurity
- infection
- Down syndrome

Table 31.1 Neonatal seizure chart

Type	Affected neonates
Subtle	
Apnoea usually seen with abnormal eye movements, tonic horizontal deviation, blinking, fluttering eyelids, jerking, drooling, sucking, tonic posturing or unusual movements of limbs (rowing, pedalling or swimming)	Most frequent type and most common in preterm babies
Clonic	
Jerking activity	
Multifocal or unifocal distinct from jittering	Term infants: hypoxic–ischaemic encephalopathy or inborn errors of metabolism
Focal: movement of one part	Disturbance of the entire cerebrum
Tonic	
Posturing similar to decerebrate posture in adults	Preterm babies with intraventricular haemorrhage
Myoclonic	
Single or multiple jerks of upper or lower extremities	Possible prediction of myoclonic spasms in early infancy

- metabolic problems (e.g. hypoglycaemia, hyponatraemia, inborn errors of metabolism)
- neurological problems (e.g. spinal cord injuries [sustained by difficult breech or forceps birth], myasthenia gravis related to maternal disease, myotonic dystrophy)
- endocrine disorders (e.g. hypothyroidism)
- neuromuscular disorders.

Renal/genitourinary system

- Urinary infections typically present with lethargy, poor feeding, increasing jaundice and vomiting.
- Urine that only dribbles out, rather than being passed forcefully, may be an indication of a problem with posterior urethral valves.
- Urine that is cloudy in appearance or smelly may be an indication of a urinary tract infection.
- Renal problems may present as a failure to pass urine.

469

- The normal newborn term neonate usually passes urine 4–10 hours after birth.
- Normal urine output for a term baby in the first day of life should be 2–4 ml/kg per hour.
- Urine output of less than 1 ml/kg per hour (oliguria) should be investigated.

Common causes of reduced urine output include:
- inadequate fluid intake
- increased fluid loss due to hyperthermia, use of radiant heaters and phototherapy units
- birth asphyxia
- congenital malformations
- infection.

Gastrointestinal tract

- Oesophageal atresia can be diagnosed antenatally because the fetus is unable to swallow the amniotic fluid, giving rise to polyhydramnios in the mother. If, however, the condition is not identified antenatally, the baby usually presents with copious saliva, which causes:
  - gagging
  - choking
  - pallor or cyanosis.
- In neonates who are inadvertently fed milk this may cause a severe respiratory arrest due to milk aspiration.
- Intestinal obstructions may be caused by atresias, malformations, or structural damage anywhere below the stomach.
- In the newborn period, gastrointestinal disorders often present with:
  - vomiting
  - abdominal distension
  - failure to pass stools
  - diarrhoea with or without blood in the stools.
- Vomiting in the postnatal period can be caused by factors other than gastrointestinal obstructions.
- Early vomiting may be caused by the baby swallowing meconium or maternal blood via the genital tract at birth. This can cause a gastritis, which will eventually settle. Some neonates may require a gastric lavage if the symptoms are severe.
- All vomit should be checked for the presence of bile or blood, and the baby observed for other signs such as abdominal

distension, watery or blood-stained stools and temperature instability.

- The baby who has an infection can often display signs of gastro-intestinal problems, usually poor feeding, vomiting and/or diarrhoea.
- Diarrhoea caused by gastroenteritis is usually very watery and may sometimes resemble urine.
- Loose stools can also be a feature of hyperbilirubinaemia for those neonates being treated with phototherapy.
- Some of the more commonly seen gastrointestinal problems include:
  - duodenal atresia
  - malrotation of the gut
  - volvulus
  - meconium ileus
  - necrotizing enterocolitis (NEC)
  - imperforate anus
  - rectal fistulas
  - Hirschsprung disease.

Duodenal atresia

- Duodenal atresia usually presents with bile-stained vomiting within 24–36 hours of birth.
- Abdominal distension may not be present.
- Insertion of a nasogastric tube may reveal a large amount of bile in the stomach and there may be a history of polyhydramnios and a delay in passing meconium.

Malrotation of the gut/volvulus

- This is a developmental malformation where incomplete rotation of the small bowel has taken place, giving rise to signs of obstruction.
- The neonate usually has no problems in the first few days of life, then presents with bilious vomiting and abdominal distension.

Meconium ileus

- The baby with meconium ileus often has cystic fibrosis.
- Clinical signs include:
  - marked abdominal distension
  - meconium is not passed, but occasionally small pellet-type stools, pale in colour, are mistakenly identified as bowel action.

- Vomiting gradually increases, mainly gastric secretions and feed, but later becomes bilious.

Necrotizing enterocolitis

- NEC is an acquired disease of the small and large intestine caused by ischaemia of the intestinal mucosa.
- It is more common in preterm babies, but may also occur in term neonates who have been asphyxiated at birth or those with polycythaemia and hypothermia (commonly found in SGA babies).
- NEC may present with vomiting or, if gastric emptying is being monitored, the aspirate is large and bile stained.
- The abdomen becomes distended, and stools are loose and may have blood in them.
- In the early stages of NEC, the neonate can display non-specific signs of temperature instability, unstable glucose levels, lethargy and poor peripheral circulation.
- As the illness progresses, the baby becomes apnoeic and bradycardic and may need ventilating.

Additional information about NEC can be found in Chapter 32.

Imperforate anus

- All neonates should be examined at birth to determine patency of the anus.

Rectal fistulas

- The midwife should look for the presence of meconium in the urine, or in female babies, meconium being passed per vaginum.

Hirschsprung disease

- Hirschsprung disease should be suspected in term neonates with delayed passage of meconium, certainly beyond the first 24 hours of life.
- The condition is caused by an absence of ganglion cells in the distal rectum.
- The area of aganglionosis varies and may include the lower rectum, colon and small intestine.
- An incomplete obstruction occurs above the affected segment.
- Abdominal distension and vomiting are clinical signs, with the vomit becoming bile stained if meconium is not passed.

Metabolic disorders (see Ch. 36)

Metabolic disorders, such as galactosaemia and phenylketonuria, present in the newborn period with vomiting, weight loss, jaundice and lethargy.

FURTHER READING

Balain, M., Oddie, S., 2014. Management of apnoea and bradycardia in the newborn. Paediatr. Child Health 24 (1), 17–22.

Useful website

http://www.nice.org.uk

Respiratory Problems

PATHOPHYSIOLOGY

Anatomical influences

- Neonates are susceptible to respiratory compromise resulting from the following:
  - Their stage of lung development and contributing lack of maturation in the other body systems.
  - An increased work of breathing owing to the high compliance of the neonatal lung, which results from the cartilaginous nature of the rib structure.
  - The neonatal diaphragm being more susceptible to fatigue due to the composition and location of the muscle within the neonatal chest.
  - Neonatal airways which are smaller; this generates higher resistance to airflow and a smaller area through which perfusion can occur.
  - The tendency for pulmonary blood flow to bypass areas of hypoxia, across the alveolar bed, consequently reducing alveolar perfusion.

Signs of respiratory compromise

These are listed in Box 32.1.

COMMON RESPIRATORY PROBLEMS

Pneumothorax

- Pneumothoraces are known to occur spontaneously in 1% of the newborn population either during or after birth; however, only one-tenth of this 1% will be symptomatic.
- The cause at birth is the result of the large pressures generated by the baby's first breaths. These may range up to 40–80 cm of water. This leads to alveolar distension and rupture, allowing air to leak to a number of sites of which the potential space between the lung pleura is one.

Box 32.1 **Signs of respiratory compromise**

Grunting

- An audible noise heard on expiration
- Appears when there is the partial closure of the glottis as the breath is expired
- The baby is attempting to preserve some internal lung pressure and prevent the airways from collapsing at the end of the breath

Retractions

- Chest distortions occur due to an increase in the need to create higher inspiratory pressures in a compliant chest
- Appear as intercostal, subcostal or sternal recession across the thorax
- Asynchrony
- The breathing appears as a 'see-saw' pattern as the abdominal movements and the diaphragm work out of unison
- A result of increased muscle fatigue and the compliant chest wall

Tachypnoea

- This is a compensatory rise in the respiratory rate (above 60 breaths per minute) initiated from the respiratory centre and aims to remove the hypoxia and hypercarbia

Nasal flaring

- An attempt to minimize the effect of the airways' resistance by maximizing the diameter of the upper airways
- The nares are seen to flare open with each breath

Apnoea

- Occurs as the conclusion of increasing respiratory fatigue in the term baby
- The preterm baby may experience apnoea of prematurity due to the immature respiratory centre, as well as apnoea from respiratory fatigue

- Babies receiving assisted ventilation also have an increased susceptibility to a pneumothorax due to:
  - maldistribution of the ventilated gas in the lungs
  - high ventilation settings
  - neonate–ventilator breathing interactions.

Presumptive diagnosis:

- reduced breath sounds on the affected side
- displaced heart sounds
- distorted chest/diaphragm movement with respiration.

Emergency treatment involves either a needle aspiration or the placement of a chest drain.

Transient tachypnoea of the newborn (TTN)

- TTN is frequently seen as a diagnosis of exclusion of other possible respiratory causes.
- The chest X-ray may show a streaky appearance with fluid apparent in the horizontal fissure, confirming the diagnosis and also accounting for the colloquialism of 'wet lung'.
- The most common predisposing factor for TTN is an elective caesarean section, as the thorax has not been squeezed while the baby descends along the birth canal. This results in lower thoracic pressures after birth.
- Although babies with TTN require initial care on a neonatal unit, their stay is usually of a short duration with the provision of oxygen and observation.

Infection/pneumonia

- Pneumonia in the neonate is difficult to diagnose, as secretions are difficult to obtain and the radiological appearances can be hard to distinguish.
- Pneumonia presenting before 48 hours of age has normally been acquired either at or before birth.
- Presentation after 48 hours indicates infection resulting from hospitalization.

All infants with infection require antibiotics.

Meconium aspiration syndrome

- A baby can develop meconium aspiration syndrome if stimulated to breathe or gasp, either before or after birth, if there is meconium in the airway that could be inhaled.

- The initial respiratory distress may be mild, moderate or severe, with a gradual deterioration over the first 12–24 hours in moderate or severe cases.
- The meconium becomes trapped in the airways and causes a ball-valve effect; the air can get in and the meconium blocks the airway during expiration, causing an accumulation of air behind the blockage.
- This accumulation can then lead to rupture of the alveoli and cause the baby to develop a pneumothorax.
- Where the meconium has contact with the lung tissue, a pneumonitis occurs.
- The surfactant is also broken down in the presence of meconium.
- The preceding factors combine with a previously hypoxic neonate to produce a severe disease process.
- These babies will need full intensive care and ventilation to prevent further deterioration.

Respiratory distress syndrome (RDS)

- RDS occurs as a result of insufficient production of surfactant, seen most frequently after a premature birth.
- Other disorders such as maternal diabetes or meconium aspiration syndrome can also inhibit surfactant production.
- Surfactant is produced to reduce the surface tension within the alveoli, preventing their collapse at the end of exhalation.
- It is much harder to inflate collapsed alveoli, in terms of the pressure and exertion required, than to reinflate partially collapsed alveoli.

Diagnosis involves the following:

- Increasing respiratory distress and work of breathing are noted.
- The X-ray shows a ground glass appearance across the lung fields, while severe disease is represented by a 'white-out'.

Treatment includes:

- oxygen therapy
- surfactant administration directly into the lungs
- ventilatory support for the most severely affected.

CARDIAC DISEASE

Cardiac defects (Box 32.2 and Chapter 34), while not a respiratory disease, present with respiratory symptoms.

477

Box 32.2 Cardiac lesions

Right-sided lesions

- The most frequently seen lesions are transposition of the great arteries, tetralogy of Fallot and pulmonary atresia or stenosis
- These infants typically present as 'blue' babies. On examination, there is little to note other than the presence of cyanosis
- Their respiratory distress, if present, is mild and consists of tachypnoea alone
- These babies will remain cyanotic in the presence of 100% oxygen

Left-sided lesions

- The most frequently seen left-sided lesions are hypoplastic left heart syndrome and coarctation of the aorta
- These frequently present with neonatal heart failure
- Initially, the baby may appear irritable, lethargic, sweaty and uninterested in feeding
- The presence of 'effortless' tachypnoea may be seen, characterized by the lack of any other sign of respiratory compromise; for example, no grunting is heard, there is no head bobbing and recession is minimal
- As the heart failure progresses, the infant shows signs of cardiogenic shock and will go on to require full resuscitative measures if left unsupported

CARE OF THE BABY WITH RESPIRATORY COMPROMISE

Respiratory care

The following assist in observations of the baby:
- saturation monitors
- transcutaneous monitors
- arterial catheter readings.

When satisfactory oxygenation is not being achieved, additional oxygen can be delivered:
- via a nasal cannula
- into a headbox
- from high-frequency oscillation (HFOV)
- by conventional mechanical ventilation (CMV)
- with continuous positive airway pressure (CPAP).

Some ventilation techniques, such as extra corporeal membrane oxygenation (ECMO), are available at specialized centres only.

Cardiovascular support

- Cardiac failure in a neonate is rare, as the majority of arrests are respiratory in origin.
- Neonates may require support to maintain an efficient and effective heart beat. Maintenance of an adequate blood pressure (the mean being equivalent to the gestational age) may need pharmaceutical support.
- A bradycardia (a heart rate below 80) may be a sign of various influences, such as a blocked endotracheal tube or sepsis.
- Occasionally, the transition from a fetal to an adult circulation is compromised and the baby develops persistent pulmonary hypertension of the newborn.
- Nitric oxide is the vasodilator of choice.

Nutrition and hydration

- A preterm baby has few nutritional reserves and will need supplementation soon after birth to meet the continual demand for glucose from the brain.
- Oral breast milk feeding is not possible for a sick neonate as the presence of the endotracheal tube or the absence of a suck reflex prevents oral feeding.
- The majority of neonates will receive a glucose-based intravenous infusion. This allows milk feeds to be given via a nasogastric, orogastric or nasojejunal tube, increasing the volumes as the baby's condition allows.
- Sick or immature babies need a cautious introduction to milk, whether expressed breast milk or formula feeds, as they are susceptible to necrotizing enterocolitis (NEC) as highlighted in Chapter 31.
- When it is expected to take more than 4–5 days before full feeding is established, total parenteral nutrition (TPN) is needed to ensure all nutritional requirements can be met.
- While some babies may need TPN for many weeks, it can have some undesirable side effects upon the liver, giving rise to a conjugated hyperbilirubinaemia or cholestasis.
- Prolonged TPN is sometimes needed in very immature babies with gastroschisis and those with NEC.

The causes of NEC are multifactorial:
- Delayed feeding causes a lowered immune response to potential pathogens.
- Administration of antibiotics can alter the dominant gut flora, as can formula milk.
- Bacterial infection can occur following episodes of hypoxia.
- Polycythaemia reduces the arterial blood flow through the mesenteric circulation and causes mucosal ischaemia; reperfusion leads to oedema, haemorrhage, ulceration and necrosis.

Signs and symptoms of NEC include:
- a painful distended abdomen
- blood in the stool
- poor feed tolerance
- air within the gut wall, leading to a perforation, hypovolaemic shock or disseminated intravascular coagulation.

Treatment of NEC involves:
- antibiotics and medical management initially
- surgery if there is a perforation or a failure to respond to the medical therapy.

The disease can be fatal; long-term problems for those who do recover can include short gut syndrome and gut stenosis.

A safe environment

- The baby with respiratory compromise needs all its energy to maintain satisfactory oxygenation and hence particular care is needed to:
  - protect from infection
  - maintain a thermoneutral environment
  - minimize stressors
  - detect and treat pain and distress.

The family

- The midwife and neonatal staff have important roles in assisting parental attachment and responsive parenting by maintaining regular, reliable and effective communication about the baby and giving advice on how parents can participate in the baby's care.

FURTHER READING

Bahadue, F.L., Soll, R., 2012. Early versus delayed selective surfactant treatment for neonatal respiratory distress syndrome. Cochrane

Database Syst. Rev. (11), CD001456, doi: 10.1002/14651858.CD001456.
pub2.

Reuter, S., Moser, C., Baack, M., 2014. Respiratory distress in the newborn.
Pediatr. Rev. 35 (10), 417–428.

Useful website

http://www.who.int

Trauma During Birth, Haemorrhage and Convulsions

TRAUMA TO SKIN AND SUPERFICIAL TISSUES

Skin

Damage to the skin may result from forceps blades, vacuum extractor cups, scalp electrodes and scalpels.

- Abrasions and lacerations should be kept clean and dry.
- If there are signs of infection, antibiotics may be required.
- Deeper lacerations may require closure with butterfly strips or sutures.

Superficial tissues

Trauma to soft tissue involves oedematous swellings and/or bruising. The oedema consists of serum and blood (serosanguineous fluid).

Caput succedaneum

This is an oedematous swelling under the scalp and above the periosteum (Fig. 33.1 and Box 33.1). A 'false' caput succedaneum can also occur if a vacuum extractor cup is used; the resulting oedematous transient swelling is known as a 'chignon'.

The baby will usually experience some discomfort.

Other injury

When the face presents, it becomes congested and bruised, and the eyes and lips become oedematous. In a breech presentation, the fetus will develop bruised and oedematous genitalia and buttocks.

Uncomplicated oedema and bruising usually resolve within a few days of life. However, if there is significant trauma during a vaginal breech birth, there can be serious complications such as:

- hyperbilirubinaemia
- excessive blood loss, resulting in hypovolaemia, shock, anaemia and disseminated intravascular coagulation

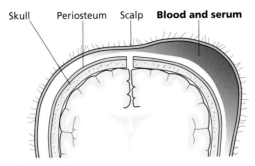

Skull   Periosteum   Scalp   **Blood and serum**

Fig. 33.1 Caput succedaneum.

Box 33.1 **Features of a caput succedaneum**

- Is present at birth
- Does not usually enlarge
- Can 'pit' on pressure
- Can cross a suture line
- Involves oedema that may move to the dependent area of the scalp
- Usually resolves by 36 hours of life
- Has no longer-term consequences

- damage to muscles, resulting in difficulties with micturition and defaecation.

Muscle trauma

Injuries to muscle result from tearing or from disruption of the blood supply.

Torticollis

- Excessive traction or twisting can cause tearing to one of the sternomastoid muscles during the birth of the anterior shoulder of a fetus with a cephalic presentation, or during rotation of the shoulders when the fetus is being born by vaginal breech. A small lump can be felt on the affected sternomastoid muscle. It appears painless for the baby. The muscle length is shortened; therefore, the neck is twisted on the affected side.

- The management of torticollis involves stretching of the affected muscle, achieved under the guidance of a physiotherapist. The swelling will usually resolve over several weeks.

Nerve trauma

Commonly, there is trauma to the facial nerve or to the brachial plexus nerves.

Facial nerve

- Damage to the facial nerve usually results from its compression against the ramus of the mandible by a forceps blade, resulting in a unilateral facial palsy. The eyelid on the affected side remains open and the mouth is drawn over to the normal side.
- If the baby cannot form an effective seal on the breast or teat, there may be some initial feeding difficulties.
- Spontaneous resolution usually occurs within 7–10 days.

Brachial plexus

- Trauma to this group of nerves usually results from excessive lateral flexion, rotation or traction of the head and neck during vaginal breech birth or when shoulder dystocia occurs.
- These injuries can be unilateral or bilateral.
- There are three main types of injury:

Erb palsy.
- There is damage to the upper brachial plexus involving the fifth and sixth cervical nerve roots.
- The baby's affected arm is inwardly rotated, the elbow is extended, the wrist is pronated and flexed, and the hand is partially closed. This is commonly known as the *waiter's tip position*.
- The arm is limp, although some movement of the fingers and arm is possible.

Klumpke palsy.
- There is damage to the lower brachial plexus involving the seventh and eighth cervical and the first thoracic nerve roots.
- The upper arm has normal movement but the lower arm, wrist and hand are affected.

There is wrist drop and flaccid paralysis of the hand with no grasp reflex.

Total brachial plexus palsy.
- There is damage to all brachial plexus nerve roots with complete paralysis of the arm and hand, lack of sensation and circulatory problems.

- If there is bilateral paralysis, spinal injury should be suspected.

All types of brachial plexus trauma will require further investigations such as X-ray and ultrasound scanning (USS), and assessment of the joints.

- Passive movements of the joints and limb can then be initiated under the direction of a physiotherapist.
- At approximately 1 month of age, magnetic resonance imaging can offer specific data on nerve damage.
- Spontaneous recovery within days to weeks is expected for most babies. Follow-up is recommended.
- Babies with no functional recovery by 6 months of age may require surgical repair.

Fractures

Fractures are rare but the most commonly affected bones are:
- clavicle
- humerus
- femur
- skull bones.

HAEMORRHAGE

Haemorrhage can be due to:
- trauma
- disruptions in blood flow

or can be related to:
- coagulopathies
- other causes.

Blood volume in the term baby is approximately 80–100 ml/kg and in the preterm baby 90–105 ml/kg; therefore, even a small haemorrhage can be potentially fatal.

Haemorrhage due to trauma

Cephalhaematoma

- A cephalhaematoma is an effusion of blood under the periosteum that covers the skull bones (Fig. 33.2 and Box 33.2).
- During a vaginal birth, if there is friction between the fetal skull and the maternal pelvic bones, such as in cephalopelvic disproportion or precipitate labour, the periosteum is torn from the bone, causing bleeding underneath.

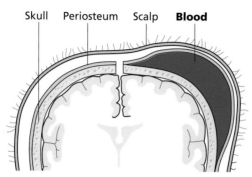

Fig. 33.2 Cephalhaematoma.

- Cephalhaematomas can also be caused during vacuum-assisted births.
- More than one bone may be affected, causing multiple cephalhaematomas to develop (Fig. 33.3).
- No treatment is necessary and the swelling subsides when the blood is reabsorbed. Erythrocyte breakdown in the extravasated blood may result in hyperbilirubinaemia.
- A ridge of bone may later be felt round the periphery of the swelling, owing to the accumulation of osteoblasts.

Subaponeurotic and subdural haemorrhage

Less common types of haemorrhage due to trauma are:
- subaponeurotic haemorrhage
- subdural haemorrhage.

These are usually associated with precipitate or difficult births or instrumental births. The most common cause of subdural haemorrhage in a term baby is a tentorial tear.

Fig. 33.3 Bilateral cephalhaematoma.

Haemorrhage due to disruptions in blood flow

Subarachnoid haemorrhage

- A primary subarachnoid haemorrhage involves bleeding directly into the subarachnoid space.
- Preterm babies, those who suffer hypoxia at birth and term babies who suffer traumatic births are vulnerable.
- A secondary haemorrhage involves the leakage of blood into the subarachnoid space from an intraventricular haemorrhage.
- The baby may have generalized convulsions from the second day of life and preterm babies may have apnoeic episodes; otherwise they appear normal and some exhibit no signs.
- If a lumbar puncture is performed, the cerebrospinal fluid will be uniformly blood stained.
- Management involves control of the consequences of asphyxia and of convulsions.
- The condition is usually self-limiting.

Germinal matrix/intraventricular haemorrhage (GMH/IVH) and intraparenchymal lesions (IPL)

These haemorrhages/lesions primarily affect babies of less than 32 weeks' gestation and those weighing less than 1500 g, although term babies can be affected.

- A small bleed can have a 'silent' onset and is only detectable on USS.

- If the haemorrhage is larger or extends, the clinical features may gradually appear and worsen. These may include apnoeic episodes, which become more frequent and severe, episodes of bradycardia, pallor, falling haematocrit, tense anterior fontanelle, metabolic acidosis and convulsions.
- The baby may be limp or unresponsive.
- If the GMH/IVH/IPL is large and sudden in onset, the baby may present with apnoea and circulatory collapse.

The care of at-risk babies is focused on prevention:

- For example, antenatal administration of steroids to the mother, artificial surfactant after birth or antibiotic therapy in the management of preterm premature rupture of the membranes.
- The neurological prognosis for babies with small haemorrhages is usually good.
- Babies who suffer a massive haemorrhage may die within 48 hours of the onset and those who survive are likely to develop significant neurological and intellectual impairment.

Haemorrhage related to coagulopathies

These haemorrhages occur because of a disruption in the baby's blood-clotting abilities.

Vitamin K deficiency bleeding

- Vitamin K deficiency bleeding (VKDB) can occur up to 12 months of age, although it more commonly occurs between birth and 8 weeks of life.
- Several proteins require vitamin K to be converted into active clotting factors.
- A deficiency of vitamin K leads to a deficiency of these clotting factors and resultant bleeding.
- Neonates are deficient in vitamin K and therefore vulnerable to VKDB.
- Early VKDB (first 24 hours) is rare and principally affects babies born to women who, during pregnancy, have taken warfarin (also known as Coumadin, Jantoven), phenobarbital or phenytoin. It is important to note that warfarin and some anti-convulsants are considered to be contraindicated during pregnancy. It is recommended that women on these medications seek preconception care.
- Classical VKDB (1–7 days) – see Box 33.3.

Box 33.3 **Babies susceptible to vitamin K deficiency bleeding**

- Those who have experienced birth trauma
- Those who have experienced asphyxia
- Those who have experienced postnatal hypoxia
- Those who are preterm
- Those who are of low birth weight
- Those who have been given antibiotic therapy
- Those who cannot maintain enteral feeding or feed poorly

- Late VKDB (1–12 months) almost exclusively occurs in breastfed babies. However, it may occur in babies who have liver disease or a condition that disrupts the absorption of vitamin K_1 from the bowel (e.g. cystic fibrosis).
- Bleeding may be evident superficially as bruising or haemorrhage from the umbilicus, puncture sites, the nose and the scalp.
- Severe jaundice for more than 1 week and persistent jaundice for more than 2 weeks are warning signs.
- Gastrointestinal bleeding is manifested as melaena and haematemesis.
- In early and late VKDB, there may be serious extracranial and intracranial bleeding.
- With severe haemorrhage, circulatory collapse occurs.
- Diagnosis is confirmed by blood tests.
- Babies who have VKDB require careful investigation and monitoring to assess their need for treatment.
- With all forms of VKDB, the baby will require administration of vitamin K_1, 1–2 mg intramuscularly.
- VKDB is a potentially fatal condition; therefore, prophylactic administration of vitamin K has become the norm in many countries (see Ch. 27).

Thrombocytopenia

- Thrombocytopenia is a low count of circulating platelets ($< 150\,000/\mu l$). Babies who are at risk are listed in Box 33.4.
- A petechial rash appears soon after birth, presenting in a mild case with a few localized petechiae.

> **Box 33.4 Babies susceptible to thrombocytopenia**
>
> - Those who have a severe congenital or acquired infection, e.g. syphilis, cytomegalovirus, rubella, toxoplasmosis or bacterial infection
> - Those whose mother has idiopathic thrombocytopenia, purpura, systemic lupus erythematosus or thyrotoxicosis
> - Those whose mother takes thiazide diuretics
> - Those who have isoimmune thrombocytopenia
> - Those who have inherited thrombocytopenia

- In a severe case, there is widespread and serious haemorrhage from multiple sites.
- Diagnosis is based on history, clinical examination and the presence of a reduced platelet count.
  - In mild cases, no treatment is required.
  - In immune-mediated thrombocytopenia, intravenous immunoglobulin administration is helpful.
  - In severe cases, where there is haemorrhage and a very low platelet count, transfusion of platelet concentrate may be required.

Disseminated intravascular coagulation (consumptive coagulopathy)

Disseminated intravascular coagulation is an acquired coagulation disorder associated with the release of thromboplastin from damaged tissue, stimulating abnormal coagulation and fibrinolysis.

Haemorrhage related to other causes

Umbilical haemorrhage

- This usually occurs as a result of a poorly applied cord ligature.
- A purse-string suture should always be inserted if umbilical bleeding does not stop after 15 or 20 minutes.

Vaginal bleeding

A small temporary discharge of blood-stained mucus occurring in the first days of life, often referred to as pseudomenstruation, is due to the withdrawal of maternal oestrogen.

Haematemesis and melaena

These signs usually present when the baby has swallowed maternal blood during birth or from cracked nipples during breastfeeding. The diagnosis must be differentiated from other serious causes.

- If the cause is swallowed blood, the condition is self-limiting, requiring no specific treatment.
- However, if the cause is cracked nipples, appropriate treatment for the mother must be implemented and attachment and positioning techniques for feeding reviewed to ensure continuation of and successful breastfeeding.

Haematuria

- Haematuria can be associated with coagulopathies, urinary tract infections and structural abnormality of the urinary tract.
- Birth trauma may cause renal contusion and haematuria.
- Occasionally, after suprapubic aspiration of urine, transient mild haematuria may be observed.
- Treatment of the primary cause should resolve the haematuria.

CONVULSIONS

- A convulsion is a sign of neurological disturbance, not a disease. It can present quite differently in the neonate and can be difficult to recognize.
- Convulsive movement can be differentiated from jitteriness or tremors in that, with the latter two, the movements:
  - are rapid, rhythmic and equal
  - are often stimulated or made worse by disturbance
  - can be stopped by touching or flexing the affected limb
  - are normal in an active, hungry baby and are usually of no consequence, although their occurrence should be documented.

  Convulsive movements:
  - tend to be slower and less equal
  - are not necessarily stimulated by disturbance
  - cannot be stopped by restraint
  - are always pathological.

Subtle convulsions include movements such as:
- blinking or fluttering of the eyelids
- staring
- clonic movements of the chin
- horizontal or downward movements of the eyes
- sucking
- drooling
- sticking the tongue out
- cycling movements of the legs
- apnoea.

Both term and preterm babies can experience subtle convulsions. These movements should be differentiated from the normal ones associated with rapid eye movement sleep.

- If the baby has tonic convulsions, there will be:
  - extension or flexion of the limbs
  - asymmetric postures of body or neck
  - altered patterns of breathing
  - maintenance of eye deviations.
- Tonic convulsions are more common in preterm babies.
- Term babies demonstrate multifocal clonic convulsions and the movements include random jerking movements of the extremities.
- Term babies also experience focal clonic convulsions in which localized repetitive clonic jerking movements are seen. An extremity, a limb or a localized muscle group can be affected.
- Myoclonic convulsions are the least common but affect term and preterm babies. The movements are single or multiple flexion jerks of the feet, legs, hands or arms, which should not be confused with similar movements in a sleeping baby.

During a convulsion, the baby may have:
- tachycardia
- hypertension
- raised cerebral blood flow
- raised intracranial pressure.

All these predispose to serious complications.

There are many conditions that cause newborn convulsions, as shown in Table 33.1.

Immediate treatment of a convulsion involves:
- seeking the assistance of a doctor
- ensuring a clear airway and adequate ventilation

Table 33.1 Selected causes of neonatal convulsions

Category	Selected causes
Central nervous system	Intracranial haemorrhage Intracerebral haemorrhage Hypoxic–ischaemic encephalopathy Kernicterus Congenital abnormalities
Metabolic	Hypo- and hyperglycaemia Hypo- and hypercalcaemia Hypo- and hypernatraemia Inborn errors of metabolism Acquired disorders of metabolism
Other	Hypoxia Congenital infections Severe postnatally acquired infections Neonatal abstinence syndrome Hyperthermia
Idiopathic	Unknown

- turning the baby to the semiprone position, with the head neither hyperflexed nor hyperextended.

The prognosis depends on the cause of convulsion, the type of convulsion and the electroencephalograph tracing.

FURTHER READING

Afsharkhas, L., Khalessi, N., Karimi Panah, M., 2015. Intraventricular hemorrhage in term neonates: sources, severity and outcome. Iran. J. Child Neurol. 9 (3), 34–39.

Ekéus, C., Högberg, U., Norman, M., 2014. Vacuum assisted birth and risk for cerebral complications in term newborn infants: population-based cohort study. BMC Pregnancy Childbirth 14, 36. doi: 10.1186/1471-2393 -14-36.

Useful website

http://www.birthinjuryguide.org

Congenital Malformations

DEFINITION AND CAUSES

By definition, a congenital malformation is any defect in form, structure or function that is present at birth. Identifiable defects can be categorized in five ways:

1. chromosome and gene malformations
2. mitochondrial DNA disorders
3. teratogenic causes
4. multifactorial causes
5. unknown causes.

Chromosome and gene malformations

Each human cell carries 44 chromosomes (autosomes) and two sex chromosomes. Each chromosome comprises a number of genes. The zygote should have 22 autosomes and one sex chromosome from each parent.

Genetic disorders (Mendelian inheritance)

Genes are composed of DNA and each is concerned with the transmission of one specific hereditary factor. Genetically inherited factors may be dominant or recessive.

- *A dominant gene* will produce its effect even if present in only one chromosome of a pair.
  - An autosomal dominant condition can usually be traced through several generations: for example, achondroplasia, osteogenesis imperfecta, adult polycystic kidney disease or Huntington chorea.
- *A recessive gene* needs to be present in both chromosomes before producing its effect: for example, cystic fibrosis or phenylketonuria.
- *In an X-linked recessive inheritance* the condition affects males almost exclusively, although females can be carriers.
  - X-linked recessive inheritance is responsible for conditions such as haemophilia A and B and Duchenne muscular dystrophy.

Mitochondrial disorders

These are inherited from the mother. Signs and symptoms are diverse but tend to occur in brain and muscles.

Teratogenic causes

A teratogen is any agent that raises the incidence of congenital malformation. The list of known and suspected teratogens is continually growing (Box 34.1).

Multifactorial causes

These stem from a genetic defect in addition to one or more teratogenic influences.

Unknown causes

Despite a growing body of knowledge, the specific cause of approximately 80% of congenital malformations remains unspecified.

Fetal alcohol syndrome/spectrum

The following characteristics are recognizable:
- a growth-restricted infant with microcephaly
- flat facies
- close-set eyes
- epicanthic folds
- small upturned nose
- thin upper lip
- low-set ears.

Being able to establish a direct link between a teratogen and a complex clinical pattern such as this is the exception rather than the rule.

Box 34.1 Known and suspected teratogens

- Prescribed drugs, e.g. anticonvulsants, anticoagulants, large amounts of vitamin A
- Drugs used in substance abuse, e.g. heroin, alcohol, nicotine
- Environmental factors, e.g. radiation and chemicals (such as dioxins, pesticides)
- Infective agents, e.g. rubella, cytomegalovirus
- Maternal disease, e.g. diabetes

GASTROINTESTINAL MALFORMATIONS

Most of the malformations affecting this system call for prompt surgical intervention.

Gastroschisis and exomphalos

- Gastroschisis (Fig. 34.1) is a paramedian defect of the abdominal wall with extrusion of bowel that is not covered by peritoneum.

Fig. 34.1 Gastroschisis showing prolapsed intestine to the right of the umbilical cord. (From Rennie & Roberton 1999, with permission of Churchill Livingstone.)

- Exomphalos or omphalocele is when the bowel or other viscera protrude through the umbilicus. These babies may have other defects, for example those involving the heart.

Immediate management of both these defects is as follows:

- Prepare for birth preferable in a regional centre where there is expert knowledge and specialized facilities.
- Prepare for neonatal resuscitation with paediatrician present at birth.
- Cover the herniated abdominal contents with clean cellophane wrap (clingfilm) or warm sterile saline swabs.
- Aspirate stomach contents.
- Reduce heat loss.
- Expedite transfer to a surgical unit.

Atresias

Oesophageal atresia

Oesophageal atresia occurs when there is incomplete canalization of the oesophagus in early intrauterine development.

- It is commonly associated with tracheo-oesophageal fistula.
- The most common type is where the upper oesophagus terminates in a blind upper pouch and the lower oesophagus connects to the trachea.
- This malformation should be suspected in the presence of maternal polyhydramnios.
- At birth the baby has copious amounts of mucus coming from the mouth.
  - The midwife should attempt to pass a wide orogastric tube but it may travel less than 10–12 cm.
  - Radiography will confirm the diagnosis.
  - The baby must be given no oral fluid. Instead the paediatrician will insert a wide-bore oesophageal tube into the upper pouch and connect it to gentle continuous suction. Usually a double-lumen 10FG tube (Replogle) is used and the baby nursed head up.
  - The neonate should be transferred immediately to a paediatric surgical unit and continuous suction must be available throughout the transfer.

Duodenal atresia

- This is persistent vomiting within 24–36 hours of birth.
- A characteristic double bubble of gas may be seen on radiological examination.

- Prognosis is good if the baby is otherwise healthy, but this condition is often associated with other problems, such as Down syndrome.

Rectal atresia and imperforate anus

- An imperforate anus should be obvious at birth but a rectal atresia might not become apparent until it is noted that the baby has not passed meconium.
- Should a baby fail to pass meconium in the first 24 hours, three other possibilities should be considered:
  - malrotation/volvulus
  - meconium ileus (cystic fibrosis)
  - Hirschsprung disease.

Pyloric stenosis

- Pyloric stenosis arises from a genetic defect which causes hypertrophy of the muscles of the pyloric sphincter.
- The characteristic clinical presentation is projectile vomiting, usually at approximately 6 weeks of age but possibly earlier.

Cleft lip and cleft palate

- Cleft lip may be unilateral or bilateral and is very often accompanied by cleft palate.
- Clefts may affect the hard palate, soft palate, or both.
- Some defects will include alveolar margins and sometimes the uvula. The palate is examined by means of a good light source rather than by digital palpation.
- If the defect is limited to unilateral cleft lip, breastfeeding is encouraged.
- Where there is the additional problem of cleft palate, arranging for the baby to be fitted with an orthodontic plate may facilitate breastfeeding but will not afford the same stimulus as nipple to palate contact.
- Cup or spoon feeding is an alternative method, and if bottle feeding there is a wide variety of specially shaped teats available to accommodate the different sizes and positions of palate defects.

Pierre Robin syndrome

- Pierre Robin syndrome is characterized by micrognathia (hypoplasia of the lower jaw), abnormal attachment of muscles controlling the tongue, which allows it to fall backward and occlude the airway, and a central cleft palate.

- To maintain a clear airway the baby is nursed prone and may require the insertion of an oral airway.
- Nasal and nasopharyngeal constant positive airways pressure may be necessary for some time after birth. This is one of the few exceptions to the rules given in the 'Back to sleep' campaign aimed at reducing cot deaths.
- There is a high risk of aspiration occurring when feeding. Suction catheter and oxygen equipment should be ready to hand. An orthodontic plate may be fitted to facilitate feeding.

MALFORMATIONS RELATING TO RESPIRATION

Diaphragmatic hernia

- There is a defect in the diaphragm, which allows herniation of abdominal contents into the thoracic cavity.
- The extent to which lung development is compromised as a result depends on the size of the defect and the gestational age at which herniation first occurred.
- At birth:
  - the baby is cyanosed
  - difficulty is experienced in resuscitation
  - heart sounds may be displaced to the right
  - the abdomen may have a flat or scaphoid appearance.
- Chest X-ray confirms the diagnosis.
- Continuous gastric suction should be commenced.
- Prognosis relates to the degree of pulmonary hypoplasia.
- There is also the possibility of coexistent anomalies, such as cardiac or skeletal defects.

Choanal atresia (Fig. 34.2)

- The condition describes a unilateral or bilateral narrowing of the nasal passage(s) with a web of tissue or bone occluding the nasopharynx.
- Tachypnoea and dyspnoea are cardinal features, particularly when a bilateral lesion is present.
- Diagnosis rests on the following criteria:
  - The baby mouth breathes and finds feeding impossible without becoming cyanosed.

499

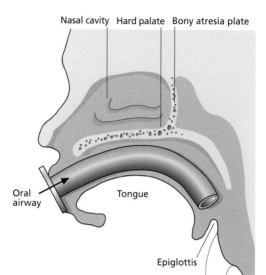

Fig. 34.2 Choanal atresia. A bony plate blocks the nose. (From Rennie & Roberton 1999, with permission of Churchill Livingstone.)

- Nasal catheters cannot be passed into the pharynx.
- If a mirror or cold spoon is held under the nose, no steam will collect.
- The baby's colour will improve with crying.
- Maintaining a clear airway is essential; an oral airway may have to be used to effect this.

Laryngeal stridor

- This is a noise made by the baby, usually on inspiration; exacerbated by crying.
- Most commonly, the cause is laryngomalacia, which is due to laxity of the laryngeal cartilage.
- The stridor may take up to 2 years to resolve.
- If it is accompanied by signs of dyspnoea or feeding problems, further investigations such as bronchoscopy or laryngoscopy become necessary to rule out a more sinister cause.

CONGENITAL CARDIAC DEFECTS

Postnatal recognition

- Clinically, babies with cardiac anomalies can be divided into two groups:
  - cyanotic
  - acyanotic congenital heart disease.

Cardiac defects presenting with cyanosis

Defects included in this group are listed in Box 34.2.

- The persistence of central cyanosis (that is, cyanosis of the lips and mucous membranes), tachypnoea and tachycardia may be the first signs that a cardiac defect is present.
- If there is cyanosis, administration of oxygen to these babies will be ineffective in improving their colour and oxygen saturation monitoring will show no improvement.
- Indeed, giving 100% oxygen may encourage closure of the ductus arteriosus, the patency of which is literally a lifeline for some of these babies.

Acyanotic cardiac defects

Anomalies subsumed under this heading are listed in Box 34.2.

Box 34.2 Cyanotic and acyanotic congenital heart disease

Conditions presenting with cyanosis

- Transposition of the great vessels
- Pulmonary atresia
- Tetralogy of Fallot
- Tricuspid atresia
- Total anomalous pulmonary venous drainage
- Univentricular/complex heart

Conditions presenting without cyanosis

- Persistent ductus arteriosus
- Ventricular or atrial septal defect
- Coarctation of the aorta
- Aortic stenosis
- Hypoplastic left heart syndrome.

Signs of cardiac failure

- Subtle signs of cardiac failure include:
  - tachypnoea
  - tachycardia
  - incipient cyanosis, especially following the exertion of crying or feeding.
- These signs will become more evident, sometimes dramatically so, with the closure of the ductus arteriosus if either coarctation of the aorta or hypoplastic left heart syndrome is present. Detailed examination may disclose heart murmurs and diminution or absence of femoral pulses in both conditions. In this event, resuscitation with prostaglandin usually stabilizes the baby and allows time for further assessment.
- Coarctation of the aorta is usually amenable to surgical correction, whereas hypoplastic left heart syndrome has a poor long-term outcome.
- Persistent ductus arteriosus, ventricular septal defects and atrial septal defects seldom entail medical or surgical intervention in early neonatal life, but do require careful follow-up for signs of developing heart failure; surgery or interventional cardiology may be necessary at a later stage.
- Not all heart murmurs heard at the first examination are significant.

CENTRAL NERVOUS SYSTEM MALFORMATIONS

Anencephaly

- This major malformation describes the absence of the forebrain and vault of the skull. It is a condition that is incompatible with sustained life, but occasionally such a baby is born alive.

Spina bifida

- Spina bifida results from failure of fusion of the vertebral column.
- There is no skin covering the defect, allowing protrusion of the meninges (meningocele). The meningeal membrane may be flat or appear as a membranous sac with or without cerebrospinal fluid but it does not contain neural tissue (Fig. 34.3).
- *Meningomyelocele* involves the spinal cord (see Fig. 34.3).
  - This lesion may be enclosed or the meningocele may rupture and expose the neural tissue.

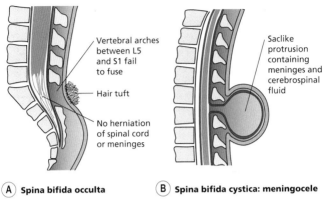

(A) **Spina bifida occulta**

Vertebral arches between L5 and S1 fail to fuse

Hair tuft

No herniation of spinal cord or meninges

(B) **Spina bifida cystica: meningocele**

Saclike protrusion containing meninges and cerebrospinal fluid

(C) **Spina bifida cystica: myelomeningocele**

Saclike protrusion is filled with cerebrospinal fluid, meninges, nerve roots, and spinal cord

Fig. 34.3 Various forms of spina bifida. (After Gould B E, Dyer R, 2010, with permission.)

- Meningomyelocele usually gives rise to neural damage, producing paralysis distal to the defect and impaired function of urinary bladder and bowel. The lumbosacral area is the most common site for these to present, but they may appear at any point along the vertebral column.
- An *encephalocele* is at the level of the base of the skull, and may contain brain tissue.

503

- Immediate management involves covering open lesions with a non-adherent dressing.

Spina bifida occulta

- Spina bifida occulta (see Fig. 34.3) is the most minor type of defect where the vertebra is bifid.
- There is usually no spinal cord involvement.
- A tuft of hair or sinus at the base of the spine may be noted on first examination of the baby.

Hydrocephalus

- This condition arises from a blockage in the circulation and absorption of cerebrospinal fluid, which is produced from the choroid plexuses within the lateral ventricles of the brain.
- The large lateral ventricles increase in size and eventually compress the surrounding brain tissue.
- It often accompanies the more severe spina bifida lesions because of a structural defect around the area of the foramen magnum known as the Arnold–Chiari malformation.
- Hydrocephaly may either be present at birth or develop following surgical closure of a myelomeningocele.
- In the absence of myelomeningocele, aqueduct stenosis is the most common cause of hydrocephalus.
- The risk of cerebral impairment may be minimized by the insertion of a ventriculoperitoneal shunt. As the baby grows, this will need to be replaced.
- Signs of increased intracranial pressure include:
    - large tense anterior fontanelles
    - splayed skull sutures
    - inappropriate increase in occipitofrontal circumference
    - sun-setting appearance to the eyes
    - irritability or abnormal movements.

Microcephaly

The occipitofrontal circumference is more than 2 standard deviations below normal for gestational age. The disproportionately small head may be associated with intrauterine infection, for example rubella, fetal alcohol syndrome or some trisomic disorders. Most babies will be mentally impaired with evidence of cerebral palsy and often seizures.

MUSCULOSKELETAL DEFORMITIES

Polydactyly and syndactyly

- In polydactyly, the extra digit(s) may be fully formed or may simply be extra tissue attached by a pedicle.
- Syndactyly (webbing) more commonly affects the hands. It can appear as an independent anomaly or as a feature of a syndrome such as Apert syndrome.

Limb reduction anomalies

Postulated or presumptive causes include:
- amniotic band syndrome
- environmental teratogens
- iatrogenic trauma, perhaps at the time of chorionic villus sampling
- failure of formation (arrest of development; e.g. thalidomide, an antiemetic).

Talipes

- Talipes equinovarus (club foot) is when the ankle is bent downwards (plantar flexed) and the front part of the foot is turned inwards (inverted).
- Talipes calcaneovalgus describes the opposite position where the foot is dorsiflexed and everted.
- Possible causes are:
  - multiple pregnancy
  - macrosomic fetus
  - oligohydramnios
  - association with spina bifida
  - family history
  - gender: statistically, more boys than girls are born with talipes.
- In the mildest form the foot may easily be turned to the correct position and exercised in this way several times a day. More severe forms will require manipulation, splinting and/or surgical correction.

Developmental hip dysplasia

- Congenital hip dysplasia is more commonly found where there has been a history of oligohydramnios or breech presentation.

- It more often occurs in primigravida pregnancies and in a higher percentage of girls.
- The left hip is more often affected than the right.
- The dysplastic hip may present in one of three ways:
  - dislocated
  - dislocatable
  - subluxation of the joint.
- Examination of the hips is by Ortolani or Barlow test.
- It is usual for the baby to have a splint or harness, such as the Pavlik harness, that will keep the hips in a flexed and abducted position of approximately 60°.

Achondroplasia

- Achondroplasia is an autosomal dominant condition where the baby is generally small with a disproportionately large head and short limbs.

Osteogenesis imperfecta

- This autosomal dominant disorder of collagen production has at least four forms and leads to unduly brittle bones in the affected fetus and infant.

ABNORMALITIES OF THE SKIN

Vascular naevi

- These defects in the development of the skin can be divided into two main types, which commonly overlap.

Capillary malformations

- These are due to defects in the dermal capillaries.
- The most commonly observed are stork marks. These are usually found on the nape. They are generally small and will fade. No treatment is necessary.

Port wine stain

- This is a purple–blue capillary malformation affecting the face. It does not regress with time; laser treatment and the skilful use of cosmetics will help to disguise it.
- Should the malformation appear to mimic the distribution of a branch of the trigeminal nerve, further malformations in the

meninges may be suspected. This is known as Sturge–Weber syndrome.

Capillary haemangiomata ('strawberry marks')

- Capillary haemangiomata are not usually noticeable at birth but appear anywhere as red raised lesions in the first few weeks of life.
- They are more common in preterm infants and especially in girls.
- Although the lesion will grow bigger for the first few months, it will then regress and usually disappear completely by the age of 5–6 years.
- No treatment is normally required.

Pigmented naevi (melanocytic)

These are brown, sometimes hairy, marks on the skin which vary in size and may be flat or raised. A percentage of this type of birthmark may become malignant. Surgical excision may be recommended to preempt this.

GENITOURINARY SYSTEM

At birth the first indications that there is an abnormality of the renal tract may be:
- a single umbilical artery in the umbilical cord
- the abnormal facies associated with Potter syndrome
- no passage of urine within 24 hours
- constant dribbling urine
- poor urine stream.

Dribbling of urine is a sign of nerve damage such as occurs with neural tube defects, whereas a poor urine stream may indicate lower urinary tract obstruction (posterior urethral valve).

Posterior urethral valve(s)

- This is a malformation affecting boys.
- The presence of valves in the posterior urethra prevents the normal outflow of urine.
- Back pressure from the distended bladder will ultimately cause hydronephrosis.
- Treatment normally involves surgical intervention.

Polycystic kidneys

- These are likely to cause problems during the birth due to an increase in abdominal girth.
- On abdominal examination, the kidneys will be palpable.
- Radiological or ultrasound investigations confirm the diagnosis.
- The prognosis is poor, with renal failure the likely outcome.

Hypospadias

- The urethral meatus opens onto the undersurface of the penis.
- The meatus can be placed at any point along the length of the penis and in some cases, will open onto the perineum.
- This malformation often coexists with chordee, in which the penis is short and bent and the foreskin is only present on the dorsal side.
- Some babies will require surgery in the neonatal period to 'release' the chordee and enlarge the urethral meatus.

Cryptorchidism

- Undescended testes may be unilateral or bilateral.
- If on examination of the baby after birth the scrotum is empty, the undescended testes may be found in the inguinal pouch.

Ambiguous genitalia

- If there is any doubt, a gender must not be assigned to the baby.
- Examination of the baby may reveal any of the signs listed in Box 34.3.
- There are a number of causes of ambiguous genitalia, all of which need expert clarification.

Box 34.3 **Signs of ambiguous genitalia**

- Small hypoplastic penis
- Chordee
- Bifid scrotum
- Undescended testes
- Enlarged clitoris
- Incompletely separated or poorly differentiated labia

Congenital adrenal hyperplasia

- One of the reasons for ambiguous genitalia is an autosomal recessive condition called congenital adrenal hyperplasia.
- The adrenal gland is stimulated to overproduce androgens because of a deficiency of an enzyme called 21-hydroxylase, which is necessary for normal steroid production from cholesterol.
- The condition is not always recognized in boys in the neonatal period.

Intersex

- This is where the internal reproductive organs are at variance with the external appearance of the genitalia.
- Ultrasound examination will help identify the nature of internal reproductive organs.
- True hermaphroditism is extremely rare.
- Following chromosomal studies to determine genetic make-up, hormone assays and consideration of the potential for cosmetic surgery, the decision of gender attribution is made.

COMMONLY OCCURRING SYNDROMES

Trisomy 21 or Down syndrome

- This arises as a non-disjunction process in the majority.
- Unbalanced translocation occurs in approximately 2.5% of cases, usually between chromosomes 14 and 21.
- Mosaic forms also occur.
- There is no difference in clinical appearance, the features of which are listed in Box 34.4, Not all the manifestations listed need be

---

Box 34.4 Clinical appearance in Down syndrome

- Widely set and obliquely slanted eyes
- Small nose
- Thick rough tongue
- Small head with flat occiput
- Squat broad hands with incurving little finger
- Wide space between thumb and index finger
- Single palmar (simian) crease
- Brushfield spots in the eyes
- Generalized hypotonia

---

present and any of them can occur alone without implying chromosomal aberration.

- Babies born with Down syndrome also have a higher incidence of cardiac anomalies, leukaemia and hypothyroidism.
- The intelligence quotient is below average, at 40–80.
- Investigations indicated include karyotyping and echocardiography, because of the increased risk of congenital heart disease.
- Some centres offer diagnosis within 2 days using fluorescent in situ hybridization (FISH) techniques.

Trisomy 18 (Edward syndrome)

- This condition is found in approximately 1 in 5000 births.
- An extra 18th chromosome is responsible for the characteristic features.
- The lifespan of these children is short and the majority die during their first year.
  - The head is small with a flattened forehead, a receding chin and frequently a cleft palate.
  - The ears are low set and maldeveloped.
  - The sternum tends to be short.
  - The fingers often overlap each other and the feet have a characteristic rocker-bottom appearance.
  - Malformations of the cardiovascular and gastrointestinal systems are common.

Trisomy 13 (Patau syndrome)

- An extra copy of the 13th chromosome leads to multiple malformations.
- These children have a short life, only 5% living beyond 3 years.
- Affected infants are small and are microcephalic.
- Midline facial malformations, such as cleft lip and palate, are common and limb defects are frequently seen.
- Brain, cardiac and renal malformations may coexist with this trisomy.

Potter syndrome

- This collection of features is due to the compressive effects of oligohydramnios in renal agenesis or severe hypoplasia.
  - The baby's face will have a flattened appearance, with low-set ears, an anti-mongoloid slant to the eyes with deep epicanthic folds and a beaked nose.

- These babies are usually severely asphyxiated at birth because they have lung hypoplasia.
- It is a syndrome incompatible with sustained life.

Turner syndrome (XO)

- In this monosomal condition, only one sex chromosome exists: an X.
  - The child is a girl with a short, webbed neck, widely spaced nipples and oedematous feet.
  - The genitalia tend to be underdeveloped and the internal reproductive organs do not mature.
  - The condition may not be diagnosed until puberty fails to occur.
  - Congenital cardiac defects may also be found.
  - Mental development is usually normal.

Klinefelter syndrome (XXY)

- This is a malformation that affects boys.
- It is not normally diagnosed until pubertal changes fail to occur.

FURTHER READING

De-Regil, L.M., Peña-Rosas, J.P., Fernández-Gaxiola, A.C., Rayco-Solon, P., 2015. Effects and safety of periconceptional oral folate supplementation for preventing birth defects. Cochrane Database Syst. Rev. (12), CD007950. doi: 10.1002/14651858.CD007950.pub3.

Useful websites

http://www.who.int. Useful factsheets on congenital anomalies can be accessed via this link.

http://www.birthdefects.org/parent-services/support-groups

Jaundice and Infection

Jaundice is the yellow discoloration of the skin and sclera that results from raised levels of bilirubin in the blood (hyperbilirubinaemia).

CONJUGATION OF BILIRUBIN

- Bilirubin is a waste product from the breakdown of haem, most of which is found in red blood cells (RBCs).
- Ageing, immature or malformed RBCs are removed from the circulation and broken down in the reticuloendothelial system (liver, spleen and macrophages), and haemoglobin becomes the by-products of haem: globin and iron.
  - Haem is converted to biliverdin and then to unconjugated bilirubin.
  - Globin is broken down into amino acids that are reused by the body to make proteins.
  - Iron is stored in the body or used for new red blood cells.

Two main forms of bilirubin are found in the body:

1. Unconjugated bilirubin is fat soluble and cannot be excreted easily either in bile or urine.
2. Conjugated bilirubin has been made water soluble in the liver and can be excreted in either faeces or urine.

Three stages are involved in the processing of bilirubin:

- transport
- conjugation
- excretion.

Transport

Unconjugated bilirubin is transported in the plasma to the liver, bound to the plasma protein albumin. If not attached to albumin, it can be deposited into extravascular fatty and nerve tissues in the body. The skin and the brain are the two most common sites.

- Staining of the skin is known as *jaundice*.
- Damage to the brain as a result of bilirubin staining and toxicity is known as *kernicterus*.

Conjugation

- Once in the liver, bilirubin is combined with glucose and *glucuronic acid*, and conjugation occurs in the presence of oxygen.
- *Uridine diphosphoglucuronyl transferase* (UDP-GT or glucuronyl transferase) is the major enzyme involved in bilirubin conjugation.
- The conjugated bilirubin is now water soluble and available for excretion.

Excretion

- The conjugated bilirubin is excreted via the biliary system into the small intestine, where it is catabolized by normal intestinal bacteria to form urobilinogen, then oxidized into orange-coloured urobilin.
- Most of the conjugated bilirubin is excreted in the faeces but a small amount is excreted in urine.

JAUNDICE

In term neonates, jaundice appears when serum bilirubin concentrations reach 85–120 μmol/L (5–7 mg/dl).

Physiological jaundice

This type of jaundice:
- *never* appears before 24 hours of life
- *usually* fades by 1 week of age.

Bilirubin levels *never* exceed 200–215 μmol/L (12–13 mg/dl).

Causes

- Neonatal physiological jaundice is the result of a discrepancy between RBC breakdown and the baby's ability to transport, conjugate and excrete unconjugated bilirubin.
- Neonates also have increased beta-glucuronidase enzyme activity in the gut, which hydrolyses conjugated bilirubin back into the unconjugated state.
- If feeding is delayed, bowel motility is decreased, further compromising excretion of unconjugated bilirubin.

Exaggerated physiological jaundice in breastfed infants

- The exact mechanisms are unknown.
- A reliable diagnosis can only be made by excluding pathological causes.
- Cessation of breastfeeding is unnecessary.
- Early-onset jaundice. It is thought that low fluid and calorie intake during colostrum production causes a slower intestinal transit time, which increases exposure to *beta-glucuronidase*; this in turn adds more unconjugated bilirubin to the system.
- Prolonged jaundice occurs for unknown reasons in some healthy breastfed babies.

Exaggerated physiological jaundice in preterm babies

- This is characterized by bilirubin levels of 165 μmol/L (10 mg/dl) or greater by day 3 or 4, with peak concentrations on days 5–7 that return to normal over several weeks.
- Preterm babies are more at risk of kernicterus. Contributing factors include:
  - a delay in the expression of the enzyme UDP-GT
  - shorter red cell life
  - complications such as hypoxia, acidosis and hypothermia that can interfere with albumin-binding capacity.

Midwifery practice and physiological jaundice

It is important to distinguish between healthy babies with a normal physiological response who need no active treatment and those who require serum bilirubin testing. Transcutaneous bilirubinometry reduces the number of blood tests. Parents should be advised to report:

- excessive sleepiness
- reluctance to feed
- decrease in the number of wet nappies
- pale stools and yellow or orange urine.

Early, frequent feeding assists newborns to cope with an increased bilirubin load.

Pathological jaundice

Pathological jaundice in newborns usually appears within 24 hours of birth, and is characterized by a *rapid rise* in serum bilirubin. Criteria are listed in Box 35.1.

> ### Box 35.1 **Diagnosis of pathological jaundice**
>
> - Jaundice within the first 24 hours of life
> - A rapid increase in total serum bilirubin > 85 μmol/L (5 mg/dl) per day
> - Total serum bilirubin > 200 μmol/L (12 mg/dl)
> - Conjugated (direct-reacting) bilirubin > 25–35 μmol/L (1.5–2 mg/dl)
> - Persistence of clinical jaundice for 7–10 days in term babies, or 2 weeks in preterm babies

Causes

- The underlying aetiology of pathological jaundice is some type of interference with bilirubin production, transport, conjugation or excretion.
- Any disease or disorder that increases bilirubin production or that alters the transport or metabolism of bilirubin is superimposed upon normal physiological jaundice.

Production

- Factors that increase haemoglobin destruction also increase bilirubin levels.
- Causes of increased haemolysis include:
  - Rhesus anti-D, anti-A, anti-B and anti-Kell and ABO blood group incompatibility
  - haemoglobinopathies – sickle cell disease and thalassaemia
  - spherocytosis – fragile RBC membrane
  - extravasated blood – cephalhaematoma and bruising
  - sepsis – can lead to increased haemoglobin breakdown
  - polycythaemia – blood contains too many red cells, as in maternofetal or twin-to-twin transfusion.

Transport

Factors that lower blood albumin levels or decrease albumin-binding capacity include:

- hypothermia, acidosis or hypoxia (can interfere with albumin-binding capacity)
- drugs that compete with bilirubin for albumin-binding sites (e.g. aspirin, sulphonamides and ampicillin).

515

Conjugation

As well as immaturity of the neonate's enzyme system, other factors can interfere with bilirubin conjugation in the liver:

- Dehydration, starvation, hypoxia and sepsis (oxygen and glucose are required for conjugation).
- TORCH infections (toxoplasmosis, others, rubella, cytomegalovirus, herpes).
- Other viral infections (e.g. neonatal viral hepatitis).
- Other bacterial infections, particularly those caused by *Escherichia coli*.
- Metabolic and endocrine disorders that alter UDP-GT enzyme activity (e.g. Crigler–Najjar disease and Gilbert syndrome).
- Other metabolic disorders, such as hypothyroidism and galactosaemia.

Excretion

Factors that can interfere with bilirubin excretion include:

- hepatic obstruction caused by congenital anomalies
- obstruction from increased bile viscosity
- saturation of protein carriers needed to excrete conjugated bilirubin into the biliary system
- infection, other congenital disorders and idiopathic neonatal hepatitis (can also cause an excess of conjugated bilirubin).

HAEMOLYTIC JAUNDICE

- Rhesus (RhD) isoimmunization causes haemolytic disease of the newborn (HDN).
- Few antibodies to blood group antigens other than those in the Rh system cause severe HDN; fetal transfusion is unusual for multiple maternal antibody isoimmunization without anti-D.
- ABO incompatibility is possibly the most frequent cause of mild to moderate haemolysis in neonates.

Rhesus-D incompatibility

- RhD incompatibility can occur when a woman with Rh-negative blood type is pregnant with a fetus with Rh-positive blood type.
- The placenta normally prevents fetal blood entering the maternal circulation. However, during pregnancy or birth, small amounts of fetal Rh-positive blood cross the placenta and enter the circulation of the mother, who has Rh-negative blood.

- The woman's immune system reacts by producing anti-D antibodies that cause sensitization.
- In subsequent pregnancies, these maternal antibodies can cross the placenta and destroy fetal erythrocytes.
- Usually, sensitization occurs during the first pregnancy or birth, leading to extensive destruction of fetal RBCs during subsequent pregnancies.
- Rh isoimmunization can result from any procedure or incident where maternal blood leaks across the placenta or from the inadvertent transfusion of Rh-positive blood to the woman (with good practice safeguard checks in place the latter should never happen).

Prevention of Rh-D isoimmunization

This is by routine antenatal anti-D immunoglobulin (Ig) prophylaxis, within 72 hours of birth or after any other sensitizing event. Anti-D Ig is a human plasma-based product that prevents the production of anti-D antibodies by the mother.

Administration of anti-D Ig

- Anti-D Ig is administered to Rh-negative women who are pregnant with, or have given birth to, an Rh-positive baby.
- It destroys any fetal cells in the mother's blood before her immune system produces antibodies.
- The process for non-sensitized women is set out in Box 35.2.

Dose of anti-D Ig

Research evidence for the optimal dose is still limited but the doses listed in Box 35.3 are recommended.

Ethical and legal issues

- Anti-D Ig is a human plasma-based product.
- To give informed consent to its use, women need to know the possible consequences of treatment, as opposed to non-treatment, with anti-D Ig.

Management of RhD isoimmunization

Effects of RhD isoimmunization

- Destruction of fetal RBCs results in anaemia, possibly oedema and congestive cardiac failure.

517

Box 35.2 Administration of anti-D Ig to non-sensitized women

1. Women who are Rh-negative are screened for Rh antibodies (indirect Coombs test). A negative test shows an *absence* of antibodies or sensitization

2. Blood is retested at 28 weeks of pregnancy. In countries where antenatal prophylaxis is routine (at 28 and 34 weeks' gestation), the first injection of anti-D Ig is given just after this blood sample is taken

3. Where a policy of routine antenatal anti-D Ig prophylaxis is *not* in place, blood is retested for antibodies at 34 weeks of pregnancy

4. When anti-D Ig prophylaxis is given at 28 weeks, blood is not retested, as it is difficult to distinguish passive anti-D Ig from immune anti-D

5. Following the birth, cord blood is tested for confirmation of Rh type, ABO blood group, haemoglobin and serum bilirubin levels and the presence of maternal antibodies on fetal red cells (direct Coombs test). Again, a negative test indicates an absence of antibodies or sensitization. The postnatal dose of anti-D Ig is *still given* if passive anti-D Ig is present

6. A Kleihauer acid elution test is also carried out on an anticoagulated maternal blood sample immediately after birth to estimate the number of fetal cells in a sample of maternal blood

7. Anti-D Ig must always be given as soon as possible, and in any case within 72 hours of any sensitizing event and the birth. Anti-D Ig is injected into the deltoid muscle, from which absorption is optimal

---

- Fetal bilirubin levels also increase as more red cells are destroyed, with possible neurological damage as bilirubin is deposited in the brain.
- Lesser degrees of destruction result in haemolytic anaemia, whereas extensive haemolysis can cause hydrops fetalis and death in utero.

Antenatal monitoring and treatment of RhD isoimmunization

Depending on the severity of Rh isoimmunization, monitoring and treatment can include the following:

- Women who are Rh-negative are screened for Rh antibodies (indirect Coombs test). A positive test indicates the *presence* of antibodies or sensitization.

Box 35.3 Recommended dosages of anti-D Ig

- 500 IU anti-D Ig at 28 and 34 weeks' gestation for women in their first pregnancy
- At least 500 IU for all non-sensitized Rh-negative woman following the birth of a Rh-positive infant
- 250 IU following sensitizing events *up to* 20 weeks' gestation
- At least 500 IU following sensitizing events *after* 20 weeks' gestation
- Larger doses for traumatic events and procedures such as caesarean birth, stillbirths and intrauterine deaths, abdominal trauma during the third trimester, or manual removal of the placenta (dose calculated on 500 IU of anti-D Ig suppressing immunization from 4 ml of RhD-positive red blood cells)
- Larger doses for any other instance of inadvertent transfusion of Rh-positive red blood cells, e.g. from an incorrect blood transfusion of Rh-positive blood platelets

---

- RBCs obtained by chorionic villus sampling (using an immune rosette technique) can be Rh phenotyped as early as 9–11 weeks' gestation.
- Maternal blood is retested frequently to monitor any increase in antibody titres. Sudden and unexpected rises in serum anti-D levels can result in hydrops fetalis.
- If antibody titres remain stable, ongoing monitoring is continued.
- If antibody titres increase, Doppler ultrasonography of the middle cerebral artery peak systolic velocity is used rather than amniocentesis to detect fetal anaemia.
- Changes in fetal serum bilirubin levels are observed.
- The fetus is closely monitored by ultrasonography for oedema and hepatosplenomegaly.
- Intravenous immunoglobulin (IVIG) has the potential to maintain the fetus until intrauterine fetal transfusion (IUT) can be performed. IVIG works by blocking Fc-mediated antibody transport across the placenta, blocking fetal red cell destruction and reducing maternal antibody levels.
- IUT can be used from approximately 20 weeks of gestation to reduce the effects of haemolysis until the fetus is capable of survival outside the uterus.

- A planned early birth depends on the ongoing severity of the haemolysis and the condition of the fetus.

Postnatal treatment of RhD isoimmunization

- Babies with mild to moderate haemolytic anaemia and hyperbilirubinaemia may require careful monitoring but less aggressive management.
- Babies with hydrops fetalis are pale and have oedema and ascites; alternatively, they may be stillborn.
- Management of surviving infants aims to prevent further haemolysis, reduce bilirubin levels, remove maternal Rh antibodies from the baby's circulation and combat anaemia.
- In some cases, phototherapy can be effective but exchange transfusion is often required, and packed cell transfusion may be needed to increase Hb levels.
- Infants are at risk of ongoing haemolytic anaemia.

ABO incompatibility

ABO isoimmunization usually occurs when the mother is blood group O and the baby is group A, or less often group B.

- Type A and B blood has a protein or antigen not present in type O blood.
- Individuals with type O blood develop antibodies throughout life from exposure to antigens in food, Gram-negative bacteria or blood transfusion, and by the first pregnancy may already have high serum anti-A and anti-B antibody titres.
- Some women produce IgG antibodies that can cross the placenta and attach to fetal red cells and destroy them.
- First and subsequent babies are at risk; however, the destruction is usually much less severe than with Rh incompatibility.
- ABO incompatibility is also thought to protect the fetus from Rh incompatibility as the mother's anti-A and anti-B antibodies destroy any fetal cells that leak into the maternal circulation.

Treatment aims to:

- prevent further haemolysis
- reduce bilirubin levels
- combat any anaemia.

As with other causes of haemolysis, if babies require phototherapy it is usually commenced at a lower range of serum bilirubin levels (140–165 µmol/L or 8–10 mg/dl). Babies with a high serum bilirubin level may require exchange transfusion.

MANAGEMENT OF JAUNDICE

Phototherapy

- Phototherapy is used to prevent the concentration of unconjugated bilirubin in the blood from reaching levels where neurotoxicity may occur.
- The neonate's skin surface is exposed to high-intensity light, which photochemically converts fat-soluble unconjugated bilirubin into water-soluble bilirubin that can be excreted in bile and urine.
- Treatment may be intermittent or continuous, with phototherapy interrupted only for essential care.

Indications for phototherapy

The commencement of phototherapy is based on serum bilirubin levels and the individual condition of each baby, particularly when jaundice occurs within the first 12–24 hours.

Side-effects of phototherapy

- Hyperthermia, increased fluid loss and dehydration.
- Damage to the retina from the high-intensity light.
- Lethargy or irritability, decreased eagerness to feed, loose stools.
- Rashes and skin burns.
- Alterations in infant state and neurobehavioural organization.
- Isolation and lack of usual sensory experiences, including visual deprivation.
- A decrease in calcium levels, leading to hypocalcaemia.
- Low platelet counts and increased red cell osmotic fragility.
- Bronze baby syndrome, riboflavin deficiency and DNA damage.

Care of the baby needing phototherapy

See Box 35.4.

Exchange transfusion

- Excess bilirubin is removed from the baby during a blood exchange transfusion. With HDN, sensitized erythrocytes are replaced with blood compatible with both the mother's and the infant's serum.
- With the exception of very premature babies and Rh incompatibility, exchange transfusion may now only be used when there is a risk of kernicterus.

Box 35.4 **Care of the baby needing phototherapy**

Temperature

- Maintain a warm thermoneutral environment
- Observe for hypothermia or hyperthermia

Eyes

- Protect with eye shields, ensuring they do not occlude the nose and are not tight

Skin

- Clean with warm water and observe frequently for rashes, dryness and excoriation
- Creams and lotions are not used

Hydration

- Fluid intake and stool and urine output are monitored

Neurobehavioural status

- Observe sleeping and waking states, feeding behaviours, responsiveness, response to stress, and interaction with parents and other carers

Calcium levels

- Hypocalcaemia may be indicated by jitteriness, irritability, rash, loose stools, fever, dehydration and convulsions

Bilirubin levels

- Levels are usually estimated daily

NEONATAL INFECTION

Modes of acquiring infection

- Through the placenta (transplacental infection).
- From amniotic fluid.
- From their passage through the birth canal.
- From carers' hands, contaminated objects or droplet infection after birth.

Vulnerability to infection

- Newborns are immunodeficient and prone to a higher incidence of infection.

- Preterm babies are even more vulnerable, as they have less well-developed defence mechanisms at birth (transfer of IgG mainly occurs after 32 weeks' gestation) and are more likely to experience invasive procedures.
- Full immunocompetence requires both innate (natural) and acquired immune responses.
- At birth the baby has some immune protection from the mother but immunoglobulins are deficient.
- Maternal exposure and transfer of IgG across the placenta limit antibody levels. However, breastfeeding increases the baby's immune protection through the transmission of secretory IgA in breast milk.
- During the early weeks of life, the baby also has deficiencies in both the quantity and the quality of neutrophils.

Management of infection

Individual risk factors for infection

These include:
- a maternal history of prolonged rupture of membranes
- chorioamnionitis
- pyrexia during birth
- offensive amniotic fluid.

Physical assessment

This can include observation of:
- temperature instability
- lethargy or poor feeding, dehydration, starvation, hypothermia, acidosis or hypoxia
- bradycardia or tachycardia, and any apnoea
- urine and stool output and any vomiting
- central nervous system signs that require a complete neurodevelopmental examination.

Investigations

See Box 35.5.

Management

The overall aim of management is to provide prompt and effective treatment that reduces the risk of septicaemia and life-threatening septic shock. Good management includes:

> **Box 35.5 Investigation of neonatal infection**
>
> - A complete blood cell count
> - Testing of specimens of urine and meconium for specific organisms
> - Swabs from the nose, throat and umbilicus, and from any rashes, pustules or vesicles to test for specific organisms
> - Magnetic resonance imaging, computed tomography scans and chest X-rays
> - A lumbar puncture to enable examination of cerebrospinal fluid (CSF)
> - Testing of amniotic fluid, placental tissue and cord blood for specific organisms

- caring for the baby in a warm thermoneutral environment and observing for temperature instability
- good hydration and the correction of electrolyte imbalance, with demand feeding if possible and intravenous fluids as required
- prompt systemic antibiotic or other drug therapy and local treatment of infection
- ongoing monitoring of the baby's neurobehavioural status
- reducing separation of mother and baby
- providing evidence-based information, support and reassurance to parents
- encouraging breastfeeding or expressing of milk, and informing women of the important role of breast milk in fighting infection.

Infections acquired before or during birth

The effects of sexually transmissible and reproductive tract infections are presented in Chapter 15. Others of importance to midwives are discussed in the following section.

Toxoplasmosis

- Toxoplasmosis is caused by *Toxoplasma gondii*, a protozoan parasite found in uncooked meat and cat and dog faeces.
- Infected neonates may be asymptomatic at birth, but can later develop retinal and neurological disease. Maternal–fetal transmission results from poor hygiene.

- Those with subclinical disease at birth can develop seizures, significant cognitive and motor deficits and reduced cognitive function over time.

Varicella zoster

- Varicella zoster virus is a highly contagious DNA virus of the herpes family, transmitted by respiratory droplets and contact with vesicle fluid; it causes varicella (chickenpox).
- It has an incubation period of 10–20 days and is infectious for 48 hours before the rash appears until vesicles crust over.

Incidence and effects during pregnancy

- Maternal deaths have been associated with varicella infection during pregnancy.
- Fetal sequelae from primary maternal infection vary with the length of gestation at the time of the infection (Box 35.6).

Rubella

- For most immunocompetent children and adults (including pregnant women), the rubella virus causes a mild and insignificant illness that is spread by droplet infection.

Incidence and effects during pregnancy

- If primary rubella infection occurs during the first 12 weeks of pregnancy, maternal–fetal transmission rates are high. First-trimester infection can have the results listed in Box 35.7.
- Babies with congenital rubella are highly infectious and should be isolated from other infants and pregnant women (but not from their own mothers).
- Babies should always be followed up for several years, as some problems may not become apparent until they are older.

Ophthalmia neonatorum

- Ophthalmia neonatorum is a notifiable condition.
- It presents with a purulent discharge from the eyes of an infant within 21 days of birth.
- The condition is usually acquired during vaginal birth and causative organisms include:
  - *Staphylococcus aureus*
  - *Streptococcus pneumonia*
  - *Haemophilus influenza*

Box 35.6 Fetal sequelae of maternal infection with varicella zoster

Maternal infection during the first 20 weeks of pregnancy

- 2% risk of fetal varicella syndrome
- Symptoms can include skin lesions and scarring in a dermatomal distribution, eye problems such as chorioretinitis and cataracts, and skeletal anomalies, in particular limb hypoplasia
- Severe neurological problems may include encephalitis, microcephaly and significant developmental delay
- Approximately 30% of babies born with skin lesions die in the first months of life

Maternal chickenpox from 20 weeks' gestation up to almost the time of birth (at least)

- A milder form of neonatal varicella that does not result in negative sequelae for the neonate.

Maternal infection after 36 weeks and particularly in the week before the birth to 2 days after

- Infection rates of up to 50%
- Approximately 25% of those infected will develop neonatal clinical varicella (or varicella infection of the newborn)
- Newborns are also at risk of contracting varicella from mothers or siblings in the postnatal period
- Most affected babies will develop a vesicular rash and approximately 30% will die
- Other complications of neonatal varicella include clinical sepsis, pneumonia, pyoderma and hepatitis

Box 35.7 Sequelae of first-trimester infection with rubella

- Spontaneous abortion
- Cataracts
- Sensorineural deafness
- Congenital heart defects
- Microcephaly
- Meningoencephalitis
- Dermal erythropoiesis
- Thrombocytopenia
- Significant developmental delay

- *Escherichia coli*
- *Klebsiella*
- *Pseudomonas*
- *Chlamydia trachomatis*
- *Neisseria gonorrhoeae.*

A swab must be taken for culture and sensitivity testing, and a doctor notified immediately. Chlamydial and gonococcal infections can cause:

- conjunctival scarring
- corneal infiltration
- blindness
- systemic spread.

Treatment includes:

- local cleaning and care of the eyes with normal saline
- appropriate drug therapy for the baby and also the mother if required.

Candida

- Candida is a Gram-positive yeast fungus that has a number of strains, including *C. albicans*, *C. parapsilosis*, *C. tropicalis* and *C. lusitaniae*.
- *C. albicans* is responsible for most fungal infections, including thrush in infants.
- Infection can affect the mouth (oral candidiasis), skin (cutaneous candidiasis) and other organs (systemic candidiasis).

Some infections acquired after birth

Eye infections

- Mild eye infections are common in babies and can be treated with routine eye care and antibiotics if required.
- Other more serious conditions must be excluded.

Skin infections

- Most neonatal skin infections are caused by *S. aureus*.
- In newborn infants the most likely skin lesions are septic spots or pustules, found either as a solitary lesion or clustered in the umbilical and buttock areas.
    - For the well neonate with limited pustules, management includes regular cleansing with an antiseptic solution.
    - Antibiotic therapy is given for more extensive pustules.

Meningitis

- Neonatal meningitis is an inflammation of the membranes lining the brain and spinal column caused by organisms such as:
  - *E. coli*
  - *group B streptococci*
  - *Listeria monocytogenes*
  - (more unusually) *Candida* and herpes.
- Very early signs may be non-specific, followed by those of meningeal irritation and raised intracranial pressure, such as:
  - increasing lethargy
  - irritability
  - bulging fontanelles
  - crying
  - tremors
  - twitching
  - severe vomiting
  - alterations in consciousness
  - diminished muscle tone.
- Diagnosis is usually confirmed by examination of cerebrospinal fluid (CSF).
- Very ill babies will require intensive care, intravenous fluids and antibiotic therapy.
- Long-term neurological complications can occur in surviving infants.

Respiratory infections

These may be minor (nasopharyngitis and rhinitis) or more severe (pneumonia).

Gastrointestinal tract infections

In the newborn these can include gastroenteritis or the more severe necrotizing enterocolitis. Causative organisms for gastroenteritis include:

- rotavirus
- *Salmonella*
- *Shigella*
- a pathogenic strain of *E. coli*.

The secretory IgA in breast milk offers important protection against these organisms, particularly rotavirus. The correction of fluid and electrolyte imbalance is an urgent priority.

Umbilical infection

- Signs can include localized inflammation and an offensive discharge.
- Untreated infection can spread to the liver via the umbilical vein and cause hepatitis and septicaemia.

Treatment may include:

- regular cleansing
- the administration of an antibiotic powder
- appropriate antibiotic therapy.

Urinary tract infections

Urinary tract infections can result from bacteria such as *E. coli*, or less often from a congenital anomaly that obstructs urine flow. The signs are usually those of an early non-specific infection. Diagnosis is usually confirmed through laboratory evaluation of a urine sample.

FURTHER READING

Hansen, T.W.R., 2016. Kernicterus in neonatal jaundice—finding the needle in the haystack. Pediatr. Crit. Care Med. 17 (3), 266–267.

Schrag, S.J., 2016. Maternal immunization to prevent neonatal group B streptococcal disease: new progress and promise. Obstet. Gynecol. 127 (2), 199–201.

Useful website

https://www.nice.org.uk/Guidance/ta156. Guidance on routine anti-D prophylaxis can be accessed from this website.

Metabolic Disturbances, Inborn Errors of Metabolism, Endocrine Disorders and Drug Withdrawal

METABOLIC DISTURBANCES

Glucose homeostasis

Following birth there is a fall in glucose concentration. At the same time, endocrine changes (decrease in insulin and a surge of catecholamines and release of glucagon) result in an increase in:

- *glycogenolysis* (breakdown of glycogen stores to provide glucose)
- *gluconeogenesis* (glucose production from the liver)
- *ketogenesis* (producing ketones, an alternative fuel)
- *lipolysis* (release of fatty acids from adipose tissue), bringing about an increase in glucose and other metabolic fuel.

Problems arise in the newborn when:

- there is a lack of glycogen stores to mobilize (i.e. preterm and intrauterine growth-restricted [IUGR] babies)
- there is excessive insulin production (infants of diabetic mothers)
- infants are sick and have a poor supply of energy and increased requirements.

Hypoglycaemia

The definition of hypoglycaemia is controversial. Currently a cut-off value in the newborn is 2.6 mmol/L. Signs of hypoglycaemia are listed in Box 36.1.

Newborns at risk of neurological sequelae of hypoglycaemia

- Preterm babies (of less than 37 weeks).
- Babies who are IUGR (less than third centile for gestation).
- Babies of diabetic mothers.
- Sick term babies (e.g. septic or following perinatal hypoxia–ischaemia).
- Babies with inborn errors of metabolism.

Box 36.1 **Signs of hypoglycaemia**

- Lethargy
- Poor feeding
- Seizures
- Decreased consciousness level
- Jitteriness (although this is common in the newborn and is not indicative on its own)

Diagnosis, prevention and treatment of hypoglycaemia

Healthy term babies tolerate low blood glucose concentrations in the initial period (24–48 hours post-birth) without ill effects as they are able to utilize alternative fuels such as ketone bodies, lactate or fatty acids through a process referred to as counter-regulation. Breastfed babies are a group who are particularly likely to have low blood glucose concentrations, probably because of the low energy content of breast milk in the first few postnatal days. Because of their ability to compensate, clinically well, appropriately grown term babies who are feeding do not require monitoring of their glucose concentration. Doing so would result in many neonates being inappropriately treated.

- Babies at risk of neurological sequelae should be monitored and hypoglycaemia prevented by:
  - adequate temperature control – keep the babies warm
  - early feeding (within 1 hour of birth) with 100 ml/kg per day if formula feeding
  - frequent feeding (3 hourly or less)
  - blood glucose check immediately before the second feed and then 4–6 hourly.
- Providing there are no symptoms, there is no advantage to checking the blood glucose concentration earlier than 4–6 hourly, as it is likely to be low and the appropriate treatment at that stage is to feed the baby.
- If there are symptoms, the glucose should be checked and treatment given immediately, including timely and appropriate referral to a paediatrician.

Breastfed babies require intelligent management in this situation because it is important to avoid unnecessary supplementary feeding with formula milk. It is essential to promote responsive and successful breastfeeding. Therefore, it is important to support the woman and observe a complete breastfeed to provide positive feedback regarding

531

positioning and attachment as well as the baby's feeding cues. The challenge is to balance the decision between protecting breastfeeding and ensuring the baby's nutritional needs are not compromised. The UNICEF baby friendly standard makes the case for a guideline on the prevention and management of neonatal hypoglycaemia developed by the interprofessional team to ensure acceptance and compliance. This guidance can be viewed at: http://www.unicef.org.uk

The dangers associated with significant hypoglycaemia in at-risk babies must not be trivialized.

If the blood glucose concentration is < 2.6 mmol/L, then feed should be given at an increased volume and decreased frequency (2 hourly or even hourly). Measures must be taken to support and protect breastfeeding as this will maximize the woman's future lactation. To this end breast milk can be expressed to be given as a cup feed or via a nasogastric tube. If the blood glucose concentration remains low despite these measures and there is an adequate feed volume intake, then paediatric review is necessary as intravenous treatment with dextrose will be required. It is important in this situation that enteral feeding is continued, as feed contains much more energy than 10% glucose and promotes ketone body production and metabolic adaptation.

If the blood glucose concentration is > 2.6 mmol/L before the second and the third feed, then glucose monitoring can be discontinued but feeding should continue at 3-hourly intervals.

In infants where enteral feeding is contraindicated for some reason, then intravenous 10% dextrose at least 60 ml/kg per day should commence.

Hyperglycaemia

Hyperglycaemia occurs predominantly in preterm and severely IUGR babies. It is also seen in term neonates in response to stress, especially following perinatal hypoxia. In general, no treatment is required.

Electrolyte imbalances in the newborn

Postnatal weight loss, fluid and electrolyte changes

All babies lose weight due to a loss of extracellular fluid. Weighing in the first few days is only needed when babies are unwell or if there are concerns about intake and fluid and electrolyte balance.

Sodium

- Sodium is normally excreted via the kidney, controlled by the renin–angiotensin system. This control mechanism is functional in the preterm infant but loss of sodium may occur because of renal tubule unresponsiveness.
- Term breast milk has relatively little sodium (< 1 mmol/kg per day), showing that the normal newborn can preserve sodium via the kidney in order to maintain growth.
- Normal sodium requirements are 1–2 mmol/kg per day in term neonates and 3–4 mmol/kg per day in those born preterm.
- The normal serum sodium concentration is 133–146 mmol/L.
- Changes in serum sodium reflect changes in sodium and water balance.
- Birth weight is important to assess changes in sodium concentration.

Hyponatraemia

- Hyponatraemia is due to either fluid overload or sodium depletion.
- Hyponatraemia in the presence of weight gain represents fluid overload.
- A low sodium with inappropriate weight loss represents sodium depletion.

The latter may be due to inadequate intake or excessive losses.

Hypernatraemia

- Hypernatraemia in the presence of a loss of weight suggests dehydration.
- When there is weight gain, hypernatraemia is due to fluid and sodium overload.

Potassium

- Potassium is the major intracellular cation.
- Abnormalities in serum potassium concentration can cause significant arrhythmias.
- Potassium concentrations can be severely affected by measurement technique and any haemolysis of the blood sample, especially from capillary sampling, is likely to lead to a falsely high value.

Calcium

- Calcium metabolism is closely linked to phosphate metabolism.
- Preterm babies need much higher concentrations of phosphate and calcium. These are given as intravenous supplements, by supplementing breast milk with fortifier or by giving specific preterm milk.
- High serum calcium concentrations are unusual but there are rare, important causes of low serum calcium.
- The normal serum concentration is 2.2–2.7 mmol/L but this must be interpreted with the serum albumin concentration, as serum calcium is bound to albumin; therefore, a low albumin concentration will lead to a falsely low serum value.
- Calcium concentrations fall within 18–24 hours of birth as the baby's supply of placental calcium ceases, but accretion into bone continues.

INBORN ERRORS OF METABOLISM

- Inborn errors of metabolism (IEM) are rare inherited disorders occurring in approximately 1 in 5000 births. They result mainly from enzyme deficiencies in metabolic pathways leading to an accumulation of substrate, which in turn causes toxicity.
- Early diagnosis and institution of therapy can reduce morbidity.
- It has been estimated that 20% of infants presenting with sepsis in the absence of risk factors have an IEM.
- Inheritance is usually autosomal recessive and the following factors should be explored:
  - affected sibling
  - previous stillbirth/neonatal death
  - parental consanguinity
  - symptoms associated with feeding, fasting or a surgical procedure
  - improvement when feeds stopped and relapse on restarting.
- Clinical examination is usually normal. The features in Box 36.2 indicate that an underlying IEM should be seriously considered.
- Principles of emergency medical management are:
  - to reduce load on affected pathways by removing toxic metabolites and stimulating residual enzyme activity;
  - to treat hypoglycaemia, ensure adequate ventilatory support and hydration are maintained, convulsions are treated and

significant metabolic acidosis is treated with intravenous sodium bicarbonate, and electrolyte abnormalities are corrected.

- Antibiotics are frequently given, as infection may have precipitated metabolic decompensation; dialysis may be required.

Box 36.2 Clinical features of inborn errors of metabolism

- Septicaemia
- Jaundice/liver disease
- Hypoglycaemia
- Severe hypotonia
- Metabolic acidosis
- Unusual body odour
- Convulsions
- Dysmorphic features
- Coma
- Abnormal hair
- Cataracts
- Hydrops fetalis
- Cardiomegaly
- Diarrhoea

Phenylketonuria (PKU)

- An autosomal recessive disorder (incidence of 1 in 10 000 in the UK).
- Caused by absence or reduction of an enzyme in the liver that converts phenylalanine to tyrosine (phenylalanine hydroxylase).
- Babies are well at birth but begin to be affected during the first few weeks.
- Diagnosed by blood test, 5–8 days after birth; this is collected on the Neonatal Screening Test Card.
- Untreated, PKU leads to severe mental disability (IQ < 30) due to build-up of phenylpyruvic acid.
- It is treated by a diet specifically restricted in phenylalanine. Affected women need to return to a strict diet in pregnancy.

Galactosaemia

- An autosomal recessive disorder (incidence of 1 in 60 000).
- Caused by an absence or severe deficiency of the enzyme galactose-1-phosphate uridyltransferase (Gal-1-PUT) that converts galactose to glucose.

- As milk's main sugar, lactose, contains glucose and galactose, babies with this condition rapidly become affected.
- Build-up of galactose-1-phosphate is harmful and can quickly cause cataracts and brain injury.
- It is treated with lactose-free formula.

Diagnosis

- Indicative if there are signs of liver failure and renal impairment.
- Considered if babies have unresponsive hypoglycaemia and prolonged/severe jaundice.
- Urine-reducing substances (i.e. galactose) are present but the urine test for glucose is negative.
- Assay is made of the enzyme level (Gal-1-PUT) within red blood cells.

ENDOCRINE DISEASE IN THE NEWBORN

Thyroid disorders

- The thyroid gland hormones have an effect on the metabolic rate in most tissues, and are essential for normal neurological development.
- Thyroid-stimulating hormone (TSH) is produced by the anterior pituitary gland and this stimulates production of T3 and T4 by the thyroid gland with a feedback mechanism to the anterior pituitary.

Hypothyroidism

- Abnormalities in gland formation, defects in hormone synthesis and rarely secondary pituitary causes.
- Babies tend to be macrosomic and to have a large posterior fontanelle, coarse features and often an umbilical hernia.
- Untreated babies develop impaired motor development, growth failure, a low IQ, impaired hearing and language problems.
- Screening is by measuring TSH (high) on a blood spot taken along with the screening test for PKU at 5–8 days of age.
- Screening does not detect pituitary causes, as they have a low TSH.

Hyperthyroidism

- Rare and due to maternal Graves disease.
- Can lead to preterm labour, low birth weight, stillbirth and fetal death.

- Symptoms are uncommon and may be present at birth or delayed till 4–6 weeks. These include:
  - irritability
  - jitteriness
  - tachycardia
  - prominent eyes
  - sweating
  - excessive appetite and weight loss.
- Babies with symptoms are treated with antithyroid medication.

Adrenal disorders

The adrenal cortex produces three groups of hormones:

1. glucocorticoids
2. mineralocorticoids
3. sex hormones.
   - Glucocorticoids regulate the general metabolism of carbohydrates, proteins and fats on a long-term basis and modify metabolism in times of stress.
   - Mineralocorticoids regulate sodium, potassium and water balance.
   - The sex hormones are responsible for normal development of the genitalia and reproductive organs.

Adrenocortical insufficiency

- Causes are congenital hypoplasia, adrenal haemorrhage, enzyme defects and can be secondary to pituitary problems.
- Diagnosis rests on symptomatic hypoglycaemia, poor feeding, vomiting, poor weight gain and prolonged jaundice.
- Babies may have hyponatraemia, hypoglycaemia, hyperkalaemia and acidosis.
- Treatment is by intravenous therapy with glucose and electrolytes; replacement of corticosteroid and mineralocorticoid hormones is then required.

Adrenocortical hyperfunction

- This may occur in the form of congenital adrenal hyperplasia due to deficiency of the enzymes responsible for hormone production within the adrenal gland.
- The most common enzyme deficiency results in an excess of androgenic hormones, but a deficiency of glucocorticoid and mineralocorticoids often also occurs.

- These disorders can cause ambiguous genitalia (virilization of females or inadequate virilization of males) and symptoms of adrenal insufficiency (vomiting, diarrhoea, vascular collapse, hypoglycaemia and hyponatraemia, hyperkalaemia).
- Treatment is by replacement of glucocorticoid and mineralocorticoid hormones.
- Virilized girls may also require surgical intervention to correct the genital abnormalities.

Pituitary disorders

- Pituitary insufficiency is rare. It may occur in association with other abnormalities, particularly midline developmental defects.
- Presentation is with signs of glucocorticoid deficiency (hypoglycaemia), prolonged jaundice or signs of hypothyroidism.
- Growth hormone deficiency generally causes hypoglycaemia but no other signs in the newborn.
- Treatment is with replacement of the missing hormones.

Parathyroid disorders

- The parathyroid glands are responsible for control of calcium metabolism, but abnormalities of the parathyroids are rare causes of hypocalcaemia or hypercalcaemia in the newborn.
- When hypoparathyroidism does occur, it may be familial or may occur in association with deletions of chromosome 22 (22q11 deletion or DiGeorge syndrome).

EFFECTS OF MATERNAL DRUG ABUSE/USE DURING PREGNANCY ON THE NEWBORN

- Opiates and other drugs cross the placenta.
- Withdrawal may be manifested before birth.

Withdrawal symptoms

- Each drug has a different half-life and this leads to different patterns of withdrawal symptoms.
- In general, methadone produces symptoms for longer periods than heroin, but benzodiazepines may also contribute to this.

The symptoms most frequently seen are listed in Box 36.3.

- Infants assessed for signs of drug withdrawal using a scoring system are less likely to be inappropriately treated and may have a shorter hospital stay.

Box 36.3 Common symptoms of drug withdrawal

- Jitteriness, irritability and constant high-pitched crying
- Often, failure to settle between feeds
- Hyperactivity
- Often, voracious feeding, although some infants have poor sucking
- Vomiting (common)
- Diarrhoea and an irritant nappy rash (common)
- Sneezing and yawning
- Episodes of high temperature in the absence of infection
- In rare circumstances, seizures

- Although it is important not to overtreat with drugs, babies who are withdrawing may appear to be in discomfort that needs to be relieved.
- The long-term effects of withdrawal symptoms are also unclear.
- The most useful sign is whether infants settle and sleep between feeding. If they do, then pharmacological treatment may be unnecessary.

Treatment

- Breastfeeding can be encouraged, as long as there is no evidence of HIV or ongoing drug use that precludes this (cocaine, heroin). This includes methadone, as long as the dose is less than 20 mg/day.
- A quiet environment with reduced light and noise is helpful in keeping stimuli to a minimum.
- Swaddling as a comfort measure might be useful providing the baby is closely observed.
- Feeds may need to be given frequently. These infants will often take large volumes of milk; this is acceptable as long as vomiting is not a problem.
- Rocking and cradling are also useful adjuncts to treatment.

Pharmacological treatment

The two most commonly used treatments are:
1. oral methadone
2. oral morphine.

539

> **Box 36.4 Some harmful effects of cocaine**
>
> - Significant fetal growth restriction
> - Brain injury due to haemorrhage or infarction
> - Abnormalities of brain development
> - Limb reduction defects
> - Gut atresias
> - Small head size and developmental scores

These appear to control withdrawal seizures much more effectively. They can be given in increasing doses if necessary until symptoms are controlled and then the dose may gradually be reduced.

- If feeding and settling do not improve or profuse watery stools and profuse vomiting continue, other treatment needs to be considered.
- Alternative medication may sometimes be useful: for example, clonazepam for benzodiazepine use or chloral hydrate as a general sedative.

Cocaine

The effects of cocaine on the newborn are different. It can produce significant withdrawal symptoms but these are often less severe and less troublesome than with other drugs. However, it is associated with many other harmful effects on the fetus (Box 36.4).

FURTHER READING

Manktelow, B.N., Smith, L.C., Seaton, S.E., et al. on behalf of the MBRRACE-UK Collaboration, 2016. MBRRACE-UK perinatal mortality surveillance report. UK perinatal deaths for births from January to December 2014. Available at: http://www.npeu.ox.ac.uk (accessed 22 August 2016).

Public Health England, 2016. NHS newborn blood spot screening programme: guidelines for newborn blood spot sampling – quick reference guide. Available at: http://www.gov.uk (accessed 22 August 2016).

Useful websites

National Perinatal Epidemiology Unit. Available at: http://www.npeu.ox .ac.uk. MBRRACE-UK (Mothers and Babies: Reducing Risk Through Audits and Confidential Enquiries Across the UK) reports can be accessed via this website.

The National Society for Phenylketonuria. Available at: http://www.nspku.org

http://www.newbornscreening.org

http://www.unicef.org.uk

Complementary Therapies and Maternity Care

- In western society, complementary and alternative medicine (CAM) are synonymous terms used to describe a wide array of disciplines that are health related but are considered to be outside the mainstream practice of conventional medicine.

- CAM is still an evolving discipline in the context of maternity care. Not surprisingly there is a paucity of credible research on which to base practice. CAM may be used by women during pregnancy, labour and postpartum as a means of relaxation to ease tension, stress and anxiety, as well as to manage nausea, pain and discomfort as highlighted by Fig. 37.1.

- Women may request the presence of a CAM practitioner at the birth. They should ensure that the therapist has a sound underpinning knowledge and full comprehension of the physiology of pregnancy, as well as the pathological conditions that may arise. Additionally, they must be conversant with conventional maternity services and have personal professional indemnity insurance cover.

- When a midwife wishes to incorporate some aspect of CAM within her own practice, she must continue to work within the parameters laid down by her regulatory body, for example, the Nursing and Midwifery Council (UK). She must also be guided by the local guideline and policy of her employing organization if she is not an independent midwife.

ACUPUNCTURE

- Acupuncture is based on the principle that the body has Qi or 'energy' lines, called meridians, flowing through it from top to hand or toe. The majority pass through a major organ, after which the meridian is named.

- There are 12 major meridians, and 365 points on these in total. These points can be stimulated to release and rebalance the energies, either by the insertion of acupuncture needles or by other means.

Promotion of wellbeing/form of relaxation therapy
in pregnancy, labour and postpartum

To help manage
discomfort of
pregnancy, e.g.
nausea, backache,
constipation

To help manage pain/
discomfort in the
postnatal period, e.g.
engorged breasts,
perineal trauma

Fig. 37.1 Use of CAM in Maternity Care.

- Sometimes thumb pressure is applied to the points (called acupressure, or the similar practice of *shiatsu*, the Japanese equivalent); on other occasions, heat is applied via moxa sticks (e.g. moxibustion for breech presentation).
- Alternatively, suction can be used if the points are covered with special cups (cupping).
- Acupuncture needles may also be stimulated by mild electric pulsations; this is similar to transcutaneous nerve stimulation (TENS), which is used for pain relief in labour.
- Certain acupuncture points are contraindicated during pregnancy as they may trigger uterine contractions.
- Some antenatal conditions respond well to acupuncture or acupressure, including many of the physiological symptoms of pregnancy. In labour, acupuncture may facilitate progress and ease pain, anxiety and tension.

HOMEOPATHY

- Homeopathy uses minute, highly diluted doses of substances that, if given in the full dose, would actually cause the symptoms being treated.
- Most homeopathic medicines are in tablet form but they do not work pharmacologically and will not interact with prescribed drugs, although certain drugs may inactivate the homeopathic tablet.
- Homeopathy is not, however, completely harmless.

Only one remedy should normally be taken at a time. Studies into the use of arnica (arnica montana) have been inconclusive but it has been found to be useful in postnatal trauma management.

HERBAL MEDICINE

- There is a common misconception that just because herbal remedies are natural they are automatically safe.
- There are many herbal remedies that should be avoided during pregnancy or breastfeeding because they may induce uterine bleeding or miscarriage, or have other systemic effects on the mother or fetus.
- Popular herbal remedies such as St John's wort and raspberry leaf tea should be used with caution.

AROMATHERAPY

- Aromatherapy is the use of highly concentrated essential oils extracted from plants.
- Essential oils enter the body by a variety of means, depending on the method of administration.
- The most frequently used modes of entry are:
  - via the skin (i.e. massage; oils added to bath water; compresses or creams)
  - via the mucous membranes (i.e. pessaries or suppositories)
  - via the respiratory tract (i.e. inhalations and vaporizers).

All essential oils act in the same way as pharmaceutical drugs, being absorbed, metabolized and excreted via the same pathways; they are therefore likely to interact with prescribed medications.

Safety (see Box 37.1)

Essential oils can be very therapeutic when used appropriately, but also have the potential to be toxic if incorrectly administered or abused. There are many oils that should be avoided during pregnancy, although some may be used in labour.

Box 37.1 **'Rules' for the correct administration of essential oils during pregnancy and childbirth**

The person administering the essential oil must be adequately and appropriately trained and aware of:
- uses and effects
- precautions and contraindications
- possible complications and side-effects

The correct essential oil should be prescribed and administered:
- to the correct person
- at the correct time
- in the correct dose
- by the correct route
- in the correct frequency
- with an accurate and contemporaneous record in the notes

OSTEOPATHY AND CHIROPRACTIC

- Both forms of treatment involve rebalancing of the neuromusculoskeletal system.
- Disorders, trauma or alterations in the body structure can cause imbalances in the whole system, which in turn can lead to a predisposition to other conditions.
- Osteopaths are concerned with mobility of joints and employ soft tissue massage prior to manipulation.
- Chiropractors deal with relative positions of joints. Different manipulative techniques are used and most chiropractors use more X-rays to aid diagnosis (although not for pregnant women).
- Craniosacral therapy, or cranial osteopathy, uses gentle manipulation of the bones of the skull, meningeal membranes and nerve endings in the scalp. It has been found to be useful for infants with colic.

REFLEXOLOGY

- Reflexology, or reflex zone therapy, involves a precise manipulation of the feet, which are thought to represent a map of the whole body. Every part of the body is reflected on one or both feet and therefore if specific parts of the feet are worked on, other areas of the body can be treated.
- Reflexology is a powerful therapy that can be very effective when used appropriately, although there are some contraindications, precautions and possible complications of treatment.
- Reflexology can be performed on the hands, as well as the tongue, face and back. It is widely thought to work along the meridians used in acupuncture.

FURTHER READING

Hall, H., McKenna, L.G., Griffiths, D.L., 2012. Midwives' support for complementary and alternative medicine: a literature review. Women Birth 25 (1), 4–12. doi: 10.1016/j.wombi.2010.12.005.

Levett, K.M., Smith, C.A., Dahlen, H., 2016. The complementary therapies for labour birth study. Making sense of labour and birth – experiences of women, partners and midwives of complementary medicine antenatal course. Midwifery doi: 10.1016/j.midw.2016.06.011.

Tiran, D., 2016. Aromatherapy in midwifery: a cause for concern. MIDIRS Digest 26 (2), 141–144.

Useful websites

British Acupuncture Council. Available at: http://www.acupuncture.org.uk

Research Council for Complementary Medicine UK. Available at: http:// www.rccm.org.uk

Australian Government, Therapeutic Goods Administration. Available at: https://www.tga.gov.au/complementary-medicines

Drugs (Medicines)

This section contains some of the common drugs used in pregnancy and birth, but it is acknowledged that many maternity units will use different medications to those listed.

Class of drug	Drug	Use and risk/ contraindications
Anaesthetic	**Lidocaine hydrochlctoride**	Local anaesthetic used for perineal infiltration and nerve blocks
	Bupivicaine hydrochloride	Epidural and spinal anaesthesia Contraindicated in hypovolaemia and local sepsis
Analgesia	**Non-steroidal anti-inflammatory drugs (NSAIDs)** (e.g. ibuprofen, indometacin, diclofenac)	Relatively safe in the first trimester but have the potential to cause fetal renal dysfunction, premature closure of the ductus arteriosus, necrotising enterocolitis and intracerebral haemorrhage Safe in breastfeeding
	Opiate analgesics (e.g. pethidine, morphine, diamorphine, codeine)	With long-term use there is a risk of neonatal withdrawal after birth Risk of respiratory depression with large doses in labour
	Paracetamol	Recommended first-line analgesic agent in pregnancy Overdose can be potentially lethal to the mother and/or fetus

Continued

Class of drug	Drug	Use and risk/ contraindications
	Aspirin	Risk of maternal, fetal and neonatal bleeding with analgesic dose (e.g. 600 mg every 6 hours); therefore contraindicated in pregnancy Low-dose (75 mg daily) aspirin is used for treatment of recurrent miscarriage, thrombophilias (inherited risk of thromboembolism) and prevention of pre-eclampsia and intrauterine growth restriction Causes antiplatelet effect for around 10 days after administration and may prolong the bleeding time; therefore may be discontinued 3–4 weeks prior to expected birth
Antacid drugs	**Ranitidine**	To reduce the acidity of stomach acid in high-risk labours and prior to caesarean section or general anaesthetic
Antibiotics		To treat infection Caution should be exercised with some drugs during pregnancy
	Aminoglycosides (e.g. gentamicin, netilmicin)	Risk of ototoxicity but often used in serious maternal infection where benefit outweighs risk
	Chloramphenicol	Risk of 'grey baby syndrome' when used in second and third trimesters
	Erythromycin	Used if woman is penicillin sensitive Enhances effect of anticoagulants

Class of drug	Drug	Use and risk/ contraindications
	Metronidazole	Used to treat or prevent anaerobic infection Avoid large single doses when breastfeeding
	Penicillins	Not known to be harmful, trace amounts in breast milk
	Quinolones (e.g. ciprofloxacin, ofloxacin)	Risk of arthropathy in fetus – most of the evidence for this obtained from animal studies
	Tetracyclines (e.g. tetracycline, oxytetracycline, doxycycline)	Risk of discolouration and dysplasia of fetal bones and teeth, cataracts when used in second and third trimesters
Anticoagulants		History of a previous thromboembolic problem, an acute event, a known thrombophilia or heart valve replacement
	Heparin	Heparin does not cross the placenta and is not excreted into breast milk Given intravenously or subcutaneously Effectiveness is monitored by measuring the activated partial thromboplastin time (APTT) Side effects include bleeding and bruising at the injection site, heparin-induced thrombocytopenia
	Low molecular weight (LMW) preparations (e.g. enoxaparin, dalteparin, tinzaparin)	Have a more predictable anticoagulant response and are usually given by once-daily subcutaneous injection

Continued

Class of drug	Drug	Use and risk/ contraindications
	Warfarin	Women on warfarin should be converted to heparin as soon as they become pregnant and will continue on heparin throughout pregnancy Considered safe in breastfeeding The dose required is very variable and is judged by monitoring the INR (international normalised ratio) in the blood
Anticonvulsants	**Carbamazepine** **Oxcarbazepine** **Phenytoin** **Valproate**	Increased risk of teratogenicity, particularly neural tube defects (NTDs) Benefits of treatment should outweigh risks Folic acid 5 mg should be taken daily Risk of neonatal bleeding; prophylactic vitamin K is recommended for mother before birth in addition to the neonatal dose Small amounts in breast milk
	Magnesium sulphate	Treatment of eclampsia Can be given intramuscularly or intravenously Care should be taken to avoid magnesium toxicity; clinical signs are loss of the patellar reflexes, a feeling of flushing, somnolence, slurred speech, respiratory difficulty and, in extreme cases, cardiac arrest The 'antidote' to magnesium sulphate is calcium gluconate

Class of drug	Drug	Use and risk/ contraindications
Antiemetics	**Cyclizine hydrochloride Metoclopramide**	Non-pharmacological therapies should be tried first Not known to be harmful but use with caution in pregnancy and breastfeeding
Antihypertensive drugs		Pre-existing hypertension, pregnancy-induced hypertension or pre-eclampsia
	ACE inhibitors (e.g. captopril, enalapril, lisinopril)	Contraindicated in pregnancy
	Beta-blockers (e.g. propranolol, atenolol, labetalol)	May cause intrauterine growth restriction, neonatal hypoglycaemia and bradycardia Considered safe in breastfeeding Contraindicated in women with asthma
	Calcium channel blockers (e.g. nifedipine, nicardipine)	Risk of serious hypotensive reactions, especially in association with magnesium sulphate Slow-release formulations should be used Risk of headache Small amounts in breast milk; avoidance recommended
	Hydralazine	Given by slow bolus injection or by infusion Avoid before third trimester Considered safe in breastfeeding
	Methyldopa	Given in 2–4 divided doses from a starting dose of 250 mg three times daily, up to a total of 3 g daily Considered safe in pregnancy and breastfeeding

Continued

Class of drug	Drug	Use and risk/contraindications
Bronchodilators		To treat or prevent an asthma attack Are all considered safe
	Inhaled bronchodilators (e.g. salbutamol, salmeterol, ipratropium), **inhaled cromoglicate, inhaled and oral corticosteroids and theophyllines**	
Corticosteroids	**Prednisolone**	Pre-existing maternal disease such as asthma, rheumatoid arthritis and other inflammatory diseases Crosses the placenta in relatively small quantities; is considered safe for use in pregnancy Women who are on long-term steroid treatment should receive extra corticosteroids in labour, usually given as intravenous hydrocortisone
	Betamethasone and dexamethasone	Fetal lung maturation in actual or threatened preterm delivery Are generally given as intramuscular injections in divided doses over 24–48 hours; the most significant effect is noticed if 48 hours have elapsed between administration of the drug and birth
Diuretics	e.g. furosemide, bendroflumethiazide	Contraindicated in pregnancy

Class of drug	Drug	Use and risk/ contraindications
Drugs for diabetes mellitus	**Bovine insulin Metformin Sulphonylureas (oral hypoglycaemic agents)** (e.g. glibenclamide, gliclazide)	Glycaemic control Avoid in pregnancy or use with caution
	Synthetic human insulins or pork-derived insulins	May be used in pregnancy
Folic acid		To reduce the risk of NTDs Recommended dose 400 μg daily Women at risk of NTDs and those taking antiepileptic drugs, 5 mg daily
Hypnotics	**Benzodiazepines** (e.g. temazepam)	Avoid regular use during pregnancy and breastfeeding
Iron preparations		To treat iron deficiency anaemia
	Oral iron (e.g. ferrous gluconate or ferrous sulphate)	May cause gastrointestinal disturbance – constipation, diarrhoea, indigestion, black stools
	Parenteral preparations	Avoid in first trimester
Aperients	e.g. **Lactulose**	Considered safe in pregnancy and breastfeeding
Oxytocics		To aid uterine contractility, either in induction of labour or in augmentation of labour, or postpartum for prevention or treatment of uterine atony

Continued

Class of drug	Drug	Use and risk/ contraindications
	Syntocinon	In labour, generally given by intravenous infusion so the amount given can be titrated against its effect It takes 20–30 minutes for oxytocin to reach a steady state and the rate of infusion should therefore not be increased at time intervals of less than 30 minutes Should not be administered within 6 hours of vaginal prostaglandins For treatment and prevention of postpartum haemorrhage, larger doses can be given either by slow intravenous or intramuscular bolus or by intravenous infusion Can cause water retention and hyponatraemia
	Ergometrine	Treatment and prevention of postpartum haemorrhage Can cause nausea, vomiting and hypertension Contraindicated in women with pre-eclampsia/hypertensive disorder and cardiac disease Can be given intramuscularly or intravenously Has a sustained action, up to 2–3 hours
	Syntometrine (oxytocin 5 IU/ml with ergometrine 0.5 mg)	Active management of the third stage of labour Given intramuscularly Has the advantage of the speed of action of oxytocin (within 3 minutes) and the sustained action of ergometrine The disadvantage is the side effect profile of ergometrine

Class of drug	Drug	Use and risk/ contraindications
Prostaglandins	**Prostaglandin E$_2$** Dinoprostone	Induction of labour Given by the vaginal route in the form of gel, tablets, slow-release pessary Oxytocin should not be given within at least 6 hours of prostaglandin because of the risk of uterine hyperstimulation
Tocolytics		To stop uterine activity
	Beta-sympathomimetics (e.g. ritodrine, terbutaline, salbutamol)	Associated with significant maternal side effects, such as tachycardia, palpitations, tremor, nausea, vomiting, headaches, thirst, restlessness, chest pain and breathlessness Blood sugar levels may rise Great care should be taken when administering these drugs and the lowest possible dose should be given
	Calcium channel blockers (e.g. nifedipine)	These have the advantage of oral administration and fewer side effects than some of the other agents Profound maternal hypotension is a risk
	Magnesium sulphate	First line drug in the management of severe pre-eclampsia/eclampsia. Common side effects include flushing, nausea, vomiting, palpitations and headaches Magnesium levels need to be monitored to avoid toxicity

Continued

555

Class of drug	Drug	Use and risk/contraindications
	NSAIDs (e.g. indometacin)	Maternal side effects include gastrointestinal bleeding, peptic ulceration, thrombocytopenia, allergic reactions and impaired renal function Fetal side effects when used in the long term include oligohydramnios, fetal renal impairment, premature closure of the ductus arteriosus, intraventricular haemorrhage and necrotising enterocolitis
	Oxytocin antagonists (e.g. atosiban)	A new class of drug that appears to have fewer side effects

An Aid to Calculations Used in Midwifery Practice

Relationship between SI or metric units are related by a factor of 1000 as illustrated in the table below:

Larger unit	Common abbreviation	Smaller unit	Common abbreviation
1 litre	L	1000 millilitres	ml
1 kilogram	kg	1000 grams	g
1 gram	g	1000 milligrams	mg
1 milligram	mg	1000 micrograms	mcg
1 mole	m	1000 millimoles	mmol

In midwifery practice it is important that midwives have a working knowledge of mathematics in order to undertake numerical calculations accurately, especially from a risk management perspective.

SIMPLE FORMULA FOR CONVERSION

To convert from one unit to another, divide or multiply by 1000
Converting from LARGER units, e.g. kilograms to SMALLER units, i.e. grams, multiply by 1000.
Converting from SMALLER units, e.g. micrograms to LARGER units, i.e. milligrams, divide by 1000.

Example:

2 g (larger units) converted to mg (smaller units) =

$$2 \times 1000 = 2000 \text{ mg}$$

When calculating the quantity of a medicine to be administered, always begin by converting prescription dose and stock volume to the same unit (i.e. grams or milligrams).

Example:

To calculate tablets, the formula is:

$$\frac{\text{dose to be given}}{\text{stock strength per tablet}} = \text{quantity of tablets}$$

A prescription requires 1 gram of a medicine to be administered, the stock strength is 500 milligrams per tablet:

$$1 \text{ gram} = 1000 \text{ milligrams}$$

$$\frac{1000 \text{ milligrams}}{500 \text{ milligrams}} = 2 \text{ tablets}$$

CONCENTRATION

Expressed as weight of the medicine per volume of solution, e.g. mg/ml, g/l, μg/ml.

This is calculated by dividing the total weight of the medicine by the volume of the solution.

Example:

To calculate the concentration of a medicine in an infusion labelled 500 mg in 250 ml glucose 5% concentration:

$$\frac{\text{total weight of medicine}}{\text{total volume of solution}} = \frac{500 \text{ mg}}{250 \text{ ml}} = 2 \text{ mg/ml}$$

PROPORTION

It is often necessary to calculate how much of a mixture you need to administer to give the required dose e.g. this may apply to the administration a liquid like a syrup or intramuscular injection.

A simple method of calculating the dose is using the following formula:

$$\text{Dose to be given} = \frac{\text{What you want x Volume you have}}{\text{What you have got}}$$

Or expressed in another way the formula to use is:

$$\frac{\text{dose to be given}}{\text{stock strength}} \times \frac{\text{stock volume}}{1} = \text{amount of mixture to be given}$$

Example

A prescription requires 2 g of a medicine to be given; the stock volume is 500 mg in 10 ml:

$$2\,g = 2000\,mg$$

$$\frac{2000}{500} \times \frac{10}{1} = 40\,ml$$

CALCULATION OF INFUSION RATES

Intravenous (IV) infusion rates may be prescribed as:
1. the volume of fluid to be infused over a specified period of time, *or*
2. the amount of a drug to be administered over a specified period of time

To calculate the volume of fluid to be infused over a specified period of time, the formula is:

$$\frac{\text{total volume of fluid to be given(in ml)}}{\text{time(in hours)}} = \text{ml/hour}$$

Example

a. 1 litre of normal saline 0.9% to be given over 8 hours:

$$1\,L = 1000\,mL$$

$$\frac{1000}{8} = 125\,ml/hour$$

To manually calculate the drip rate, the formula is:

$$\frac{\text{volume} \times \text{number of drops per ml}}{\text{time in minutes}}$$

Using the above example and a standard giving set which delivers 20 drops per ml:

$$\frac{125 \times 20}{60} = 41.67\,\text{drops per minute}$$

559

As drops can only be given as a whole number, 0.49 is rounded down and 0.50 rounded up. The rate is therefore 42 drops per minute.

b. If a prescription requires a drug in solution to be administered, the formula is:

$$\frac{\text{weight of drug}}{\text{volume of solution}}$$

Example

$$\frac{500 \text{ mg}}{100 \text{ ml}} = 5 \text{ mg/ml}$$

If the prescription requires 15 mg/hour, the drip rate would then be calculated as in the example given in a. above to deliver 3 ml of the solution per hour.

CALCULATING INFANT FEEDING FORMULA

When calculating feeding regimes for neonates who require a specified intake, this is based on:
- weight of the baby
- age, i.e. number of days old
- required feeding pattern, i.e. frequency of feeds (e.g. 1, 2, 3 or 4 hourly)
- daily nutritional requirements:
  - day 1: 60 ml/kg
  - day 2: 90 ml/kg
  - day 3: 120 ml/kg
  - day 4: 150 ml/kg, etc.

The formula to calculate volume of milk per feed is:

$$\frac{\text{weight in kg} \times \text{ml/kg/day}}{\text{number of feeds in 24 hours}}$$

Example

A preterm baby weighing 2 kg is 2 days old and he requires 2-hourly feeds:

$$\frac{2 \times 90}{12} = \frac{180}{12} = 15 \text{ ml per feed}$$

FORMULA FOR CALCULATING BODY MASS INDEX (BMI)

$$\text{Body Mass Index} = \frac{\text{Weight (kg)}}{\text{Height (m)}^2}$$

Example:

To calculate the BMI, the midwife needs to multiple the height measurement of the woman by itself (i.e. height squared).

Example:

A woman attends antenatal clinic for her booking appointment. She weighs 105 kg, and is 1.6 m tall.

$$1.6 \times 1.6 = 2.56$$

$$105 \div 2.56 = 41$$

The BMI is 41.

Normal Values in Pregnancy

Laboratory or physical measurements are presented as a range representing the average in a particular population. The physiological changes of pregnancy may affect what is considered 'normal' for the non-pregnant population. In addition, 'normal' values in pregnancy might be different at different gestations and hence care must be taken when deciding whether a test result(s) is actually abnormal for the woman/fetus concerned. A large sample of women having a straightforward physiological pregnancy is necessary to produce accurate pregnancy value ranges and hence there can be small variations from book to book.

UNITS OF MEASUREMENT

Care needs to be taken in the interpretation of units of measurement as abbreviations are used and represent very different amounts. In addition, values might be expressed in SI or traditional units. For example:
- g = grams
- mg = milligrams
- mmol = millimoles
- L = litres
- dl = decilitres (N.B. prefix 'd' signifies 10).

WEIGHT GAIN IN PREGNANCY

Average weight gain during pregnancy is about 12.5 kg; however, this varies according to the woman's pre-pregnancy body mass index (BMI) which is weight/height^2. Those women with a low BMI are expected to gain more weight, whereas those women who are obese should gain less.

Category	Pre-pregnant BMI
Low (underweight)	< 18.5
Normal	18.5–24.9
High (overweight)	25.0–29.9
Obese	> 29.9

Obesity is often subdivided into the following categories:
- Class I: BMI of 30 to < 35
- Class II: BMI of 35 to < 40
- Class III: BMI of 40 or higher. Class 3 obesity is sometimes categorized as 'extreme' or 'severe' obesity. The term morbid obesity is also used.

Source: Center for Disease Control and Prevention. Available at: https://www.cdc.gov/obesity/adult/defining.html

BIOCHEMISTRY

Test/units	Non-pregnant typical range	Pregnant typical range	Comments
Alanine transaminase (ALT) IU/L	6–40	Range lowers slightly in late pregnancy	Raised levels indicate liver damage
Alkaline phosphatase IU/L	40–120	Doubled by late pregnancy	Usually elevated in third trimester due to placental production of enzyme
Bile acids μmol/L	< 5	< 12	Values of total bile acids ≥ 14 μmol/L are viewed as abnormal, indicating cholestasis
Bilirubin (total) μmol/L	5–22	2–19	Little change from non-pregnant range
Creatinine μmol/L	44–80	80 approx. is upper limit of normal in late pregnancy	Lower in mid-pregnancy but rises towards term

Test/units	Non-pregnant typical range	Pregnant typical range	Comments
Potassium mmol/L	3.5–5.3	Unchanged	Unchanged in pregnancy
Albumin g/L	41–53	23–42	Total protein and albumin are both lower in pregnancy
Urea mmol/L	2–7	Usually ≤ 4.6	Lower in pregnancy
Uric acid µmol/L	150–333	Lowest values in second trimester, 10 × gestational age in weeks is approx. upper limit of normal	Increases with gestation, although lower levels than non-pregnant

HAEMATOLOGY

Note: pregnancy is a hypercoagulable state and prothrombin, partial thromboplastin and thrombin times are slightly faster than controls.

Test/units	Non-pregnant typical range	Pregnant	Comments
Clotting time	12 min	8 min	Observe whether blood is clotting or oozing from venepuncture sites in high-risk groups
Fibrin degradation products µg/ml	Mean 1.04	High values in third trimester and especially around time of birth	
Fibrinogen g/L	2–5	By term 3.7–6.2	Marked increase in pregnancy, especially in third trimester and around time of birth

Continued

Test/units	Non-pregnant typical range	Pregnant	Comments
Haematocrit L/L	0.35–0.47	0.31–0.35	Lower in pregnancy
Haemoglobin g/dl	11.5–16.5	10.0–12.0 Should be ≤ 10 in third trimester	Good iron stores needed to maintain pregnancy levels Fall in first trimester whether or not iron and folate taken
Platelets × 10^9 L	165–415	Slight decrease in normal pregnancy Lower limit of 'normal' = 120	No functional significance
White cell count × 10^9 L	3.5–9	6–17 Higher values up to 25.0 around time of birth	Normal increase in pregnancy. Rise in infections

Appendix | 4 |

Glossary of Selected Terms

Abortion Termination of pregnancy before the fetus is viable, i.e. before 24 weeks' gestation in the UK. Age of viable may be different in other countries.

Abruptio placenta Premature separation of a normally situated placenta. Term normally used from viability (24 weeks).

Aetiology The science of the cause of disease.

Amenorrhoea Absence of menstrual periods.

Amniotic fluid embolism A rare maternity emergency resulting in cardio-respiratory collapse triggered by the escape of amniotic fluid through the wall of the uterus or placental site into the maternal circulation, leading to a life-threatening allergic reaction (anaphylactic shock) in the mother.

Amniotomy Artificial rupture of the amniotic sac.

Anhedonia Inability to experience pleasure.

Antigen A substance which stimulates the production of an antibody.

Anuria Producing no urine.

Atresia Closure or absence of an usual opening or canal.

Augmentation of labour Intervention to correct slow progress in labour, e.g. use of intravenous oxytocic agent.

Basal body temperature The temperature of the body when at rest.

Bicornuate uterus A structural malformation of the uterus.

Bishop score Rating system to assess suitability of cervix for induction of labour.

Cardiotocograph Measurement of the fetal heart rate and uterine activity on a machine that is able to provide a paper print of the information it records.

Cephalopelvic disproportion Disparity between the size of the woman's pelvis and the fetal head.

Chloasma (or melasma) Pigmentation of the face, which affects at least half of all pregnant women.

Choanal atresia (Bilateral) membranous or bony obstruction of the nares; baby is blue when sleeping and pink when crying.

Conjoined twins Identical twins where separation is incomplete so their bodies are partly joined together and vital organs may be shared.

Diastasis symphysis pubis A painful condition in which there is an abnormal relaxation of the ligaments supporting the pubic joint, also referred to as pelvic girdle pain.

Dichorionic twins Twins who have developed in their own separate chorionic sacs.

Disseminated intravascular coagulation/coagulopathy A rare life-threatening condition that develops secondary to a primary complication such as major postpartum haemorrhage where there is inappropriate blood clotting in the small blood vessels. This can affect blood flow throughout the blood vessels and ultimately result in organ damage.

Dizygotic (dizygous) Formed from two separate zygotes.

Dyspareunia Painful or difficult intercourse experienced by the woman.

Echogenic bowel Bright appearances of bowel, equivalent to the brightness of bone. Also associated with intra-amniotic bleeding and fetal swallowing of blood-stained liquor.

Echogenic foci in the heart Bright echoes from calcium deposits in the fetal heart, often the left ventricle. These do not affect cardiac function.

Ectopic pregnancy An abnormally situated pregnancy, most commonly in a uterine tube.

Embryo reduction (see Fetal reduction).

Endocervical Relating to the internal canal of the cervix.

Epicanthic folds A vertical fold of skin on either side of the nose which covers the lacrimal caruncle. They may be common in Asian babies, but may indicate Down syndrome in other ethnic groups.

Epulis (pregnancy) Swelling of the gums.

Erb palsy Paralysis of the arm due to the damage to cervical nerve roots 5 and 6 of the brachial plexus.

Erythematous Reddening of the skin.

Erythropoiesis The process by which erythrocytes (red blood cells) are formed. After the 10th week of gestation, erythropoiesis production rises and seems to be involved in red cell production in the bone marrow during the third trimester.

External cephalic version (ECV) The use of external manipulation on the pregnant woman's abdomen to convert a breech to a cephalic presentation.

False-negative rate The proportion of affected pregnancies that would not be identified as high risk. Tests with a high false-negative rate have low sensitivity.

False-positive rate The proportion of unaffected pregnancies with a high-risk classification. Tests with a high false-positive rate have low specificity.

Fetal reduction The reduction in the number of viable fetuses/embryos in a multiple (usually higher multiple) pregnancy by medical intervention.

Fetofetal transfusion syndrome (twin-to-twin transfusion syndrome, TTTS) Condition in which blood from one monozygotic twin fetus transfuses into the other via blood vessels in the placenta.

Fetus papyraceous A fetus that dies in the second trimester of the pregnancy and becomes compressed and parchment-like.

Fibroid Firm, benign tumour of muscular and fibrous tissue.

Fraternal twins Dizygotic (non-identical).

Fundal height The distance between the top part of the uterus (the fundus) and the top of the symphysis pubis (the junction between the pubic bones). This assessment is undertaken to assess the increasing size of the uterus antenatally and decreasing size postnatally.

Haematuria Blood in the urine.

Haemostasis The arrest of bleeding.

HELLP syndrome A condition of pregnancy characterized by haemolysis, elevated liver enzymes and low platelets.

Homeostasis The condition in which the body's internal environment remains relatively constant within physiological limits.

Hydatidiform mole A gross malformation of the trophoblast in which the chorionic villi proliferate and become avascular.

Hydropic vesicles Fluid filled sacs, or blisters.

Hypercapnia An abnormal increase in the amount of carbon dioxide in the blood.

Hyperemesis gravidarum Protracted or excessive vomiting in pregnancy.

Hypertrophy Overgrowth of tissue.

Hypovolaemia Reduced circulating blood volume due to external loss of body fluids or to loss of fluid into the tissues.

Hypoxia Lack of oxygen.

Induction of labour Intervention to stimulate uterine contractions before the onset of spontaneous labour.

Intraepithelial Within the epithelium, or among epithelial cells.

Intrahepatic cholestasis of pregnancy (ICP) An idiopathic condition of abnormal liver function.

Leucorrhoea Normal vaginal discharge in pregnancy.

Lochia The discharge from the genital tract in the postpartum period. The term is plural and there are three different types of lochia (rubra, serosa and alba).

Løvset manoeuvre A manoeuvre for the delivery of shoulders and extended arms in a breech presentation.

Macrosomia Large baby.

Malposition A cephalic presentation other than normal well-flexed anterior position of the fetal head, e.g. occipitoposterior.

Malpresentation A presentation other than the vertex, i.e. face, brow, compound or shoulder. (Breech may be included in this category).

Mauriceau–Smellie–Veit manoeuvre A manoeuvre to deliver a breech baby which involves jaw flexion and shoulder traction.

McRoberts manoeuvre A manoeuvre to rotate the angle of the symphysis pubis superiorly and release the impaction of the anterior shoulder in shoulder dystocia. The woman brings her knees up to her chest.

Midwife-led care Midwives or a midwife take the lead role in care of a woman or group of women.

Miscarriage Spontaneous loss of pregnancy before viability (see Abortion).

Monoamniotic twins Twins who have developed in the same amniotic sac.

Monochorionic twins Identical twins who have developed in the same chorionic sac.

Monozygotic (monozygous) Formed from one zygote (identical twins).

Multifetal reduction (see Fetal reduction).

Naegele's rule Method of calculating the expected date of birth.

Neoplasia Growth of new tissue.

Neutral thermal environment (NTE) The range of environmental temperature over which heat production, oxygen consumption and nutritional requirements for growth are minimal, provided the body temperature is normal.

Oedema The effusion of body fluid into the tissues.

Oligohydramnios Abnormally small amount of amniotic fluid in pregnancy.

Oliguria Producing an abnormally small amount of urine.

$PaCO_2$ Measures the partial pressure of dissolved carbon dioxide (CO_2). This dissolved CO_2 has moved out of the cell and into the bloodstream. The measure of a $PaCO_2$ accurately reflects the alveolar ventilation.

569

PaO$_2$ Measures the partial pressure of oxygen in the arterial blood. It reflects how the lung is functioning but does not measure tissue oxygenation.

Pemphigoid gestationis (previously known as herpes gestationis) is a rare autoimmune skin condition of pregnancy that more commonly occurs during the 2nd and 3rd trimesters. It has no association to the herpes virus hence the term pemphigoid gestationis is more appropriate. It is characterized by an urticarial rash that develop into blisters.

Perinatal WHO defines this period as: commencing at 22 completed weeks (154 days) of gestation and ending seven completed days after birth. Perinatal and maternal health are closely linked.

pH A solution's acidity or alkalinity is expressed on the pH scale, which runs from 0 to 14. This scale is based on the concentration of H$^+$ ions in a solution expressed in chemical units called moles per litre (mol/l). When the fetus is hypoxic the increased acid produced raises the acidity of the blood and the pH falls.

Placenta accrete Abnormally adherent placenta into the muscle layer of the uterus.

Placenta increta Abnormally adherent placenta into the perimetrium of the uterus.

Placenta percreta Abnormally adherent placenta through the muscle layer of the uterus.

Placenta praevia A condition in which some or all of the placenta is attached in the lower segment of the uterus.

Placental abruption (see Abruptio placenta).

Polyhydramnios An excessive amount of amniotic fluid in pregnancy. Also referred to as hydramnios.

Polyp Small growth.

Porphyria An inherited condition of abnormal red blood cell formation.

Postnatal period The period after the end of labour during which the attendance of a midwife upon the woman and baby is required, being not less than 10 days and for such longer periods as the midwife considers necessary.

Postpartum After labour.

Pre-eclampsia A condition peculiar to pregnancy, which is characterized by hypertension, proteinuria and systemic dysfunction.

Primary postpartum haemorrhage A blood loss in excess of 500 ml or any amount which adversely affects the condition of the mother within the first 24 hours of birth.

Progestogen Synthetic progesterone used in hormonal contraception.

570

Prostaglandins Locally acting chemical compounds derived from fatty acids within cells. They ripen the cervix and cause the uterus to contract.

Proteinuria Protein in the urine.

Pruritus Itching.

Ptyalism Excessive salivation.

Puerperal fever/pyrexia A rise in temperature in the puerperium. This is poorly defined in the literature but is assumed to be based on the definition of pyrexia which is a rise above the normal body temperature. Where pyrexia is used as a clinical sign of importance, the elevation in temperature is generally taken as being 38°C and above or 37.5°C on at least two consecutive occasions.

Puerperal sepsis Infection of the genital tract following childbirth; still a major cause of maternal morbidity and mortality especially where it is undetected, detected late and/or untreated.

Puerperium A period after childbirth where the uterus and other organs and structures which have been affected by the pregnancy are returning to their non-gravid state. Usually described as a period of 6–8 weeks.

Quickening First point at which the woman recognizes fetal movements in early pregnancy.

Retraction Process by which the uterine muscle fibres shorten after a contraction. Unique to uterine muscle.

Rubin manoeuvre A rotational manoeuvre to relieve shoulder dystocia. Pressure is exerted over the fetal back to adduct and rotate the shoulders.

Sandal gap Exaggerated gap between the first and second toes.

Secondary postpartum haemorrhage An 'excessive' or 'prolonged' vaginal blood loss which is usually defined as occurring from 24 hours to 6 weeks after the birth.

Selective fetocide The medical destruction of an abnormal twin fetus in a continuing pregnancy.

Shoulder dystocia Failure of the shoulders to spontaneously traverse the pelvis after birth of the head.

Speculum (vaginal) An instrument used to open the vagina.

Subinvolution The uterine size appears larger than anticipated for days postpartum, and may feel poorly contracted. Uterine tenderness may be present.

Surfactant Complex mixture of phospholipids and lipoproteins produced by type 2 alveolar cells in the lungs that decreases surface tension and prevents alveolar collapse at end expiration.

Symphysis pubis dysfunction (see Diastasis symphysis pubis).

Talipes A complex foot deformity, affecting 1/1000 live births and is more common in males. The affected foot is held in a fixed flexion (equinus) and in-turned (varus) position. It can be differentiated from positional talipes because the deformity in true talipes cannot be passively corrected.

Teratogen An agent believed to cause congenital malformations, e.g. thalidomide.

Torsion Twisting.

Uniovular Monozygotic.

Unstable lie After 36 weeks' gestation, a lie that varies between longitudinal and oblique or transverse is said to be unstable.

Uterine involution The physiological process that starts from the end of labour that results in a gradual reduction in the size of the uterus until it returns to its non-pregnant size and location in the pelvis.

Vanishing twin syndrome The reabsorption of one twin fetus early in pregnancy (usually before 12 weeks).

Vasa praevia A rare occurrence in which umbilical cord vessels pass through the placental membranes and lie across the cervical os.

Withdrawal bleed Bleeding due to withdrawal of hormones.

Zygosity Describing the genetic make-up of children in a multiple birth.

Index

Page numbers followed by "*f*" indicate figures, "*t*" indicate tables, and "*b*" indicate boxes.

complementary feeds, 442–445
contraindications to, 441–442
    cancer, 441
    HIV infection, 442
    medication, 441
    surgery, 441
difficulties, 440–441
feeding behaviour, 434–435
first feed, 433
'let-down' reflex, 428
management of, 433–445
'milk ejection' reflex, 428
with one breast, 436
pausing in, 434
problems with, 437–441
supplementary feeds, 442–445
in third stage of labour, 273
timing and frequency of feeds in, 434–435
weaning from breast, 442
Breathing, increased work of, 464
Breech extraction, 320
Breech presentation, 311–326, 312f–313f
abdominal examination of, 314
antenatal diagnosis of, 314–315
antenatal management of, 315–316
causes of, 312–313
complications of, 326
diagnosis during labour in, 315
management of, 317–326, 319b
persistent, 316
types of, 311
ultrasound examination of, 315
vaginal examination of, 315, 315f
X-ray examination of, 315
Brim
diameters of, 5–7, 6f
    anteroposterior, 5–6
    oblique, 7
    transverse, 7
pelvic, 4
Brow presentation, 47, 309–311
abdominal palpation and, 310
causes of, 310
complications in, 311

conversion to, from occipitoposterior position, 306
diagnosis in, 310–311
management of labour of, 311, 311b
Brown fat, in newborn, 400
Bruising, 462b–463b
Bullous impetigo, 462b–463b
Burns Marshall method, in breech birth, 321–322, 322f
Buttocks
distending the perineum, 320
internal rotation of, 317
restitution of, 317
BV. see Bacterial vaginosis (BV)

C

Caesarean section(s), 335–340
anaesthesia in, 337–338
in breech presentation, 316
care following regional block, 339
cephalopelvic disproportion, evidence of, 295
cervical dystocia and, 296
complications associated with, 338
elective, 316, 336, 336b
emergency, 336, 337b
immediate care for, 338–339
observations, 338–339
positioning of woman in, 336
postnatal ward and, 339–340
postoperative care in, 338–340
preparation of, 335–337
previous, vaginal birth following, 296
in shoulder presentation, 328
vaginal birth after, 336–337
wounds, 378
Calcium, 431
electrolyte imbalances in newborn, 534
Cancer, 150–151
breastfeeding contraindication, 441
of cervix, 119
Candida, neonatal infections and, 527